S0-AMP-807

THE ACUTE STROKE

CONTEMPORARY NEUROLOGY SERIES AVAILABLE:

Fred Plum, M.D., *Editor-in-Chief*
J. Richard Baringer, M.D., *Associate Editor*
Sid Gilman, M.D., *Associate Editor*

THE ACUTE STROKE

VLADIMIR HACHINSKI, M.D., F.R.C.P.(C)

Professor of Neurology
Department of Clinical Neurological Sciences
University of Western Ontario
London, Canada

JOHN W. NORRIS, M.D., F.R.C.P.

Associate Professor of Medicine (Neurology)
University of Toronto
Toronto, Canada

 F. A. DAVIS COMPANY·PHILADELPHIA

ST. PHILIP'S COLLEGE LIBRARY

Copyright © 1985 by F. A. Davis Company

All rights reserved. This book is protected by copyright. No part of it may be reproduced, stored in a retrieval system, or transmitted in any form or by any means, electronic, mechanical, photocopying, recording, or otherwise, without written permission from the publisher.

Printed in the United States of America

NOTE: As new scientific information becomes available through basic and clinical research, recommended treatments and drug therapies undergo changes. The author(s) and publisher have done everything possible to make this book accurate, up-to-date, and in accord with accepted standards at the time of publication. However, the reader is advised always to check product information (package inserts) for changes and new information regarding dose and contraindications before administering any drug. Caution is especially urged when using new or infrequently ordered drugs.

Library of Congress Cataloging in Publication Data

Hachinski, Vladimir.
  The acute stroke.

  (Contemporary neurology series; 27)
  Includes bibliographies and index.
  1. Cerebrovascular disease.   I. Norris, John W.
II. Title.   [DNLM: 1. Cerebrovascular Disorders.
W1 C0769N v.27 / WL 355 H117a]
  RC388.5.H33 1985   616.8′1   85-6880
  ISBN 0-8036-4502-3

PREFACE

This book represents our joint and equal effort to provide a comprehensive, reasoned, and orderly approach to stroke. Most books on stroke consist of edited collections of different experiences, and often unreconciled viewpoints. This book is largely based on our prospective data from the MacLachlan Acute Stroke Unit in Toronto, where patients are systematically assessed and managed by the same stroke care team. Children with stroke and patients with subarachnoid hemorrhage are not admitted to the Toronto Unit and therefore are not discussed.

This book aims to meet the needs of a variety of readers and situations. After introductory chapters on basic epidemiology, stroke care and pathophysiology, the book outlines the care of the stroke patient, from diagnosis through management, to prognosis and prevention. The headings, illustrations, and conclusions allow selective reading for those seeking a synopsis of stroke management. Medical practitioners and students, specialty trainees, and all those caring for stroke patients may find this book useful. As a synthesis and interpretation of our own data and the literature, we are largely addressing neurologists and other colleagues in the field of stroke. While present knowledge does not always warrant firm conclusions, we consider an evolving scheme preferable to weaving bland summaries from the contradictory literature on stroke. "Truth is more likely to arise from error than from confusion" (Francis Bacon).

VH
JWN

ACKNOWLEDGMENTS

Among our many debts of gratitude, none is greater nor more deserved than that owing to the late Colonel Graham MacLachlan. First as a patient and then as a patron, fund raiser, and friend, his indefatigable efforts made possible the establishment of the acute stroke unit that bears his name. This book reflects the experience gained in that Unit and is dedicated to his memory, in the hope that advances in knowledge, therapy, and prevention will make the need for acute stroke care increasingly obsolete.

Bette Shurvell was Stroke Data Coordinator throughout the developmental phase of the Unit, and her diligent and meticulous management of clinical and laboratory data, and later their evaluation, was critical to many of our publications. Cecily Ziliotto was instrumental in data acquisition and processing, often against prevailing odds.

Our colleagues have earned our appreciation, including Dr. John Edmeads, Head of the Division of Neurology at Sunnybrook Medical Centre, who kindly allowed his patients in the Unit to be evaluated by us. Drs. Perry Cooper and Ted Kassel at Sunnybrook Medical Centre and Drs. Allan Fox, David Pelz, and Fernando Viñuela at University Hospital helped us with the radiologic illustrations, and Marie Lehman drew most of the original diagrams.

Our Stroke Research Fellows also made important contributions to the development of our standardized approach to stroke care by their active participation, discussion, and arguments. We therefore thank Drs. Raul Rudelli, Miklos Vilaghy, Joseph D'Alton, and Brian Chambers.

The queries, challenges, and suggestions of many neurology and internal medicine residents resulted in improvements in the Toronto Unit protocol. Without the interest and labor of the Sunnybrook nursing staff, the evaluation of much of the data would not have been feasible.

We acknowledge our debt to various funding sources. Dr. Hugh Barber, Chairman of the Stroke Steering Committee, Sunnybrook Medical Centre, ensured that our early research projects were funded from that source. Grants from the Medical Research Council of Canada, the Heart and Stroke Foundation of Ontario, and Ontario Ministry of Health paid for much of the work presented in this book. Dr. Hachinski enjoyed personal support from the Heart and Stroke Foundation of Ontario, first as Senior Research Fellow, and now as Research Associate.

Colleagues at home and abroad patiently read and commented on manuscript chapters, despite schedules replete with more pressing obligations. These include Drs. Henry Barnett, Sandra Black, Lou Caplan, Brian Chambers, Miller Fisher, Allan Fox, Andrew Kertesz, Harold Merskey, Dave Sackett, Bo Siesjö, and Phil Wolf. What errors remain prove that we did not always follow their good advice.

Barbara Huth's devotion to the book and her gift for clarity, logic, and language made her an indispensable and appreciated partner. Our secretaries, Clare Forbes, Zahir Hussain, and Ruth Donovan, and the volunteer work of Carole Gaily, ensured the completion of the book.

Lastly and warmly, we thank our families, for this book was written on their time.

VH
JWN

CONTENTS

Chapter 1

THE PROBLEM

Nothing is constant except change.
Heraclitus

Stroke is the most common serious neurologic problem in the world.[1] In Japan and parts of China,[2] it kills more people than any other disease and, despite declining incidence,[3] remains the third commonest cause of death in North America and most European countries.[4] The National Survey of Stroke in the United States identified 414,000 new victims of stroke annually. Added to previous cases, this amounts to a prevalence of 1.7 million. The estimated cost, including direct care costs and loss of earnings, exceeds 7 billion dollars per year.[5] This merely reflects the financial cost; the human costs are immeasurable.

Atherosclerosis, hypertension, and heart disease rank as the most important risk factors for stroke.[6] Atherosclerosis underlies most ischemic stroke throughout the world. Variations in incidence reflect the age of the population more than changes in the pathologic process, though the pattern of involvement varies. The Japanese,[4] some African populations,[7] and American blacks[8] have a high incidence of stroke and a relatively lower incidence of ischemic heart disease. By contrast, North American whites have a relatively higher incidence of atherosclerotic heart disease than stroke, while both ischemic stroke and ischemic heart disease occur commonly in Finland.[4]

Hypertension represents the greatest but most treatable risk factor for all types of stroke. It predisposes to intracerebral hemorrhage and accelerates and complicates atherosclerosis. Ischemic heart disease, which may result from atherosclerosis and hypertension, is an index of and a risk factor for stroke. Nonatherosclerotic heart disease is also increasingly recognized as an important cause of stroke.[9] Smoking, a

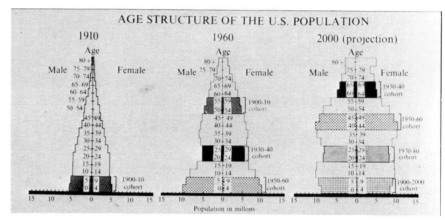

FIGURE 1. Age structure of the U.S. population. (From Editorial: *Life as a wonderful one-hoss shay*. Nature 298:779, 1982, with permission.)

strong contributor to ischemic heart disease, is only a weak risk factor for stroke.[6]

Lifestyle may also be important. Urbanization and industrialization curtail physical activity, increase stress, and change eating habits toward high-calorie, high-lipid diets. Resultant obesity, hypertension, and diabetes raise the risk for stroke.[6] Diabetes occurs not only in the overfed but also in the undernourished. In several poorer countries, pancreatic calcification is a notable cause of diabetes among the young.[7] As living standards and life expectancy rise in developing countries, more of the population will reach an age at which strokes become common, a trend also present in developed countries (Fig. 1). Mounting evidence implicates lifestyle as a powerful determinant in the development of circulatory disorders and suggests an increasingly important role for behavior modification in their prevention.[10]

HISTORIC PERSPECTIVE

Sudden episodes of loss of consciousness or paralysis have been recognized since antiquity. An acute loss of all movement and sensation was termed "apoplexy," whereas "paralysis" referred to chronic conditions with partial impairment of movement or sense.[11,12] In the 17th century, Wepfer established that stroke could be caused by intracerebral hemorrhage or by "fibrous masses" (atheroma) or clotted blood in the carotid or vertebral arteries stopping the flow of "vital spirits" into the brain.[13] In a series of clinicopathologic studies, Morgagni confirmed that apoplexy could be hemorrhagic or "serous." He said that his teacher Valsalva "had planned . . . to make many experiments about the cause of apoplexy. For instance, whether it could be artificially brought on by throwing into the carotid arteries of beasts this or that thing; whether these arteries being tied the animal would nevertheless feel."[12] Unfortunately, neither Valsalva nor Morgagni carried out these experiments.

In the early 19th century, Leon Rostan established that cerebral softening was "the most frequent cerebral lesion" and that it was not due to inflammation, as was then believed:[12,14]

That hardening of the arteries leads to softening of the brain was not implied before the 1830s, and even then far from being generally believed. There was the beginning of the notion that stroke is primarily the result of vascular as opposed to blood disease, and mechanical rather than inflammatory.[12]

Virchow and his pupils established the morphologic basis for the concepts of thrombosis and embolism in the mid-1800s. He was first to propose the concept of "ischemic apoplexy," which he believed to be most frequently caused by embolism.

It was not until the mid-20th century that the widespread use of arteriography and clinical pathologic studies, particularly those of Miller Fisher, established the modern basis of understanding ischemic and hemorrhagic cerebrovascular disease.[12,13] In 1950, cerebral angiography was coming into general use, isotope brain scanning had yet to gain prominence, and CT scanning had not been invented. The importance of hypertension as a cause of stroke was unrecognized, and the role of anticoagulants and antiplatelet agents in its prevention unknown.[15] Carotid artery surgery was first attempted in 1954,[16] and cerebral microvascular surgery became possible with the advent of the operating microscope. In the past three decades, stroke has changed from being a diagnosable but untreatable condition to being a field of therapeutic opportunities.

TERMINOLOGY AND CLASSIFICATION

Terminology

Cerebrovascular terminology reflects cerebrovascular thinking—and sometimes a lack of thinking. "Cerebrovascular accident" (CVA) has gained undeserved currency and implies precision it does not have. While "cerebrovascular" appropriately describes most strokes, cerebral arteries are frequently passive recipients of cardiac emboli, a situation better termed "cardiovascular." Strokes result from identifiable, often predictable causes and are rarely "accidents." "CVA" is a pseudoscientific characterization of stroke that substitutes labeling for understanding and invites confusion between the sides of the brain and body. "Left-sided CVA" means a left-hemisphere lesion to some and left hemiplegia to others. "CVA" more often than not stands for "confused vascular analysis."[17]

"Stroke" conveys the suddenness and potential devastation of vascular disease without pedantic or etiologic pretenses. It has an old, noble ancestry as a conceptual descendant of the Greek "apoplexia," and is a semantic relative of the German "Schlaganfall" and the French "coup de sang." The Oxford dictionary defines "stroke" as "an attack of disease; an apoplectic or (now more usual) paralytic seizure, 1599." Dr. Samuel Johnson wrote "he has had a stroke, like of an apoplexy" (*Dictionary of the English Language*, 1755). "Apoplexy" is the older, more learned term, but it has come to imply hemorrhage; and thus the lay term "stroke" is

ST. PHILIP'S COLLEGE LIBRARY

preferable to describe a sudden neurologic deficit of presumed vascular origin.

"Transient ischemic attack" (TIA) also lacks precision. Patients are seldom examined during an attack and, although investigations suggest an etiology, no later investigation can confirm the clinical suspicion of a TIA. Consequently, the diagnosis is only clinical and presumptive rather than proven.

Other proposals do not improve the simple terminology outlined above.[18] "Reversible ischemic neurologic deficit" (RIND) has been suggested for neurologic impairments persisting beyond 24 hours but resolving within a week. Despite the "reversible" nature of the deficit, most of these patients probably have small cerebral infarcts. Ladurner and colleagues found that 76 percent of patients with RIND had hypodense lesions on CT scan, suggesting clinical recovery rather than ischemic reversibility.[19] Further, 18 percent of patients with transient ischemic attacks, which, by definition, last less than 24 hours, showed evidence of cerebral infarction on CT scan.

"Partial nonprogressive stroke" (PNP) would be a useful term if one could be sure at assessment that the stroke is indeed "nonprogressive." Actually, about one third of strokes progress after the patient's admission to the hospital.[20]

"Stroke-in-evolution" reflects a worsening, dynamic situation. Unfortunately, the term has become closely associated with the idea of stroke worsening because of progression of thrombosis, whereas the actual causes of neurologic deterioration are many. An equivalent term, free from preconception, is needed, such as "deteriorating stroke."[20]

Classification

Before 1948, the International Classification of Diseases (ICD) (America) only cited the generic term "cerebrovascular disease," which included dementia attributed to "generalised cerebral arteriosclerosis," the majority really representing Alzheimer's disease.[21]

The 1977 edition of the ICD marks a regression rather than an improvement.[22] Among the five rubrics for cerebrovascular disease are Code 436 "acute but ill-defined cerebrovascular disease," Code 437 "other and ill-defined cerebrovascular disease," and Code 438 "late effects of cerebrovascular disease."[23] "Ill-defined" is apt. Exhaustively precise classification may be as confusing as frustrating vagueness. An expert committee has suggested a pathophysiologic classification of three pages, an anatomic classification of five and one half pages, and a pathologic classification of eight pages for cerebrovascular diseases[24]—a proposal more appropriate for research and reference than for everyday practice.

A simple categorization applies to the vast majority of patients with cerebrovascular disease. Initial diagnoses should be "presumed stroke" or "presumed TIA," implying other possibilities. Localizing the lesion narrows the etiologic possibilities and prevents premature diagnostic conclusions. After considering the etiology, the physician should then

TABLE 1. Suggested Classification of Stroke

A. Presumed stroke
   Presumed TIA
   Other
	By cause
	   Ischemia
	      Extracranial vascular disease
	      Embolism

B. Anatomic classification
   By axial location
      Supratentorial
         Lobar (specify)
         Centrencephalic (specify)
      Infratentorial
         Cerebellar (specify)
         Brainstem (specify)
   By vascular territory
      Carotid (specify)
      Vertebrobasilar (specify)
	Other
	   Hemorrhage
	      Hypertension
	      Amyloid angiopathy
	      Vascular malformation
	      Other
	
	D. Management classification
	   TIA and minor stroke
	   Major stroke
	   Deteriorating stroke
	   Young stroke

C. Etiologic classification
   By result
      Cerebral infarct
         Arterial
         Arteriolar (lacunar)
         Venous
      Cerebral hemorrhage
         Intraparenchymal
         Subarachnoid	

decide to which of four major stroke management categories the patient belongs (Table 1):

1. *TIA and Minor Stroke.* These patients are at high risk of stroke, yet have no lasting neurologic deficit. Complete neurologic investigation is justified, in most cases including cerebral angiography or, if indicated, a search for possible cardiac sources of emboli.

2. *Major Stroke.* These patients have a stable, usually severe, deficit. Invasive investigations seldom prove rewarding. Patients may be candidates for active, prompt rehabilitation, though sometimes compassionate inaction is more appropriate. The brain harbors intellect and personality and, when these are destroyed or irreparably damaged, death may be preferable to mere biologic survival.

3. *Deteriorating Stroke.* Up to one third of acute stroke patients deteriorate neurologically, owing to cerebral or systemic causes after admission to the hospital.[20,25] The term "deteriorating stroke" is proposed to encourage a search for the cause of this decline. Deteriorating stroke calls for prompt investigation and specific action directed toward the most likely cerebral or systemic factor. Cerebral edema or progressing "thrombosis" is too often only the presumed cause, resulting in inappropriate therapy.

4. *Young Stroke.* In persons below 45 years, stroke is due to a wide variety of causes,[26] many of them remediable. Young patients with stroke also have better powers of recovery, so investigation for the cause should be exhaustive.

All diagnoses are not of equal value. Whenever possible, the clinical diagnosis should refer to supporting laboratory evidence. If a CT scan, angiography, autopsy, or other highly specific test has been performed, the results should be stated. At times, the diagnosis of stroke remains presumptive and the location speculative. In these cases it becomes particularly important to give the evidence and state the doubt rather than casting them into an "ill-defined cerebrovascular" category.

EPIDEMIOLOGY

The problems of identification of stroke in epidemiologic studies include the difficulty of diagnosing "silent" and nonhemiplegic strokes and the reciprocal relationship between the incidence of cardiovascular and cerebrovascular disease.[27] "Silent" strokes may occur in the frontal lobes, basal ganglia, and cerebral white matter. Even when symptoms such as visual impairment are detected, they may not be attributed to a cerebrovascular lesion. Only 70 percent of stroke patients present with hemiplegia[28] so that, unless a careful neurologic examination is carried out, many other types of stroke can be missed or misinterpreted.

In a population having a high incidence of cardiovascular disease, fewer people may survive to have a stroke. Conversely, when mortality from heart disease is low, more subjects may live into the decades when stroke is commonest. This seesaw relationship between cardiovascular and cerebrovascular disease should enter into the evaluation of risk factors for both conditions.[27]

Geography

Both the incidence and the quality of reporting vary in different parts of the world (Fig. 2).[4] The incidence of stroke can also vary within a country. In the United States, for example, the highest incidence is in the southeastern states and the lowest incidence in the midwestern states.[29]

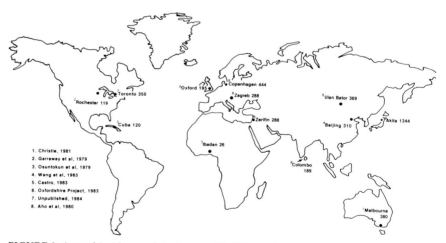

FIGURE 2. Annual incidence of stroke, per 100,000 population. Figures from different studies are not strictly comparable. (Compiled from data in references 7, 42, and 49 to 54.)

ACUTE STROKE

6

Bancalari and associates[30] studied the incidence of hospital-confirmed strokes in two Peruvian cities situated at heights of 3720 and 4500 meters, respectively, and in Lima, which is approximately at sea level. Despite the polycythemic levels of the hematocrit in the mountain population (sometimes over 70 percent), the incidence of stroke there was lower (2.7 percent) than at sea level (15.4 percent). These results are interesting but preliminary, since the groups were not entirely comparable.

Age and Sex

We are all aging, both as individuals and as populations. In North America, Europe, the USSR, and Japan, the proportion of persons aged 65 years and older represents at least 10 percent of the population and is rising.[31] While average life expectancy in the United States has risen from 47 to 73 years of age in this century, the maximum life span has not increased.[32] The net effect is an increasing proportion of older individuals in the population (Fig. 3). The incidence of stroke rises sharply with age, and a small shift in the mean age of the population results in a relatively large increase in the incidence of stroke, which may affect the results of therapeutic trials that include different age groups.

Men over age 45 years have a greater incidence of stroke than women have. Kurtzke estimated the overall male/female ratio at 1.33,[4] a ratio similar to that of the Toronto Unit (1.22).[33]

Social Factors

Racial influences on stroke cannot be easily distinguished from those of environment, but American blacks have a higher incidence of stroke and hypertension than American whites.[8] While Japan has the world's high-

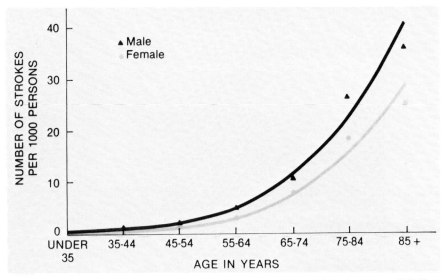

FIGURE 3. Risk of stroke, by sex and age. (From U.S. Dept. of Health, Education and Welfare, National Survey of Stroke, NIH Pub No 80-2069, 1980, with permission.)

est stroke incidence, Japanese living in Hawaii and California have fewer cerebral and more myocardial infarcts than those living in Japan.[34] Moyamoya, a cerebral arteritis of unknown origin, predominates in Japan.[35] Japanese patients with ischemic cerebrovascular disease participating in an international study of extracranial/intracranial bypass surgery most commonly had middle cerebral artery stenosis, while North American and European patients most frequently had carotid artery disease.[36]

In Nigeria, an unusually high proportion of stroke patients come from the upper and middle socioeconomic groups. Their levels of serum cholesterol, triglycerides, and phospholipids are much higher than those of the peasants, similar to unaffected members of their own social class, but lower than those of Caucasians.[7,37] The marginal caloric diet of the lower social classes may protect them from advanced atherosclerosis[7] or may keep them from reaching the age at which stroke is common. In the United States, by contrast, stroke is more common among the lower socioeconomic groups.[38]

Dietary customs acquired for a good reason may persist when the reason no longer exists. The highest stroke incidence and the highest prevalence of hypertension in Venezuela is found on the island of Nueva Esparta. Salted fish is the staple diet of most inhabitants. Although most families can afford refrigerators, they prefer salted over "dead" fish. The high salt intake may contribute to the high incidence of hypertension and stroke.[39]

Long-Term Trends

Stroke mortality has decreased for at least 30 years, especially in the past decade. The reduction in deaths from stroke for people under 65 years has been even more dramatic.[40] Some of the reduction results from changes in diagnostic fashion, such as misclassification of dementia as "cerebrovascular disease." Also, as more disease entities are described, the relative number in each category decreases.[41] Nevertheless, the magnitude and acceleration of the decrease is not entirely artifactual, since the incidence of stroke is also decreasing[42-44] while survival is increasing.[45]

The reasons for the decline in stroke probably include better diagnosis and treatment. The sharpest decline in stroke deaths coincides with recognition of the importance and treatment of hypertension.[44] In Canada, over the same period that stroke mortality dropped by 51 percent, deaths from hypertension fell by 88 percent (Fig. 4). The falling incidence of intracranial hemorrhage and lacunar infarcts[46] also coincides with better control of hypertension. Deaths from rheumatic heart disease decreased 75 percent over the period, paralleling a decline in rheumatic valvular disease and consequently of cerebral embolism. Mitral stenosis and atrial fibrillation are common sequelae of rheumatic heart disease that dispose to stroke. Control of rheumatic heart disease by improved living conditions and antibiotics has contributed to declining stroke mortality. Transient ischemic attacks are risks for cerebral infarction, and aspirin can improve the natural history of TIA.[47] The widespread use of antiplatelet agents may also be contributing inadvertently to the decline of stroke.[48] The role of carotid endarterectomy in decreasing stroke inci-

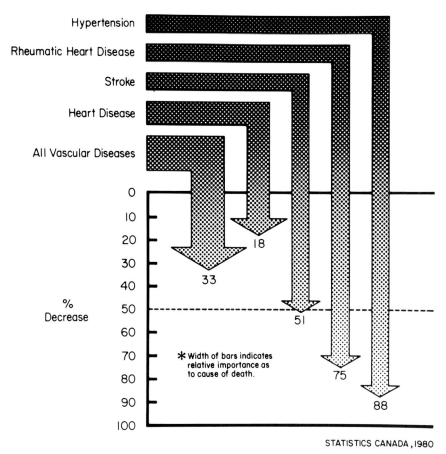

Hypertension
Rheumatic Heart Disease
Stroke
Heart Disease
All Vascular Diseases

%
Decrease

0
10
20
30
40
50
60
70
80
90
100

18
33
51
75
88

✳ Width of bars indicates relative importance as to cause of death.

STATISTICS CANADA, 1980

FIGURE 4. Mortality rates for hypertension, heart disease, and stroke for individuals aged 65 and under in Canada during 1953 to 1978. (From Barnett, HJM: *Platelet antiaggregants in stroke prevention*. In Barnett, HJM, Hirsch, J, and Mustard, JF: *Acetylsalicylic Acid, New Uses for an Old Drug*. Raven Press, New York, 1982, p 176, with permission.)

dence remains plausible but unproven, since a controlled study meeting contemporary standards has not yet been conducted.

The decline in stroke has several important implications. Any study using historic controls will show a favorable trend, reaffirming the need for coeval controlled studies. The changing nature of stroke requires continuous re-examination of knowledge, even of that gained recently. Despite present trends, cerebrovascular disease will not disappear. Even if atherosclerosis and hypertension were eliminated, genetic, inflammatory, and nonarteriosclerotic cardiovascular and cerebrovascular disease demand understanding of the cerebral circulation and skillful management of the damaged brain.

While most developed countries benefit from decreasing stroke mortality, developing countries are experiencing an increased incidence of stroke. In China, as acute infections, tuberculosis, and malnutrition come under control, cardiovascular and cerebrovascular diseases become commoner. In a district of Beijing, for example, the annual stroke mortality rate rose from 43/100,000 during the period 1955 to 1959 to 97/100,000 during 1974 to 1978. Stroke as a cause of death also moved from

THE PROBLEM

9

seventh to second place. In 8 of 12 Chinese cities studied, cerebrovascular diseases represented the leading cause of death.[2]

Stroke remains pre-eminent among neurologic problems, buffeted between decline and resurgence because of the rising mean age of the world's population.[31]

CONCLUSION

Stroke is a leading and worldwide cause of death and disability. The striking change in stroke type and incidence documented throughout the world demands a new look at stroke classification. North America, Australia, and parts of Europe have experienced a steady decline in stroke mortality, especially during the last decade—a trend threatened by an increasingly elderly and stroke-prone population. As the younger populations of developing countries urbanize and industrialize, the incidence of circulatory disorders, including stroke, may rise.

Stroke terminology and classification have not kept pace with advances in understanding. The International Classification of Diseases offers vague, overlapping categories that mix etiology, anatomy, and symptomatology in their definitions. Experts' elaborate and exhaustive classifications lack the practicality required at the bedside. We propose a simple classification combining anatomic location, nature, cause and temporal evolution of the lesion, and a management classification composed of TIA or minor stroke, major stroke, deteriorating stroke, and young stroke.

Although apoplexy has been recognized since antiquity, only in the past three decades has enough knowledge been gained to alter its course.

REFERENCES

1. LAMBO, TA: *Stroke—A worldwide health problem*. In GOLDSTEIN, M, ET AL (EDS): *Advances in Neurology*, Vol 25. Raven Press, New York, 1979, p 1.

2. WU, YK: *Epidemiology and community control of hypertension, stroke and coronary heart disease in China*. Chin Med J (Engl)92:665, 1979.

3. WHISNANT, JP: *The role of the neurologist in the decline of stroke*. Ann Neurol 14:1, 1983.

4. KURTZKE, JF: *Epidemiology of cerebrovascular disease*. In SIEKERT, RG (ED): *Cerebrovascular Survey Report*. National Institute of Neurology and Communicative Disorders and Stroke, Bethesda, MD, 1980, p 135.

5. WEINFELD, FD (ED): *The National Survey of Stroke*. Stroke 12(Suppl 1):I-71, 1981.

6. WOLF, PA, KANNEL, WB, AND VERTER, J: *Current status of risk factors for stroke*. Neurol Clin 1:317, 1983.

7. OSUNTOKUN, BO, ET AL: *Incidence of stroke in an African city: Results from the stroke registry at Ibadan, Nigeria 1973–75*. Stroke 10:205, 1979.

8. HEYMAN, A, FIELDS, WS, AND KEATING, RD: *Joint study of extracranial arterial occlusion. vi. Racial differences in hospitalized patients with ischemic stroke*. JAMA 222:285, 1972.

9. BARNETT, HJM: *Heart in ischemic stroke—A changing emphasis*. Neurol Clin 1:291, 1983.

10. HERD, JA, AND WEISS, SM (EDS): *Behavior and Arteriosclerosis*. Plenum Press, New York, 1983.

11. CLARKE, E: *Apoplexy in the Hippocratic writings*. Bull Hist Med 37:301, 1963.

12. SCHILLER, F: *Concepts of stroke before and after Virchow*. Med Hist 14:115, 1970.

13. GURDJIAN, ES, AND GURDJIAN, ES: *History of occlusive cerebrovascular disease, i. From Wepfer to Moniz*. Arch Neurol 36:340, 1979.

14. ACKERMAN, RH: *Controversies in ischemic brain disease*. Neurology (Suppl)31:160, 1981.

15. ROWLAND, LP: *Presidential address: Thirty years of progress and problems in clinical neurology.* Ann Neurol 11:327, 1982.

16. EASTCOTT, HHG, PICKERING, GW, AND ROBB, CG: *Reconstruction of internal carotid artery in a patient with intermittent attacks of hemiplegia.* Lancet 2:994, 1954.

17. HASS, WK: *Occlusive cerebrovascular disease.* Med Clin North Am 56:1281, 1972.

18. CAPLAN, LR: *Are terms such as completed stroke or RIND of continued usefulness?* Stroke 14:431, 1983.

19. LADURNER, G, ET AL: *A correlation of clinical findings and CT in ischemic cerebrovascular disease.* Eur Neurol J 18:281, 1979.

20. HACHINSKI, VC, AND NORRIS, JW: *The deteriorating stroke.* In MEYER, JS, ET AL (EDS): *Cerebral Vascular Disease 3.* Excerpta Medica, Amsterdam, 1980, p 315.

21. HACHINSKI, VC, LASSEN, NA, AND MARSHALL, J: *Multi-infarct dementia, a cause of mental deterioration in the elderly.* Lancet 2:207, 1974.

22. KURTZKE, JF: *ICD 9: A Regression.* Am J Epidemiol 109:383, 1979.

23. WORLD HEALTH ORGANIZATION: *International Classification of Diseases, Ninth Revision Conference 1975.* World Health Organization, Geneva, 1977.

24. MILLIKAN, CH, ET AL: *A classification and outline of cerebrovascular diseases II.* Stroke 6:564, 1975.

25. CARTER, AB: *Ingravescent cerebral infarction.* Q J Med 29:611, 1960.

26. HART, RG, AND MILLER, VT: *Cerebral infarction in young adults: A practical approach.* Stroke 14:110, 1983.

27. OSTFELD, AM: *A review of stroke epidemiology.* Epidemiol Rev 2:136, 1980.

28. HATANO, S: *Experience from a multicentre stroke register: A preliminary report.* Bull WHO 54:541, 1976.

29. KULLER, LH: *Epidemiology of stroke.* In SCHOENBERG, BS (ED): *Advances in Neurology,* Vol 19. Raven Press, New York, 1978, p 281.

30. BANCALARI E, ET AL: *Hospital incidence of cerebrovascular diseases in high altitude.* In MEYER, JS, ET AL (EDS): *Cerebral Vascular Disease 4.* Excerpta Medica, Amsterdam, 1983, p. 22.

31. EDITORIAL: *World Health Day 1982: Add life to years.* WHO Chron 36:68, 1982.

32. FRIES, JF: *Aging, natural death and the compression of morbidity.* N Engl J Med 303:130, 1980.

33. CHAMBERS, BR, ET AL: *Prognostic profiles in acute stroke* (abstr). Can J Neurol Sci 11:335, 1984.

34. KAGAN, A, ET AL: *Epidemiologic studies on coronary artery disease and stroke in Japanese men living in Japan, Hawaii and California: Prevalence of stroke.* In SCHEINBERG, P (ED): *Cerebrovascular Diseases.* Raven Press, New York, 1976, p 267.

35. SUZUKI, J, AND KODAMA, N: *Moyamoya disease—A review.* Stroke 14:104, 1983.

36. BARNETT, HJM, AND PEERLESS, SJ: *Collaborative EC/IC Bypass Study: The rationale and a progress report.* In MOOSSY, J, AND REINMUTH, OM (EDS): *Cerebrovascular Diseases.* Raven Press, New York, 1981, p 271.

37. OSUNTOKUN, BO: *The neurology of non-alcoholic pancreatic diabetes mellitus in Nigerians.* J Neurol Sci 11:17, 1970.

38. ACHESON, RM HEYMAN, A, AND NEFZGER, MD: *Mortality from stroke among US veterans in Georgia and five western states. 3. Hypertension and demographic characteristics.* J Chron Dis 26:417, 1973.

39. PONCE-DUCHARME, P: *Personal communication.* March, 1982.

40. BARNETT, HJM: *Platelet antiaggregants in stroke prevention: A review of rationale and results.* In BARNETT, HJM, HIRSH, J, AND MUSTARD, JF: *Acetylsalicylic Acid: New Uses for an Old Drug.* Raven Press, New York, 1982, p 175.

41. HACHINSKI, VC: *Decline of the incidence and mortality of stroke.* Stroke 15:376, 1984.

42. GARRAWAY, WM, ET AL: *The declining incidence of stroke.* N Engl J Med 300:449, 1979.

43. UEDA, K, ET AL: *Decreasing trend in incidence and mortality from stroke in Hisayama residents, Japan.* Stroke 12:154, 1981.

44. WHISNANT, JP: *The decline of stroke.* Stroke 15:160, 1984.

45. GARRAWAY, WM: *The changing pattern of survival following stroke.* Stroke 14:699, 1983.

46. FISHER, CM: *Lacunar strokes and infarctions: A review.* Neurology 32:871, 1982.

47. BARNETT, HJM: *The Canadian cooperative study of platelet-suppressive drugs in transient cerebral ischemia.* In PRICE, TR, AND NELSON, E (EDS): *Cerebrovascular Diseases.* Raven Press, New York, 1979, p 221.

48. HACHINSKI, V: *Decreased incidence and mortality of stroke.* Stroke 15:376, 1984.

49. CHRISTIE, D: *Stroke in Melbourne, Australia: An epidemiological study.* Stroke 12:467, 1981.
50. WANG, C, ET AL: *Epidemiology of cerebrovascular disease in the People's Republic of China.* Stroke 14:121, 1983.
51. CASTRO, IM: *Cerebrovascular accidents as public health problem: Possibilities of prevention.* JAMA Rev Cub Med 22:53, 1983.
52. OXFORDSHIRE COMMUNITY STROKE PROJECT: *Incidence of stroke in Oxfordshire: First year's experience of a community stroke register.* Br Med J 287:713, 1983.
53. NORRIS, JW, AND HACHINSKI, VC: Unpublished material derived from Toronto acute stroke unit data, 1984.
54. AHO, K, ET AL: *Cerebrovascular disease in the community: Results of a WHO Collaborative Study.* Bull WHO 58:113, 1980.

Chapter 2

APPROACHES TO THE PROBLEM

Every man takes the limits of his own field of vision
for the limits of the world.
Arthur Schopenhauer

Stroke patients are managed inconsistently and often poorly. In some developing countries, the true incidence and mode of managing stroke patients are entirely unknown.[1,2] Stroke is a medical emergency needing hospitalization, since correct treatment depends on accurate diagnosis, which requires expertise and technology only available in a hospital. Many patients are still treated at home, even in developed countries. For instance, 42 percent of 84 acute stroke patients in a single general practice in northeastern England were managed without hospital admission[3] and, as recently as 1983, Wade and Hewer[4] argued against admitting acute stroke patients to the hospital. Scarcity of beds, finances, cultural factors,[5] and the belief that hospital treatment does not change prognosis may influence hospital admission. In the hospital, patients may be looked after by a family physician, internist, geriatrician, neurologist, or other type of physician, and their quality of care is often a matter of chance. Only recently has the need for a consistent approach and a minimal level of expertise been urged.[6]

Many physicians are therapeutic nihilists concerning stroke, creating a vicious circle in which lack of knowledge retards the search for effective therapy, generating even more negative attitudes. Following a flurry of controversial reports[7–10] in the early 1970s, little has been written about stroke units. Unlike coronary care units, acute stroke units create immense problems, of an essentially geriatric population needing chronic care, which no hospital administration confronts enthusiastically. The paucity of controlled studies of the benefits of acute stroke units has not eased this situation, and conflicting and uncritical reports confuse rather than clarify. Conclusions that acute stroke units have little impact on patient care but educate the personnel[11] are unlikely to encourage their proliferation by health planners.

Acute stroke units are modeled on coronary intensive care units, yet they have not multiplied in the same way. If the benefits of coronary care units are questioned, acute stroke units are even more in dispute. Mortality is an easily defined measure of care in acute myocardial infarction. In stroke, the issues are more complex, as survival after a devastating stroke may be more grievous than death.

Intensive or acute care for stroke should not be equated with acute rehabilitation. Stroke rehabilitation units treat patients who have survived the initial, most dangerous phase of stroke. These patients often are young, are less disabled, and have good prospects of recovery. They are *not* comparable to patients in acute stroke units, in which diagnostic accuracy is higher[12] and in which cerebral rather than systemic factors[13] determine outcome.

THE RATIONALE FOR ACUTE STROKE UNITS

The three major goals of acute stroke units are:

1. To optimize patient care
2. To foster research into acute cerebrovascular disorders
3. To further education in all aspects of stroke

Acute care units provide immediate specialist care and continuous clinical observation. Commenting on the California Regional Stroke Program, Drake and colleagues stated, "The major operational emphasis of most units was on personnel and services as opposed to equipment."[10] Potentially reversible deterioration in the acute stroke patient is detected earlier by attentive nurses than by any cardiac or cerebral monitoring system yet devised.

Since vascular diseases of the brain and heart are closely related, combined cardio-cerebrovascular acute care units have been advocated. The absence of neurologic input to this otherwise favorable concept is evidenced by the absence of any data relating to the effect of such units on stroke outcome.[14]

Effective stroke units would have a major impact on health planning, since stroke is an increasing cause of mortality and long-term disability in an aging population. Unfortunately, published studies vary from anecdotal reports on small groups of patients to larger but uncontrolled studies.[9,10,14,15] The type of stroke unit must be described, since data from intensive care units,[7] combined cardio-cerebrovascular units,[14] and stroke rehabilitation units[16] are not comparable.

The benefits alleged for stroke unit patients are not valid without a comparison group, and the nonrandom allocation of control patients invites bias.[9] Comparison of outcomes in different institutions with different diagnostic criteria is also likely to be invalid.[17] The comparative study of Kennedy and coworkers, although one of the earliest,[7] remains the most reliable and convincing. "Before-and-after" studies following initiation of a stroke program[10] suffer all the drawbacks of historic controls and of retrospective studies. The conclusion that neurovascular care units reduce complication-related deaths is therefore subject to the influence of extraneous factors. The benefits of acute stroke units can only be unequivocally demonstrated by studies using random allocation of patients either to an acute stroke unit or to one providing standard medical care with equivalent assessment in both units.

THE TORONTO EXPERIENCE

The MacLachlan Acute Stroke Unit in Toronto (Fig. 5) provides acute (not intensive) care to five patients with continuous nursing observation and bedside ECG monitoring but does not include intensive respiratory support.[15] Active rehabilitation starts on admission to prevent complications that may otherwise prolong morbidity or increase mortality.[7]

Admission Criteria

Most acute stroke patients are admitted from the emergency department and, since systemic and cerebral deterioration is maximal in the first few hours, it is essential to minimize delay in admission to the unit. Patients are not excluded because of age, concurrent illness, or severity of stroke, and admission is decided on the individual case. The event should be

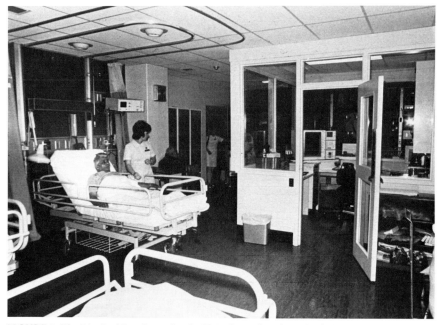

FIGURE 5. The MacLachlan Acute Stroke Unit, Sunnybrook Medical Centre, Toronto.

TABLE 2. Stroke Type and Location in 1269 Patients Admitted to the Toronto Unit, 1975–1980

	Male	Female	Total	Percentage All Stroke
Infarction				
Carotid territory	446	371	817	64
Vertebrobasilar territory	90	59	149	12
M:F = 1.25:1				
TIA				
Carotid territory	67	46	113	9
Amaurosis fugax	9	2	11	1
Vertebrobasilar territory	43	26	69	5
M:F = 1.61:1				
Hemorrhage				
Supratentorial	41	53	94	7
Infratentorial	6	10	16	1
M:F = 0.74:1				

less than 48 hours old, since highly specialized cardiac and cerebral monitoring facilities are inappropriate for patients in whom rehabilitation is the major priority. Early CT or isotope scanning identify subdural hematoma, subarachnoid hemorrhage, and cerebral tumors, which may mimic stroke.

Although completed ischemic stroke is by far the commonest cause for admission (Table 2), it is essential to admit patients with "threatened stroke," since they have the most potential for treatment. Patients with serious stroke deficits commonly die from irreversible causes, and admission priority should be directed to those whose potential for treatment and recovery is maximal, such as patients with minimal deficits or TIAs.[18]

The Standardized Approach to Acute Stroke

Initial assessment of all stroke patients by a neurologist will ensure greater diagnostic accuracy.[12,19] Management of "stroke" patients at home, while economical, ignores progress in diagnosis and management. All patients should have the opportunity for confirmation of the diagnosis.[20] The milder the stroke, the greater the chance of recovery, and the more compelling the hospital admission.

Stroke Disability Scales

A standardized assessment at regular intervals using a clinical scoring system will help to detect deterioration and monitor the course of the patient.

Numerous scoring systems have been used to evaluate the functional severity of acute stroke patients and to predict prognosis. The Glasgow Coma Scale[21] is too insensitive for stroke monitoring and omits critical variables such as aphasia. Other systems either include nonfunctional variables such as deep tendon reflexes[22] or distort the evaluation

TABLE 3. Neurologic Scoring Systems of Mathew,[26] Gilsanz,[27] and Larsson,[28] and Colleagues

Factor	Mathew et al[26] (1972)	Gilsanz et al[27] (1975)	Larsson et al[28] (1976)
Level of consciousness	0–8	0–9	0–6
Orientation	0–6	0–9	0–6
Speech	0–23	0–9	0–6
Eyefields	0–3	0–6	0–3
Conjugate deviation	0–3	0–6	0–3
Facial weakness	0–3	0–6	0–6
Motor power (each limb)	0–5	0–6	0–4
Reflexes	0–3	0–6	0–8
Sensation	0–9		0–3
Disability status scale	0–28	0–9	
Maximum score	100	75	54

by emphasizing unusual findings such as disturbed mental function.[23] Some methods score positively for absent variables such as seizures,[24] which have little effect on severity or outcome.[25]

The scales of Mathew, Gilsanz, and Larsson, and their colleagues[26–28] (Table 3) are practical and include most of the relevant variables. Their greatest limitation is oversimplification, since they equate mild deficits such as hemianopia with more severe ones such as paralysis. This was corrected by weighting each variable in the Toronto Stroke Scale and in the Canadian Neurological Scale (Tables 4 and 5; Figs. 6 and 7).[29,30]

TABLE 4. The Toronto Stroke Scoring System

1. Consciousness	alert, drowsy, stuporous, light coma, deep coma		0–4	×25	0–100
2. Paresis		face	0–3	×1	0–3
		arm	0–4	×3.5	0–14
		leg	0–4	×2.5	0–10
3. Sensory impairment		face	0–2	×1.5	0–3
		arm	0–2	×6	0–12
		leg	0–2	×4.5	0–9
4. Hemianopia			0–2	×3	0–6
5. Aphasia	none, mild, moderate, severe, total		0–4	×10	0–40
6. Higher cortical function		frontal	0–2	×12	0–48
		parietal	0–2		
7. Mental confusion			0–3	×3	0–9
8. Forced gaze			0–2	×2	0–4
9. Incoordination			0–3	×3	0–9
10. Dysarthria			0–3	×2	0–6
11. Dysphagia			0–2	×4	0–8
Maximum score					281

From Norris, JW,[29] with permission.

TABLE 5. Toronto Stroke Scale Related to Clinical Bedside Assessment

Stroke Severity (Number of Cases)		Mean Score	Standard Deviation	Range
Mild	(11)	24	18	1–50
Moderate	(24)	72	24	11–102
Severe	(7)	114	33	75–155

From Norris, JW,[29] with permission.

THE EFFECT OF ACUTE STROKE UNITS ON PATIENT CARE

Diagnostic Accuracy

Diagnostic advances may cause an apparent change in stroke mortality by excluding disorders with differing prognoses, such as postictal states. Epidemiologic studies of stroke based on death certificates suffer severe drawbacks in diagnostic accuracy,[31] and pathologic series are unrepresentative. Clinical series fall somewhere in between. The Toronto series approaches epidemiologic representativeness, since patients were referred from a well-defined catchment area and the diagnostic accuracy of the unit was evaluated in detail.[12] The reported accuracy of clinical stroke diagnosis compared with autopsy findings varies from 40 to 90 percent.[32] Diagnostic skill is primarily clinical and is more easily acquired and retained by the concentrated experience of a specialized unit.

Brain imaging techniques such as CT scanning do not substitute for clinical acumen. Although the CT scan is positive in virtually all patients with cerebral hemorrhage, it is only positive in half of cases of cerebral infarction by the second day.[33] Equally important in distinguishing cerebral hemorrhage from infarction is to identify patients with other disor-

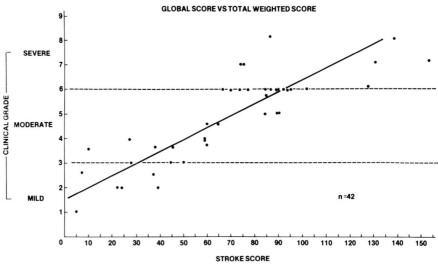

FIGURE 6. Relationship of clinical evaluation to stroke score (each point represents the initial score of one patient). (From Norris, JW,[29] with permission.)

ACUTE STROKE

18

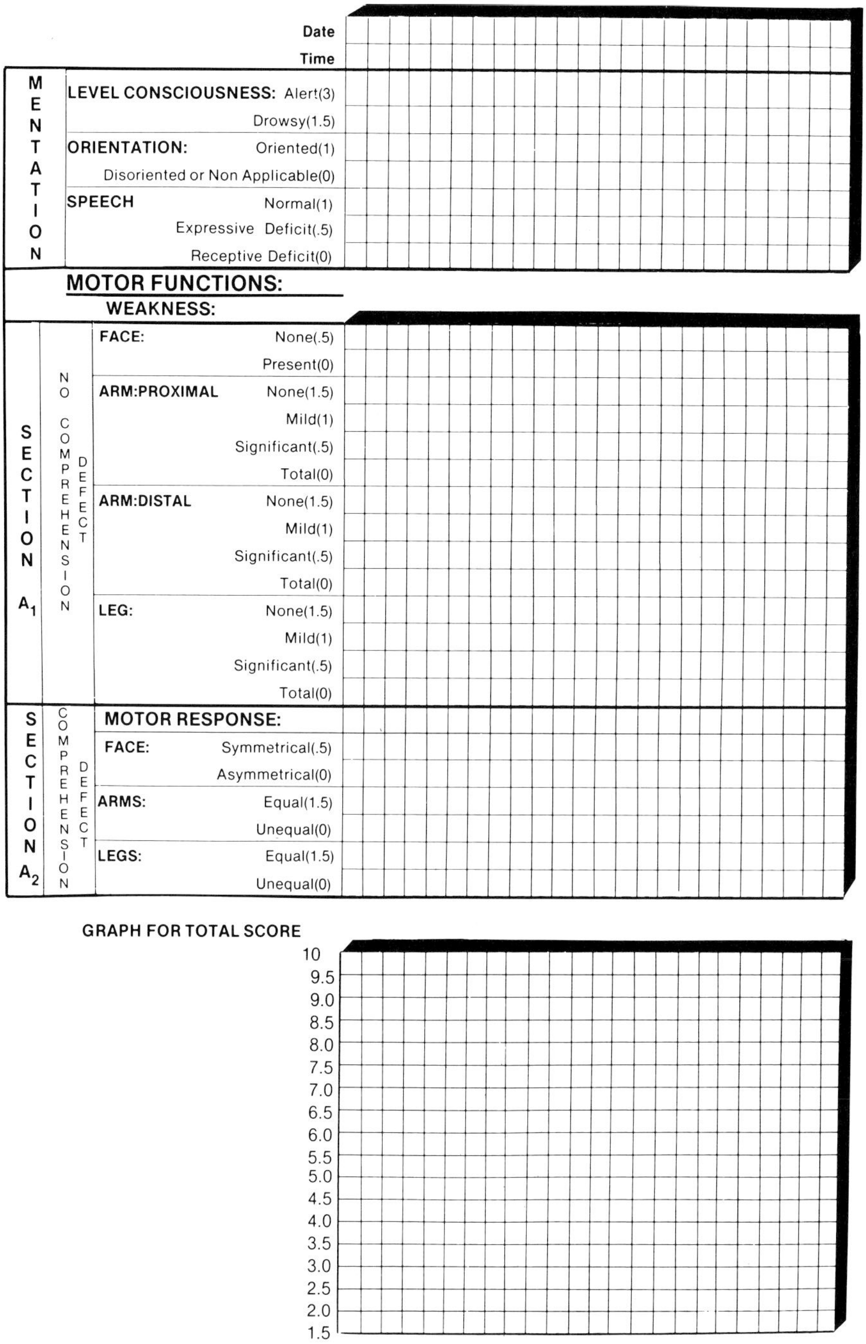

			Date	
			Time	

MENTATION

LEVEL CONSCIOUSNESS:	Alert(3)
	Drowsy(1.5)
ORIENTATION:	Oriented(1)
	Disoriented or Non Applicable(0)
SPEECH	Normal(1)
	Expressive Deficit(.5)
	Receptive Deficit(0)

MOTOR FUNCTIONS:
WEAKNESS:

SECTION A₁ — NO COMPREHENSION DEFECT

FACE:	None(.5)
	Present(0)
ARM:PROXIMAL	None(1.5)
	Mild(1)
	Significant(.5)
	Total(0)
ARM:DISTAL	None(1.5)
	Mild(1)
	Significant(.5)
	Total(0)
LEG:	None(1.5)
	Mild(1)
	Significant(.5)
	Total(0)

SECTION A₂ — COMPREHENSION DEFECT

MOTOR RESPONSE:

FACE:	Symmetrical(.5)
	Asymmetrical(0)
ARMS:	Equal(1.5)
	Unequal(0)
LEGS:	Equal(1.5)
	Unequal(0)

GRAPH FOR TOTAL SCORE

10
9.5
9.0
8.5
8.0
7.5
7.0
6.5
6.0
5.5
5.0
4.5
4.0
3.5
3.0
2.5
2.0
1.5

FIGURE 7. Observation record, Canadian Neurological Scale. Items are weighted, and the total is graphed at bottom. The greater the score, the better the preserved function. (From Côté, et al,[30] with permission.)

TABLE 6. Comparison of Mechanisms of Death During the Acute and Subacute Phases in 180 Patients With Supratentorial Stroke Admitted to the Toronto Unit

Cause of Death	Cerebral Infarction		Cerebral Hemorrhage	
	1st Wk	2nd–4th Wk	1st Wk	2nd–4th Wk
Transtentorial herniation	36	6	42	2
Pneumonia	0	28	1	2
Cardiac causes	7	17	0	2
Pulmonary embolism	0	4	0	0
Sudden death	2	8	0	0
Septicemia	1	4	0	0
Unknown	0	12	1	3
Brainstem extension of hematoma	0	0	1	1
Total	46	79	45	10

From Silver et al,[18] with permission.

ders misdiagnosed as stroke. For instance, in the pre-CT era, Carter described the difficulties of differentiating patients with acute cerebral infarction from those with cerebral tumor,[34] whereas in 1982, we found only 1 percent misdiagnosed in this way.[12]

Improving Mortality

Death in the acute phase occurs mainly from cerebral causes and in the subacute and chronic phases primarily from systemic causes (Table 6; Fig. 8).[18,35–37] The clinical effects of raised intracranial pressure from ischemic edema or cerebral hemorrhage are detected early in an acute stroke unit. Although the patient with cerebral hemorrhage may need emergency craniotomy, no effective medical or surgical treatment is available to most stroke patients, so the special facilities of an acute stroke unit may add little to management.

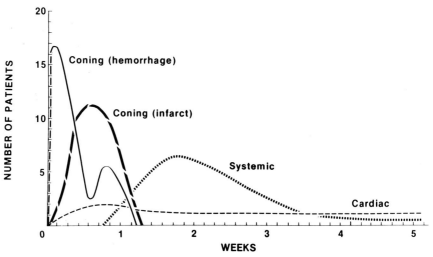

FIGURE 8. Cause of death following supratentorial infarction or hemorrhage in 180 consecutive patients admitted to the Toronto Unit. (From Silver, et al,[18] with permission.)

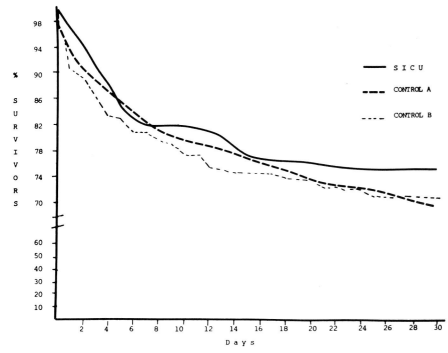

FIGURE 9. Survival curves for patients in stroke intensive care units and control hospital wards. (From Kennedy, et al,[7] with permission.)

After the first 2 weeks, death is more commonly due to pneumonia, pulmonary embolism, or ischemic heart disease,[18,36] which are reduced by early ambulation and physiotherapy. Since systemic complications influence outcome, management in the subacute and later stages may be critical. Initial data from stroke rehabilitation units supported the concept of early rehabilitation,[38] but these gains were not later maintained.[39] Kennedy and associates[7] found identical survival over 30 days in comparably ill stroke patients admitted to special stroke units compared with those admitted to routine hospital facilities (Fig. 9). They noted that "significant reduction in early stroke death must await new developments in medical and surgical therapy."[7] Unfortunately, little has changed since those prophetic words were written in 1970.

Improving Stroke Morbidity

Data on the quality of survival are scarce, because controlled studies are lacking and existing reports cannot be compared. Disability owing to brain damage (primary morbidity) should be distinguished from disability owing to complications (secondary morbidity).

Primary Morbidity

Adverse determinants of later neurologic disability[10,13,17,40,41] are:

1. Severity of initial lesion
2. Age
3. Impaired conscious state on admission

TABLE 7. Comparative Risk of
Developing Complications in
Stroke Unit Patients and Two
"Control" Stroke Groups

	0–9 Days		10–30 Days	
	Total	Dead	Total	Dead
SICU	1.0	1.0	1.0	1.0
Control A	2.54	1.93	0.763	1.39
Control B	2.13	2.5	0.808	1.36

From Kennedy et al,[7] with permission.

4. Persistent forced conjugate gaze
5. Hemispheric lesions (more favorable outcome in brainstem strokes)

None of these factors is likely to be affected by the intervention of an acute stroke unit.

Secondary Morbidity

Continuous nursing care in acute stroke units prevents and minimizes complications such as pneumonia, pulmonary embolism, thrombophlebitis, urinary tract infections and septicemia, decubiti, and sudden death (from acute myocardial infarction) (Tables 7 and 8).[7] Activities of daily living were significantly improved in patients randomly allocated on admission to a "stroke unit" (geriatric rehabilitation unit), compared with a control group admitted to a medical ward (Table 9).[38] However, the functional improvement noted at hospital discharge was lost after 1 year, and this was attributed to overprotection by the families of stroke unit patients, rather than representing a failure of the long-term effect of the rehabilitation unit.[39]

Silver and associates investigated the mechanisms of death in stroke in the Toronto Unit and found that late deaths were commonly preventable, but most of these patients had poor functional recovery (Table 10).[18] They concluded that acute stroke units should admit patients with minor neurologic deficits in whom further stroke could be prevented, rather than treating patients with irreversible and disabling brain damage. The threat of cardiac complications, including sudden death, persists for at least 30 days, striking the mildly and severely impaired alike.

TABLE 8. Increased Frequency of
Late Complications in the Three
Groups

	0–9 Days	10–30 Days
SICU	1.0	8.0
Control A	1.0	5.74
Control B	1.0	4.36

From Kennedy et al,[7] with permission.

TABLE 9. Outcome at End of Rehabilitation Stage (60 Days)

Activities of Daily Living	Stroke Unit n = 155	Medical Units n = 152
Independent	78 (50%)	49 (32%)
Dependent	47 (31%)	60 (40%)
Dead	30 (19%)	43 (28%)

From Garraway et al,[39] with permission.

The Problem of Pulmonary Embolism in Stroke

Deep venous thrombosis (DVT), with its constant threat of fatal or disabling pulmonary embolism, is a major problem in all severely immobilized patients. Added to the risk of death or pulmonary infarction is the common sequela of the postphlebitic syndrome. The reported incidence of DVT varies from 19 to 43 percent in postneurosurgical patients,[42] acute spinal injury patients,[43,44] and those with stroke.[45] If pulmonary embolism accounted for half the "sudden deaths" in the Toronto Unit (see Table 6), then it caused 5 percent (9 of 180) of stroke deaths.

The study of Kakkar and colleagues[46] illustrates the major problems of detecting and managing DVT. Thrombosis, confirmed by phlebography, developed in 30 percent of 132 postoperative patients whose legs were scanned with ^{125}I-fibrinogen. The thrombus resolved in 14 patients and remained in 26, of whom four developed pulmonary embolism. The thrombus remained localized to the calf in 19 patients, but in nine, including the four who developed pulmonary embolism, it extended into the upper leg and pelvis.

Clinical examination detects 10 to 50 percent of cases,[47,48] and all screening procedures have disadvantages. Phlebography is the most accurate but is invasive and has complications, which limits its use to confirmation.[49] ^{125}I-fibrinogen scanning detects 90 percent of distal (calf) thrombi but is much less sensitive[50] for ileofemoral thrombosis, a much commoner source of emboli. Since only 20 percent of positive-scan patients develop ascending thrombus, its clinical relevance is questionable.[51]

Although Doppler examination has a reported sensitivity of 84 percent for detection of proximal thrombi, it has never found popularity

TABLE 10. Functional Status Prior to Death in 123 Patients Dying of Noncerebral Causes

	Grade	Supratentorial		Infratentorial	
		Infarction	Hemorrhage	Infarction	Hemorrhage
I	Normal	11	1	0	0
II	Semiambulant	13	0	2	0
III	Bedridden	37	5	9	0
IV	Vegetative	22	3	16	4
	Total	83	9	27	4

From Silver et al,[18] with permission.

owing to its observer variability.[52] Impedance plethysmography (IPG) is reliable, accurate, and totally noninvasive.[53] False-positive results may occur, however, in uncooperative patients and in those with congestive heart failure or peripheral vascular disease. Since ^{125}I-fibrinogen scanning is effective for distal thrombi and IPG for proximal thrombi, their combination is probably best.

Despite the known frequency of DVT in stroke patients,[45] there have been surprisingly few attempts at pharmacologic prophylaxis. Anticoagulants reduce the incidence of DVT and pulmonary embolism in patients with risk factors such as varicose veins, obesity, and immobility.[51,54] Antiplatelet agents reduce DVT, but their effect on pulmonary embolism is questionable.[52]

Secondary bleeding into cerebral infarction is theoretically a serious consequence of low and "minidose" heparin therapy, but these have proven safe and effective prophylaxes for DVT in spinal cord trauma patients.[55] Heparin prophylaxis in acute ischemic stroke awaits identification of a subgroup at high risk of embolism.

CONCLUSION

Stroke management differs widely, from therapeutic nihilism to enthusiastic treatment with unproven remedies. Acute stroke units, by concentrating experience and education in stroke care, increase diagnostic accuracy. All stroke patients deserve hospital admission for diagnosis but not necessarily for treatment. Continuous observation and standardized neurologic assessment by skilled personnel shows more sensitivity in detection of early clinical deterioration than does any laboratory test yet devised.

Acute stroke units do not affect mortality, since early death in stroke results from untreatable swelling and destruction of the brain. They reduce systemic complications, mainly pulmonary and cardiac, decreasing late mortality and enhancing the quality of life of survivors—but they have no effect on neurologic recovery.

The cost effectiveness of these units is uncertain, since reducing mortality may result in increased morbidity. Patients with minimal lesions or threatened stroke should have first priority for admission, rather than those with devastating lesions.

REFERENCES

1. DALAL, PM: *Strokes in the young in west central India.* In GOLDSTEIN, M, ET AL (EDS): *Advances in Neurology,* Vol 25. Raven Press, New York, 1979, p 339.
2. OSUNTOKUN, BO: *Undernutrition and infectious disorders as risk factors in stroke (with special reference to Africans).* In GOLDSTEIN, M, ET AL (EDS): *Advances in Neurology,* Vol 25. Raven Press, New York, 1979, p 161.
3. WATERS, HJ, AND PERKIN, JM: *Study of stroke patients in a single general practice.* Br Med J 284:791, 1982.
4. WADE, DT, AND HEWER, RL: *Why admit stroke patients to hospital?* Lancet 1:807, 1983.
5. NDIAYE, IP, AND CHRAIBY, M: *Neurogeriatrics in Senegal.* In TERRY, RD, BOLIS, CL, AND TOFFANO, G: *Neural Aging and its Implications in Human Neurological Pathology.* Raven Press, New York, 1982, p 215.

6. CAPLAN, LR: *Treatment of cerebral ischemia—Where are we headed?* Stroke 15:571, 1984.

7. KENNEDY, FB, ET AL: *Stroke intensive care—An appraisal.* Am Heart J 80:188, 1970.

8. TAYLOR, RR: *Acute stroke demonstration project in a community hospital.* J SC Med Assoc 66:225, 1970.

9. PITNER, SE, AND MANCE, CJ: *An evaluation of stroke intensive care: Results in a municipal hospital.* Stroke 4:737, 1973.

10. DRAKE, WE, ET AL: *Acute stroke management and patient outcome: The value of neurovascular care units (NCU).* Stroke 4:933, 1973.

11. MILLIKAN, CH: *Stroke intensive care units, objectives and results.* Stroke 10:235, 1979.

12. NORRIS, JW, AND HACHINSKI, VC: *Misdiagnosis of stroke.* Lancet 1:328, 1982.

13. NORRIS, JW, ET AL: *Outcome of brainstem strokes.* In BERGUER, R, AND BAUER, RB (EDS): *Vertebrobasilar Occlusive Disease.* Raven Press, New York, 1984, p 37.

14. COOPER, SW, OLIVET, JA, AND WOOLSEY, FM: *Establishment and operation of combined intensive care unit.* NY State J Med 72:2215, 1972.

15. NORRIS, JW, AND HACHINSKI, VC: *Intensive care management of stroke patients.* Stroke 7:573, 1976.

16. BLOWER, P, AND ALI, S: *A stroke unit in a district general hospital: The Greenwich experience.* Br Med J 2:644, 1979.

17. CARPENTER, RR, AND REED, DE: *The outcome for patients with cerebrovascular disease in university and community hospitals.* Stroke 3:747, 1972.

18. SILVER, FL, ET AL: *Early mortality following stroke: A prospective view.* Stroke 15:492, 1984.

19. CALANCHINI, PR, ET AL: *Cooperative study of hospital frequency and character of transient ischemic attacks. iv. The reliability of diagnosis.* JAMA 238:2029, 1977.

20. STEINER, TJ: *Letter to the Editor: Why admit stroke patients to hospital?* Lancet 1:1379, 1983.

21. TEASDALE, G, AND JENNETT, B: *Assessment of coma and impaired consciousness, a practical scale.* Lancet 2:81, 1974.

22. BAUER, RB, AND TELLEZ, H: *Dexamethasone as a treatment in cerebrovascular disease; 2. A controlled study in acute cerebral infarction.* Stroke 4:547, 1973.

23. PATTEN, BM, ET AL: *Double-blind study of the effects of dexamethasone on acute stroke.* Neurology 22:377, 1972.

24. GILROY, J, BARNHART, MI, AND MEYER, JS: *Treatment of acute stroke with Dextran 40.* JAMA 210:293, 1969.

25. BLACK, SE, HACHINSKI, VC, AND NORRIS, JW: *Seizures after stroke* (abstr). Can J Neurol Sci 9:291, 1982.

26. MATHEW, NT, ET AL: *Double-blind evaluation of glycerol therapy in acute cerebral infarction.* Lancet 2:1327, 1972.

27. GILSANZ, V, ET AL: *Controlled trial of glycerol versus dexamethasone in the treatment of cerebral oedema in acute cerebral infarction.* Lancet 1:1049, 1975.

28. LARSSON, O, MARINOVICH, N, AND BARBER, K: *Double-blind trial of glycerol therapy in early stroke.* Lancet 1:832, 1976.

29. NORRIS, JW: *Letter to the Editor: Comment on "study design of stroke treatments."* Stroke 13:527, 1983.

30. CÔTÉ, R, ET AL: *The Canadian Neurological Scale: A pilot study in acute stroke patients.* Stroke (in press).

31. CORWIN, LI, ET AL: *Accuracy of death certification of stroke: The Framingham study.* Stroke 13:125, 1982.

32. WYLIE, CM: *Epidemiology of cerebrovascular disease.* In VINKEN, PJ, AND BRUYN, GW (EDS): *Handbook of Clinical Neurology,* Vol 11. North Holland, Amsterdam, 1972, p 183.

33. ABRAMS, HL, AND McNEIL, BJ: *Medical implications of computed tomography (CAT scanning).* N Engl J Med 298:255, 1978.

34. CARTER, AB: *Cerebral Infarction.* Pergamon Press, New York, 1964.

35. SHAW, CM, ALVORD, ED, JR, AND BERRY, RG: *Swelling of the brain following ischemic infarction with arterial occlusion.* Arch Neurol 1:161, 1959.

36. BROWN, M, AND GLASSENBERG, M: *Mortality factors in patients with acute stroke.* JAMA 224:1493, 1973.

37. BOUNDS, JV, ET AL: *Mechanisms and timing of deaths from cerebral infarction.* Stroke 12:474, 1981.

38. GARRAWAY, WM, ET AL: *Management of acute stroke in the elderly: Preliminary results of a controlled trial.* Br Med J 280:1040, 1980.

39. GARRAWAY, WM, ET AL: *Management of acute stroke in the elderly: Follow-up of a controlled trial.* Br Med J 281:827, 1980.

40. HAERER, AF, AND WOOSLEY, PC: *Prognosis and quality of survival in a hospitalized stroke population from the south.* Stroke 6:543, 1975.

41. OXBURY, JM, GREENHALL, RCD, AND GRAINGER, KMR: *Predicting the outcome of stroke: Acute stage after cerebral infarction.* Br Med J 3:125, 1975.

42. POWERS, SK, AND DEWARDS, MSB: *Prophylaxis of thrombo-embolism in the neurosurgical patient: A review.* Neurosurgery 10:509, 1982.

43. SILVER, JR: *The prophylactic use of anticoagulant therapy in prevention of pulmonary emboli in 100 consecutive spinal injury patients.* Paraplegia 12:188, 1974.

44. TATOR, C: Personal communication. March, 1984.

45. WARLOW, C, OGSTON, D, AND DOUGLAS, AS: *Deep vein thrombosis of the legs after strokes. Part 1: Incidence and predisposing factors.* Br Med J 1:1178, 1976.

46. KAKKAR, VV, ET AL: *Natural history of postoperative deep-vein thrombosis.* Lancet 2:230, 1969.

47. WATSON, N: *Anticoagulant therapy in the treatment of venous thrombosis and pulmonary embolism in acute spinal injury.* Paraplegia 12:197, 1974.

48. GALLUS, AS, ET AL: *Diagnosis of venous thrombo-embolism.* Semin Thromb Hemostas 2:203, 1976.

49. ALBRECHTSSON, U, AND OLSSEN, CG: *Thrombotic side effects of lower limb phlebography.* Lancet 1:723, 1976.

50. HULL, R: *The combined use of leg scanning and impedance plethysmography in suspected venous thrombosis.* N Engl J Med 296:1497, 1977.

51. RUSSELL, JC: *Prophylaxis of postoperative deep vein thrombosis and pulmonary embolism.* Surg Gynecol Obstet 157:89, 1983.

52. HANEL, K, ET AL: *The role of two noninvasive tests in deep venous thrombosis.* Ann Surg 6:725, 1981.

53. HULL, R, ET AL: *Impedance plethysmography using the occlusive cuff technique in the diagnosis of venous thrombosis.* Circulation 53:696, 1976.

54. KAKKAR, V: *The current status of low dose heparin prophylaxis of thrombophlebitis and pulmonary embolism.* World J Surg 2:3, 1978.

55. WATSON, N: *Anticoagulant therapy in the prevention of venous thrombosis and pulmonary embolism in the spinal cord injury.* Paraplegia 16:263, 1978.

Chapter 3

THE VASCULAR INFRASTRUCTURE

Happy is he who knows about the causes of things.
Virgil

The brain is the organ most prone to spontaneous intraparenchymal hemorrhage and the second-most liable to symptomatic ischemic infarction. Cerebral arteries are thinner than equivalent-sized arteries and, while they have an internal elastic lamina, they have little elastic tissue and scant adventitia.[1] When not affected by atherosclerosis, cerebral arteries appear almost transparent, illustrating their thinness and proneness to rupture. Since they lack vasa vasora, the bulk of the nourishment for the arterial wall comes from the lumen.

Once cerebral arteries penetrate the brain they effectively become end-arteries. They terminate in an all-pervading capillary plexus but function as end-arteries, since the collateral flow is insufficient to maintain the neural tissue should the artery occlude.[2] Capillary density is greater in grey matter than in white matter and is denser in layers IV and V of cortical grey matter than in layers I, II, III, and VI. Cortical capillary density increases with phylogenetic newness, being least dense in the archicortex, denser in the paleocortex and densest in the neocortex (Fig. 10).

All vertebrates have carotid arteries. "Carotid" derives from the Greek "ker," meaning head and referring to the arteries of stupor or sleep. Ancient Greek entertainers pulled a cord around a goat's neck and the animal collapsed. When they released the cord, the animal sprang to its feet again, to the cruel amusement of the audience. The Assyrians put their knowledge of carotid compression to another use; they pressed on the carotid arteries of adolescent boys during circumcision to minimize their pain.[3]

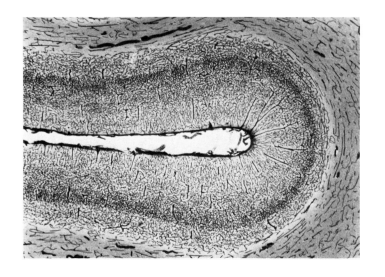

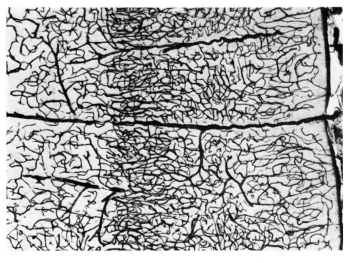

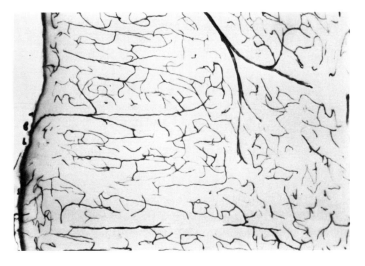

In most submammalian vertebrates, the brain's blood supply relies entirely on a pair of internal carotid arteries.[4] After penetrating the skull, each artery divides into caudal and rostral divisions. In fishes, the caudal branch predominates, supplying the medulla, cerebellum, and optic tectum. Amphibians, reptiles, birds, and mammals have progressively larger forebrains and correspondingly larger rostral divisions.[4] Humans have the largest forebrain and the most-developed rostral division of the carotid artery. Its main divisions have lengthened, curved, and branched while clinging to the expanding hemispheres, although the main arterial trunks have remained at the base.

The basilar artery is formed by the union of the caudal rami of both internal carotid arteries.[4] A pair of vertebral arteries form from enlargement of the pre-existing and anastomotic channels in the upper cervical spine and occipital region,[5] taking over the blood supply of the basilar artery in the fully developed fetus.

THE VASCULAR CENTRENCEPHALON

Penfield's "centrencephalon" indicated a theoretic site for epilepsy originating in the upper brainstem and the diencephalon.[6] The term may also prove useful in understanding the vasculature of the brain and the pathogenesis of stroke.

The medial and basal portions of the brain and brainstem are supplied by relatively short arteries penetrating the brain in the basal dorsal direction. Since these arteries arise from large basal trunks, the gradation between arterial and capillary pressure occurs over a relatively short distance, requiring the arteries to withstand high pressures. Hemorrhages tend to occur in small arteries that have undergone fibrinoid degeneration and microaneurysm formation. Microaneurysms predominate in hypertensives, particularly those over the age of 65 years.[7] Hypertrophy and hyaline degeneration also predispose the penetrating arteries to occlusion, creating small (lacunar) infarcts.[8] Lacunae can also result from atherosclerotic occlusion of the lenticulostriate artery and paramedian branches of the basilar artery.[9]

The vascular centrencephalon encompasses the major sites of lacunar infarction and hypertensive hemorrhage (Fig. 11). Functionally, arteries within the vascular centrencephalon are end-arteries. Occlusion of a centrencephalic artery usually results in a small infarct, because it supplies a limited cylinder of tissue. By contrast, the long circumferential arteries outside the vascular centrencephalon have rich anastomoses,[2] are less prone to in situ thrombosis, and are more often the recipients of emboli.[10]

←

FIGURE 10. *Top,* Capillary density is greater in grey than in white matter. Calcarine (primary visual) cortex with border of white matter, 63-year-old male, magnification ×20.

Middle, Cortical capillary density increases with phylogenetic newness, being densest in neocortex. Full width of calcarine cortex, same subject as at *top,* magnification ×80.

Bottom, Full width of presubicular cortex, 39-year-old male, magnification ×80. (From Dr. Mary Bell, Wake Forest University, with permission.)

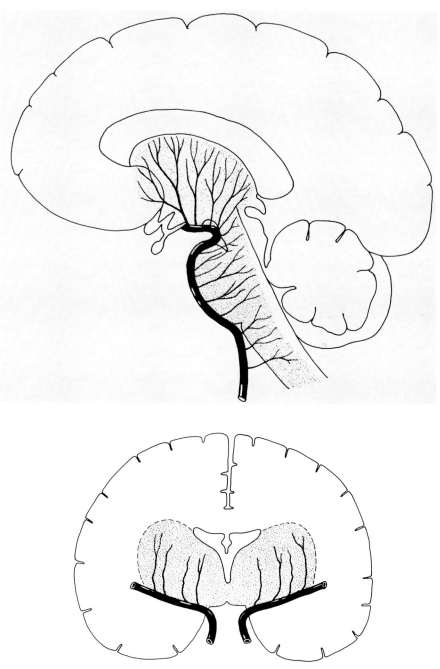

FIGURE 11. The vascular centrencephalon, the system of arteries arising from the basal arterial trunks and supplying the central phylogenetically older parts of the brain (sagittal (*top*), coronal (*bottom*), and horizontal (*top of next page*) sections).

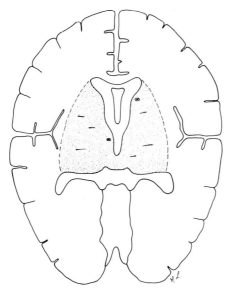

FIGURE 11. *Continued*

Rupture of a centrencephalic artery often proves devastating as it supplies compact, phylogenetically older areas of the brain. Within the vascular centrencephalon, the sharp angulation of the lenticulostriate arteries subjects their walls to considerable stress at peak systole,[11] rendering them particularly vulnerable to rupture and to massive basal ganglia hemorrhages.[12] Hemorrhage within the centrencephalon cannot be reached surgically without great risk of inflicting further damage. Hemorrhages occurring outside the centrencephalon are more accessible and may be due to a number of causes. Hemorrhage from arteriovenous malformations and amyloid angiopathy is also more common outside the centrencephalon.[13,14]

COLLATERAL CIRCULATION

Watershed Areas

The border zones of major vascular territories ("border zone network," Fig. 12) are particularly vulnerable to hypotension, because their arteries lie furthest from the parent vessel. Major watersheds occur at the borders between cerebral and cerebellar cortical vessels and in the depths of the brain between the terminal arterioles of the basal and circumferential vessels[15] (between centrencephalic and noncentrencephalic arteries).

THE IMPORTANCE OF THE BLOOD-BRAIN BARRIER

The blood-brain barrier is a complex biochemical and structural mantle investing the brain and protecting it from potentially noxious influences in the systemic circulation. It reflects the unique and sensitive metabolic requirements of cerebral function.

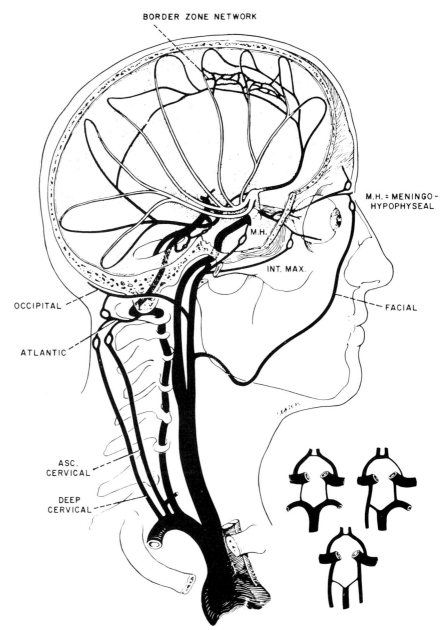

FIGURE 12. Collateral circulation of the brain. (From Fisher, CM: *The anatomy and pathology of the cerebral vasculature.* In Meyer, JS (ed): *Modern Concepts of Cerebrovascular Disease.* Spectrum, New York, 1975, p 1, with permission.)

Intravenous injection of dyes such as trypan blue stains all organs except the brain, which remains "snow-white."[16] Biochemical and electron microscopy data indicate that the major factor preventing systemic substances from entering the brain is structural.[17,18] Brain capillaries differ from systemic capillaries and impede the passage of substances into the brain for the following reasons:

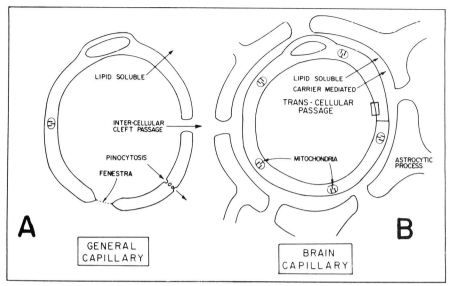

FIGURE 13. Brain capillaries (*B*) have tight endothelial junctions, scanty pinocytosis, and no fenestra, compared with general capillary (*A*). (From Oldendorf, WH: *The quest for an image of brain: A brief historical and technical review of brain imaging techniques.* Neurology 28:520, 1978, with permission.)

1. Capillary endothelial cells abut each other by tight junctions (zona occludens), preventing egress of molecules from the lumen (Fig. 13)
2. Pinocytosis (the process by which substances are normally transferred across endothelial cells by tiny vesicles) is minimal
3. Basement membrane invests the capillary tightly and completely
4. Fenestrations (holes normally present in the endothelial cells) are absent

Astrocyte foot processes invest the capillary incompletely and are probably only a minor structural barrier.[17] Transport of foreign and endogenous substances into the brain is enhanced by:[19]

1. Small size of molecules
2. High degree of lipid solubility
3. Low degree of plasma binding
4. Low degree of ionization at physiologic pH
5. Carrier-mediated transport (facilitated transfer of glucose, amino acids, and other substances) across the blood-brain barrier

The area postrema, the posterior pituitary, the pineal gland, the hypothalamus, and the subfornicular organ are devoid of a blood-brain barrier. Although these "windows" allow numerous substances easy passage into and out of the brain, they probably do not represent a significant area of "leakage."

The Effect on the Barrier of Hypoxic Ischemic Injury

Brain capillary endothelium is particularly resistant to ischemia.[20] Total circulatory arrest lasting less than 15 minutes has little effect on the blood-brain barrier, judging by the action of protein-bound dyes. Reperfusion remains possible after 1 hour of ischemia, although there is delayed opening of the barrier. The blood-brain barrier stays intact[21] after 4 hours of arterial occlusion[21] but then begins disintegrating, first water and then macromolecules leaking out.[22] The mechanism and spread of this vasogenic edema are critical to morbidity and mortality in acute stroke.

Changes in the blood-brain barrier are also critical in the pathogenesis of stroke-like syndromes and other neurologic manifestations seen in hypertensive encephalopathy. Within 90 seconds of angiotensin-induced experimental hypertension, proteins leak and astrocyte foot processes swell.[23] This increased permeability is unrelated to splitting of the tight endothelial junctions, as was previously believed, but rather to increased pinocytotic activity. Drugs such as phenothiazines protect the blood-brain barrier during this acute hypertensive crisis by modifying the endothelial cell membrane, probably by further reducing pinocytosis.[24] This therapeutic action has clinical implications beyond hypertensive encephalopathy.

Blood-brain barrier damage in cerebral infarction in humans does not appear until the second week,[25] so edema appearing earlier must result from other mechanisms. Magnetic resonance and positron emission tomography data may prove more rewarding. Understanding the exact pathogenesis and timing of acute disruption of the blood-brain barrier has enormous therapeutic implications, since death and morbidity in acute stroke result mainly from uncontrollable cerebral edema.[26–28]

CEREBRAL BLOOD FLOW AND METABOLISM

The brain is well perfused and richly oxygenated. Lipids compose about 50 percent of its dry weight, compared with 6 to 20 percent in most other organs.[29] It receives 800 ml blood and 52 ml oxygen every minute, making it the thirdmost perfused and oxygenated organ, after the kidneys and heart.[30]

Normally, the brain metabolizes only oxygen and glucose, but if starved it can satisfy up to 30 percent of its needs from ketone bodies.[31] It takes up glucose avidly and metabolizes it promptly. Glucose fulfills the brain's energy requirements through the production of adenosine triphosphate (ATP) and provides building blocks for the synthesis of all brain components except for essential fatty and amino acids.[29] Glucose metabolism occurs via three pathways: the citric acid cycle in mitochondria, the glycolytic pathway in the cellular cytoplasm, and the hexose monophosphate shunt.

Most brain energy derives from the (aerobic) citric acid cycle, metabolizing approximately 85 percent of the glucose and producing 38 moles ATP per mole of glucose. The glycolytic (anaerobic) pathway metabolizes about 15 percent of the brain's glucose, yielding only 2 moles ATP per mole of glucose. The hexose monophosphate shunt supplies no ATP but contributes pentose phosphates for the synthesis of nucleotides and lipids.[29] Little glucose is synthesized into glycogen, the brain's limited reserves of glycogen and glucose barely sufficing to fuel normal brain activity for more than 2 or 3 minutes.[32] The brain's scant energy reserves and ceaseless metabolism, even during sleep,[33,34] make it dependent on a continuous rich supply of oxygen and glucose.

Autoregulation

The brain's constant metabolic need is well served by its ability to adjust its own blood flow. This autoregulation is achieved through mechanical, biochemical, and perhaps neurogenic means. Bayliss[35] observed that the carotid artery contracts in response to stretching. Increased intraluminal pressure from a surge of blood stretches the artery, which then contracts, decreasing the lumen and diminishing blood flow. Conversely, decreasing intraluminal pressure slackens the stretch on the artery, lessens its contraction, and increases the lumen and blood flow. The limits of this autoregulation to perfusing blood pressure are well defined (Fig. 14).[36,37]

The main byproducts of the brain's activity are carbon dioxide, lactic acid, and other acidic metabolites, which decrease the perivascular pH and result in vasodilation. When cerebral metabolism decreases, fewer acidic metabolites form, the perivascular pH increases, inducing vasoconstriction and diminishing the lumen and blood flow. Adenosine, cyclic AMP, K^+, Na^+, and Ca^{++} may also play a role in biochemical regulation.[32,38] While the major cerebral arteries bear a lacework of sympathetic, cholinergic, and peptidergic nerves, their presence does not prove

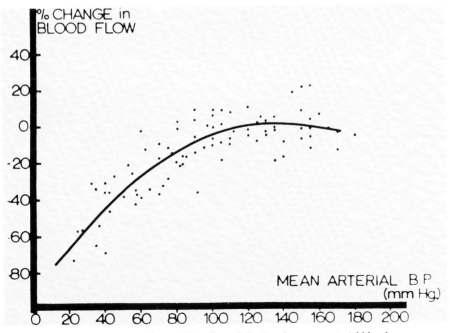

FIGURE 14. Cerebral autoregulation. The effect of altering the mean arterial blood pressure on cortical cerebral blood flow. (From Harper,[36] with permission.)

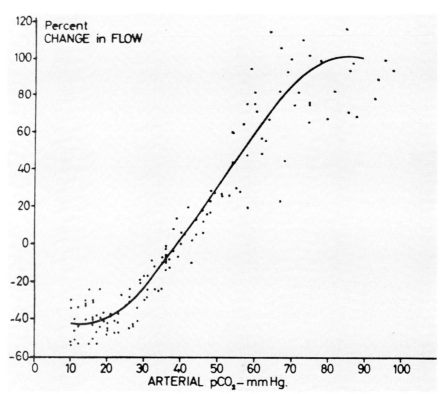

FIGURE 15. Cerebral blood flow response to changing arterial P_{CO_2}. (From Harper, AM, and Glass, HI: *Effect of alterations in the arterial carbon dioxide tension on the blood flow through the cerebral cortex at normal and low arterial blood pressures.* J Neurol Neurosurg Psychiatry 28:449, 1965, with permission.)

a neurogenic component of autoregulation.[39,40] Nonetheless, a sympathetic nerve supply seems to protect the brain during extreme increases in blood pressure.[41]

While the cerebral circulation resists changes in blood pressure, it responds exquisitely to varying carbon dioxide concentration (Fig. 15). Cerebral blood flow increases 7 percent per 1 mm Hg rise in the Pa_{CO_2}.[37] Increases in P_{O_2} vasoconstrict and decrease cerebral blood flow, whereas a fall of P_{O_2} to 40 mm Hg or lower elicits brisk vasodilation and increased brain blood flow.[42] Blood flow is constant to the brain but variable within it. Local changes in cerebral metabolism also occur with various mental activities,[44] suggesting that regional cerebral blood flow, metabolism, and function act in concert (Fig. 16).

ATHEROSCLEROSIS

Humans are particularly prone to atherosclerosis. While other animals, from pig[45] to elephant, can develop spontaneous atherosclerosis, it appears earliest and most seriously in humans. Babies can develop fatty streaks in their aorta,[46] and 45 percent of young American soldiers killed in Vietnam had some evidence of atherosclerosis.[47]

The theory of injury and repair best explains the origin, growth, and regression of atherosclerosis (Table 11).[48] Any injury to the vascular

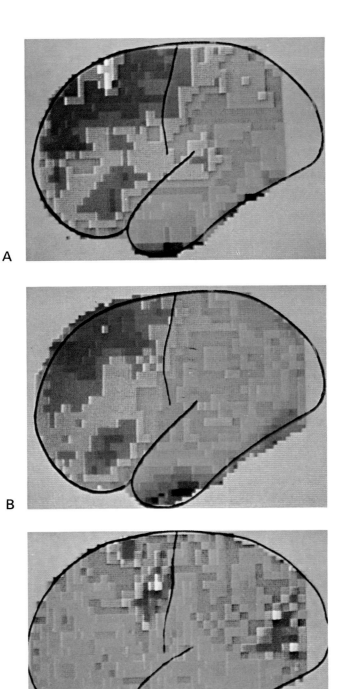

FIGURE 16. Computer-generated images of blood flow in superficial cerebral cortex, measured by intracarotid xenon-133. During rest, relatively more blood flows through the frontal areas than through the parietal or temporal regions, producing a "hyperfrontal" pattern (*A*—left hemisphere, *B*—right hemisphere). Following a moving object with the eyes increases blood flow in the visual association cortex (*C*). Listening to speech activates the temporal auditory cortex and Wernicke's area (*D*). Moving the fingers on the side opposite the hemisphere being recorded activates the hand-finger area of the central cortex and the supplementary motor area (*E*), while counting aloud increases blood flow to the mouth area of the central cortex, the supplementary motor area, and the auditory cortex (*F*). (From Lassen, et al,[43] with permission.)

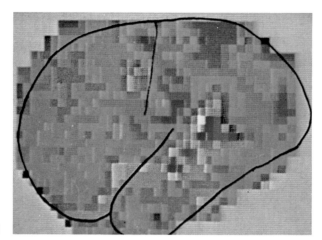

D

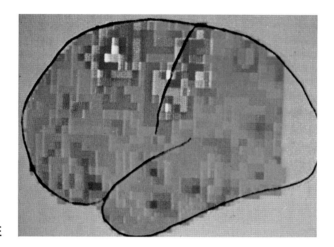

E

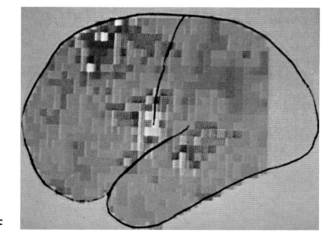

F

TABLE 11. Relation of Pathogenetic Factors to Atherosclerotic Lesions and Clinical Disease

Lesions		Factors (Instrumental and Promoting)
Early	Fatty streaks Gelatinous elevations Microthrombi	Inception	Injurious to endothelium and/or intima (mechanical, chemical, metabolic, and so on)
Advanced	Atherosclerotic plaque	Progression (Growth)	Repeated episodes of: 1. Insudation 2. Mural thrombosis 3. Hemorrhage from capillaries
Complicated	Thrombosis Ulcerations Calcification Hemorrhage	Complication	1. Local (e.g., degeneration of connective tissues, enlarging atheroma, many others) 2. Systemic (e.g., hypertension)
Terminal process	1. Occlusive thrombosis 2. Massive hemorrhage into atheroma 3. Embolism from ulcerated atheroma	Precipitation	Cigarette smoking Hypertension Hyperlipidemias Physical exertion
Clinical manifestations (referrable to):	Ischemia Infarction Hemorrhage		

From Haust and More,[46] with permission.

endothelium can induce smooth muscle proliferation, leading eventually to atherosclerosis. Platelets secrete a mitogenic factor that enhances smooth muscle proliferation, and they aggregate and facilitate the formation of thrombi, which become incorporated into the atherosclerotic lesion.[49] The role of platelets in atherosclerosis offers both problems and hope. Aspirin-induced thrombocytopenia prevented atherosclerotic lesions induced by traumatizing the aorta of rabbits fed a high-fat diet.[50] Antiplatelet agents may prove a means of minimizing or arresting the progress of atherosclerosis in humans.

Atherosclerosis develops first in the aorta, later in the coronary and lower limb arteries, and last in the cervical and cerebral arteries. Atherosclerosis occurs early at the carotid bifurcation and increases with age.[51] Although atherosclerosis and the likelihood of cerebral infarction correlate, specific predictions court error. Arterial stenoses and occlusions may be asymptomatic,[52] and blood flow falls only when the carotid lumen decreases to 2 sq mm or less.[53] Most atherosclerotic narrowing is gradual, allowing collateral flow to develop, and cerebral infarction results more commonly from sudden occlusion than from hypotension in the presence of critically stenosed arteries.[54]

CONCLUSION

The blood supply to the brain consists of basal arteries nourishing the phylogenetically older, central parts of the neural axis ("vascular centrencephalon") and larger circumferential arteries supplying the newer structures. The "vascular centrencephalon" is supplied by shorter thinner arteries, which are prone to occlusion, producing lacunar infarction, and to rupture, producing intraparenchymal hemorrhage. Centrencephalic hemorrhages commonly result from hypertension and often are surgically inaccessible. Hemorrhages outside the centrencephalon have multiple causes and are surgically more accessible.

The blood-brain barrier and autoregulation of the cerebral blood flow maintain a global homeostasis but are in constant flux focally, reflecting local neuronal activity. The brain's reliance on a continuous supply of oxygen and glucose renders it particularly vulnerable to impaired perfusion. Reversal of ischemia becomes the pivotal problem in brain recovery.

Atherosclerosis spares no one who lives long enough. Growing understanding of the dynamic nature of atherosclerosis and of the process of injury and repair provides scientific bases for its modification and eventual prevention.

REFERENCES

1. LAZORTHES, G, GOUAZE, A, AND SALAMON, G: *Vascularisation et circulation de l'encéphale*, Vol 1. Masson, Paris, 1976.
2. GILLILAN, LA: *Anatomy of the blood supply to the brain and spinal cord*. In SIEKERT, RG (ED): *Cerebrovascular Survey Report*. National Institute of Neurological and Communicative Disorders and Stroke, Bethesda, MD, 1980, p 1.
3. HILL, L: *The Physiology and Pathology of the Cerebral Circulation: An Experimental Research*. J & A Churchill, London, 1896.

4. SARNAT, HB, AND NETSKY, MG: *Evolution of the Nervous System*, ed 2. Oxford University Press, London, 1981, p 81.

5. KIER, EL: *Fetal cerebral arteries: A phylogenetic and ontogenetic study*. In NEWTON, TH, AND POTTS, DG (EDS): *Radiology of the Skull and Brain: Angiography*, Vol 2, Book 1. CV Mosby, St Louis, 1974, p 1089.

6. PENFIELD, W, AND JASPER H: *Epilepsy and the Functional Anatomy of the Human Brain*. Little, Brown & Co, Boston, 1954.

7. COLE, FM, AND YATES, P: *The occurrence and significance of intracerebral micro-aneurysms*. J Pathol Bacteriol 93:393, 1967.

8. FISHER, CM, ET AL: *Acute hypertensive cerebellar hemorrhage: Diagnosis and surgical treatment*. J Nerv Ment Dis 140:38, 1965.

9. MOHR, JP: *Lacunes*. Neurol Clin 1:201, 1983.

10. KANE, WC, AND ARONSON, SM: *Cardiac factors predisposing to embolic stroke*. Stroke 1:164, 1970.

11. PLETS, C: *Quantitative anatomy of the cerebral vascular bed*. In MINDERHOUD, JM (ED): *Cerebral Blood Flow—Basic Knowledge and Clinical Implications*. Excerpta Medica, Amsterdam, 1981, p 20.

12. ZUELCH, KJ: *Neuropathology of intracranial haemorrhage*. In LUYENDUK, W (ED): *Progress in Brain Research, Vol 30, Cerebral Circulation*. Elsevier, Amsterdam, 1968, p 151.

13. GILBERT, JJ, AND VINTERS, HV: *Cerebral amyloid angiopathy: Incidence and complications in the aging brain, i. Cerebral hemorrhage*. Stroke 14:915, 1983.

14. VINTERS, HV, AND GILBERT, JJ: *Cerebral amyloid angiopathy: Incidence and complications in the aging brain, ii. The distribution of amyloid vascular changes*. Stroke 14:924, 1983.

15. VAN DEN BERGH, R: *Centrifugal elements in the vascular pattern of the deep intracerebral blood supply*. Angiology 20:88, 1969.

16. GOLDMANN, EE: *Vitalfärbung am Zentralnerven System*. Abhandlungen der preussischen Akademie der Wissenschaften, Klasse für Mathematik, Physik und Technik, No 1, 1913, p 1.

17. POLLAY, M, AND ROBERTS, PA: *Blood-brain barrier: A definition of normal and altered function*. Neurosurgery 6:675, 1980.

18. GOLDSTEIN, GW, AND BETZ, AL: *Recent advances in understanding brain capillary function*. Ann Neurol 14:389, 1983.

19. KATZMAN, R, AND PAPPIUS, HM: *Brain Electrolytes and Fluid Metabolism*. Williams & Wilkins, Baltimore, 1973, p 49.

20. NEMOTO, EM: *Pathogenesis of cerebral ischemia-anoxia*. Crit Care Med 6:203, 1978.

21. SCHUIER, FJ, AND HOSSMANN, K-A: *Experimental brain infarcts in cats, ii. Ischemic brain edema*. Stroke 11:593, 1980.

22. O'BRIEN, MD, JORDAN, MM, AND WALTZ, AG: *Ischemic cerebral edema and the blood-brain barrier*. Arch Neurol 30:461, 1974.

23. DINSDALE, HB: *Hypertensive encephalopathy*. Neurol Clin 1:3, 1983.

24. JOHANSSON, BB, AUER, LM, AND LINDER, L-E: *Phenothiazine-mediated protection of the blood-brain barrier during acute hypertension*. Stroke 13:220, 1982.

25. TERENT, A, ET AL: *Ischemic edema in stroke, a parallel study with computed tomography and cerebrospinal fluid markers of disturbed brain cell metabolism*. Stroke 12:33, 1981.

26. SHAW, CM, ALVORD, EC, JR AND BERRY, RG: *Swelling of the brain following ischemic infarction with arterial occlusion*. Arch Neurol 1:1261, 1959.

27. NG, LKY, AND NIMMANNITYA, J: *Massive cerebral infarction with severe brain swelling*. Stroke 1:158, 1970.

28. SILVER, F, ET AL: *Early mortality following stroke: A prospective view*. Stroke 15:492, 1984.

29. COOPER, JR, BLOOM, FE, AND ROTH, RH: *The Biochemical Basis of Neuropharmacology*, ed 4. Oxford University Press, London, 1982.

30. ZIJLSTRA, WG: *Physiology of the cerebral circulation*. In MINDERHOUD, JM (ED): *Cerebral Blood Flow—Basic Knowledge and Clinical Implications*. Excerpta Medica, Amsterdam, 1981, p 34.

31. OWEN, OE, ET AL: *Brain metabolism during fasting*. J Clin Invest 46:1589, 1967.

32. PLUM, F, AND POSNER, JB: *The Diagnosis of Stupor and Coma*. FA Davis, Philadelphia, 1980.

33. TOWNSEND, RE, PRINZ, PN, AND OBRIST, WD: *Human cerebral blood flow during sleep and waking*. J Appl Physiol 35:620, 1973.

34. SOKOLOFF, L: *Circulation and energy metabolism of the brain*. In SIEGEL, GJ, ET AL (EDS): *Basic Neurochemistry*, ed 3. Little, Brown & Co, Boston, 1981, p 471.

35. BAYLISS, WM: *On the local reactions of the arterial wall to changes of internal pressure.* J Physiol (London) 28:220, 1902.

36. HARPER, AM: *Physiology of cerebral blood flow.* Br J Anaesth 37:225, 1965.

37. OLESEN, J: *Cerebral blood flow methods for measurement, regulation, effects of drugs and changes in disease.* Acta Neurol Scand 50(Suppl 57):1, 1974.

38. WINN, HR, RUBIO, GR, AND BERNE, RM: *The role of adenosine in the regulation of cerebral blood flow.* J Cereb Blood Flow Metab 1:239, 1981.

39. HEISTAD, DD, AND MARCUS, ML: *Evidence that neural mechanisms do not have important effects on cerebral blood flow.* Circ Res 42:295, 1978.

40. PURVES, MJ: *Do vasomotor nerves significantly regulate cerebral blood flow?* Circ Res 43:485, 1978.

41. MUELLER, SM, AND ERTEL, PJ: *Association between sympathetic nerve activity and cerebrovascular protection in young spontaneously hypertensive rats.* Stroke 14:88, 1983.

42. SIESJÖ, BK: *Brain energy metabolism.* John Wiley & Sons, New York, 1978.

43. LASSEN, NA, INGVAR, DH, AND SKINHØJ, DH: *Brain function and blood flow.* Sci Am 239:62, 1978.

44. PHELPS, ME, ET AL: *Study of cerebral function with positron computed tomography.* J Cereb Blood Flow Metab 2:113, 1982.

45. LUGINBUEHL, H: *Comparative aspects of cerebrovascular anatomy and pathology in different species.* In SIEKERT, RG, AND WHISNANT, JP (EDS): *Cerebral Vascular Diseases.* Grune & Stratton, New York, 1966.

46. HAUST, MD, AND MORE, RH: *Development of modern theories on the pathogenesis of atherosclerosis.* In WISSLER, RW, AND GEER, JC (EDS): *The Pathogenesis of Atherosclerosis.* Williams & Wilkins, Baltimore, 1972, p 1.

47. MCNAMARA, JJ, ET AL: *Coronary artery disease in combat casualties in Vietnam.* JAMA 216:1185, 1971.

48. HAUST, MD: *Injury and repair in the pathogenesis of atherosclerotic lesions.* In JONES, RJ (ED): *Atherosclerosis.* Springer-Verlag, New York, 1970, p 12.

49. CAPRON, L: *Athérosclérose, descriptions et mécanismes.* Rev Neurol (Paris) 139:167, 1983.

50. MOORE, S, ET AL: *Inhibition of injury induced thromboatherosclerotic lesions by anti-platelet serum in rabbits.* Semin Thromb Hemost 35:78, 1976.

51. PETERSON, RE, LIVINGSTON, KE, AND ESCOBAR, A: *Development and distribution of gross atherosclerotic lesions at cervical carotid bifurcation.* Neurology 10:955, 1960.

52. YATES, PO, AND HUTCHINSON, EC: *Cerebral infarction: The role of stenosis of the extracranial cerebral arteries.* Privy Council, Medical Research Council Special Report Series, no 300, London, p 1961.

53. BRICE, JG, DOWSETT, DJ, AND LOWE, RD: *Haemodynamic effects of carotid artery stenosis.* Br Med J 2:1363, 1964.

54. TORVIK, A, AND SKULLERUD, K: *How often are brain infarcts caused by hypotensive episodes?* Stroke 7:255, 1976.

Chapter 4

REVERSIBILITY OF CEREBRAL ISCHEMIA

Search and study out the secrets of nature by way of experiment.
William Harvey

Negative attitudes toward the management of stroke patients largely stem from the long-held belief that the clinical effects of stroke result from dead brain and are therefore irreversible. Studies of stroke outcome demonstrate a surprisingly favorable outlook in the immediate recovery phase of most cases. After the initial 20 to 25 percent death rate in the first month, most survivors of ischemic stroke return to a normal or only partially disabled life.[1,2] Knowledge of the factors contributing to this recovery originates from many sources, but a few developments merit special mention:

1. Description of the train of histopathologic events following cerebral ischemia[3]
2. The neurochemical and neurophysiologic resistance of the mammalian brain to ischemia under certain conditions[4]
3. The difference between complete and incomplete ischemia in neurocellular biochemistry and cellular energy failure[5]
4. The charting of the ischemic thresholds of cerebral perfusion, electrical activity, and ionic pump failure[6]
5. Cerebral blood flow and oxygen metabolism in the acute phase of focal cerebral ischemia as demonstrated by PET scanning[7]
6. The harmful effects of high blood glucose on the ischemic brain[8]
7. The role of calcium in the biochemical cerebral "cascade" of cellular ischemia[9]

The concept of a zone of viable but metabolically lethargic cells surrounding an area of focal cerebral infarction as an "ischemic penumbra" has moved from an attractive hypothesis to established fact.[10] Ischemic thresholds of cerebral electroactivity and cellular ionic flux within this area are reversible,[11] raising optimism for future therapy.

One of the most intriguing concepts relates to carbohydrate metabolism in acute cerebral ischemia.[8,12] Incomplete ischemia induces anaerobic glycolysis and lactic acidosis to which astrocytes are especially vulnerable. An alternative explanation, offered by Siesjö,[13] is that the excessive acidosis simply kills more neurons. This mass cell death secondarily affects glial cell membranes, so all cells die together.

Severe incomplete ischemia produces membrane failure and initiates irreversible cell damage, but this can be delayed by hypothermia, barbiturate and lidocaine coma, and paradoxically, hyperglycemia. Since the ischemic threshold of cerebral perfusion for membrane failure is as low as 8 ml/100 g/min, irreversible damage can be prevented if cerebral blood flow can be maintained above this level.[10]

THRESHOLDS OF ISCHEMIA

Some patients with dense hemiplegia make a surprisingly rapid recovery, while others with less severe deficits change little, even after many months. Little scientific basis exists for the popular concept that rapid recovery results from spare neurons being pressed into service, but there is evidence that potentially viable brain cells remain in the ischemic penumbra (Fig. 17).

Transient ischemic attacks clinically model complete reversal of focal cerebral ischemia in which cell death is absent or at least undetectable. Complete cerebral circulatory arrest bears only an approximate relationship to focal cerebral ischemia.[4] Systemic anoxia-ischemia models are

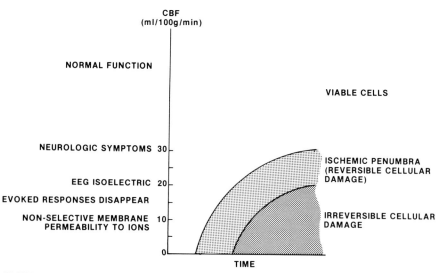

ACUTE STROKE

42   FIGURE 17. The ischemic penumbra. (Adapted from Astrup.[10])

even less reliable, since they superimpose the effects of cardiovascular failure, and the heart is more sensitive to oxygen deprivation than the brain is.[14,15] Total occlusion of all blood supply to the brain results in unconsciousness within seconds, in coma within minutes, and in death or irreversible brain damage after 5 minutes.

Experimentally, as cerebral perfusion falls, synaptic transmission, ionic pumps, and energy metabolism fail from depletion of high energy phosphates.[6] Irreversible cell damage finally occurs when the lethal

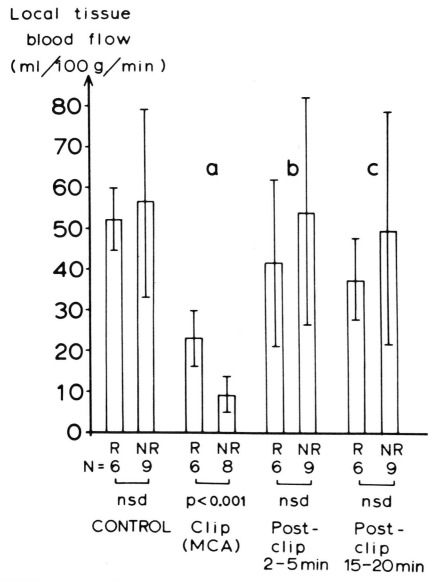

FIGURE 18. Recovery of somatosensory evoked potential correlated with regional cerebral perfusion.
    R = Recovery of evoked potentials to control level
    NR = No recovery
    NSD = No significant difference between R and NR flows
(From Branston, et al,[18] with permission.)

threshold of cerebral perfusion is reached and the ionic pumps can no longer be reactivated.

EEG changes sensitively reflect the cerebral effects of carotid clamping during surgery, at a threshold of cerebral blood flow (CBF) of 17 ml/100 g/min.[16,17] Experimentally, focal cerebral ischemia abolishes somatosensory evoked responses below CBF of 15 ml/100 g/min, but these are restored once cerebral perfusion reverts to normal (Fig. 18). Explanations for these threshold effects include synaptic depolarization secondary to massive release of cellular potassium to the extracellular space, changes in neurotransmitter metabolism, or tissue acidosis.[18]

Correlating focal CBF with somatosensory evoked potentials, and extracellular K^+ and H^+ activity, Astrup and colleagues[11] mapped a spectrum of thresholds (Fig. 19). The threshold of electrical failure was unrelated to the efflux of intracellular K^+, which had its own CBF threshold, about 50 percent below the electrical threshold and not far above that of cell death. Both the electrical failure and the potassium release from severe extracellular acidosis readily reversed when CBF increased above ischemic levels. When autoregulation failed, mean arterial blood pressure related linearly to CBF, so systemic hypotension produced deterioration from one threshold down to another, enlarging the area of impaired brain. This adverse effect reversed promptly once normotensive levels were restored, an experience well recognized in clinical practice.[11]

The ultimate limit of ischemic anoxia is probably the threshold for lactate damage in brain cells, assessed variously as 16 to 20 mmol/kg[12] to 20 to 30 mmol/kg.[19] Such severe lactic acidosis from anaerobic glycolysis is commoner in incomplete than complete ischemia. Astrocytes

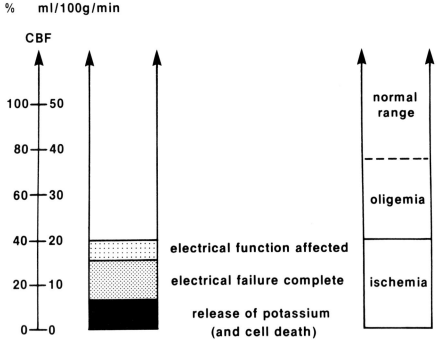

ACUTE STROKE

44 FIGURE 19. Thresholds of ischemia. (From Astrup,[11] with permission.)

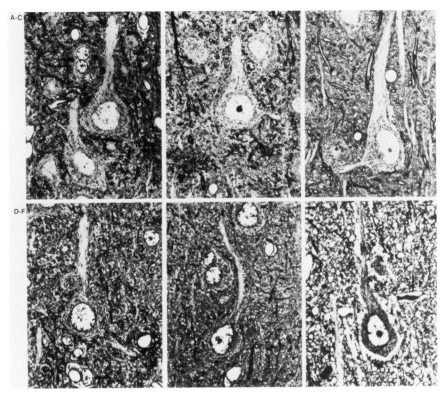

FIGURE 20. Progressive neuronal damage in postischemic rat brain, glucose-infused animals (*A–C*) compared with saline-infused controls (*D–F*). (From Kalimo, H, et al: *Brain lactic acidosis and ischemic cell damage. 2. Histopathology.* J Cereb Blood Flow Metab 1:313, 1981.)

are especially prone to the noxious effect of lactate, causing adjacent neurons to lose their metabolic support system and suffer the damage inflicted by falling oxygen levels. This leads to focal necrosis of all cellular elements (astrocytes, neurons, and vascular endothelium), unlike the more selective laminar damage caused by anoxia alone (Fig. 20).

THRESHOLDS OF CEREBRAL BLOOD FLOW AND OXYGEN METABOLISM

The Xenon Era

In 1945, Kety and Schmidt[20] derived the brain blood flow by the Fick principle, using arterial and cerebral venous nitrous oxide levels when the subject inhaled the gas. The subsequent development of regional cerebral blood flow (rCBF) techniques using gamma-emitting isotopes such as xenon-133[21,22] allowed comparisons of perfusion between ischemic and normal cortex as well as the cerebrovascular response to blood pressure, drugs, and CO_2 changes.[23] The cerebral circulation is highly sensitive to changes in arterial P_{CO_2},[24] which diffuses easily through the vascular endothelial membrane, normally impermeable to hydrogen and bicarbonate ions. Clamping the internal carotid artery of patients during carotid endarterectomy indicated a threshold of cerebral blood flow of 30 ml/100 g/min, below which neurologic deficits appeared, depending upon the duration of occlusion.[25]

An area of hyperemia sometimes seen in focal ischemia was aptly dubbed "luxury perfusion" by Lassen, who suggested that it resulted from lactic acidosis in an area of low oxygen metabolism.[26] This may be an oversimplification since marked hyperemia also occurs in hypoglycemia at an alkaline pH.[27] The uncoupling of cerebral metabolism from cerebral blood flow was later confirmed by positron emission tomography.[7] Perfusion in the ischemic area becomes passively dependent upon systemic blood pressure, owing to vasoparalysis occurring in acute infarction and in TIAs.[28]

"Intracerebral steal"[29] occurs when normal blood vessels dilate in response to hypercapnia and so steal blood from the adjacent ischemic area where the vessels are already maximally dilated. Vasodilators such as carbon dioxide and papaverine might therefore do more harm than good, since hyperperfusion of brain tissue beyond its metabolic needs is unlikely to be of benefit and, in any case, the collateral vessels are already maximally dilated.

The PET Era

The xenon-133 CBF technique had serious technical limitations. Accurate determination of CBF was confined to the cortex, leaving the perfusion of underlying white matter largely undetermined. Also, radioactivity from underlying normal brain tissue showed through the invisible "windows" of superficial areas of focal cortical ischemia, giving the impression of normal perfusion. Clearly, deeper resolution or tomographic techniques were needed.

Positron emission tomography (PET) demonstrates cerebral blood flow and metabolism three-dimensionally, can be measured in vivo, and is noninvasive. Critical thresholds for regional CBF (rCBF), oxygen extraction fraction (OER), and oxygen metabolism ($CMRO_2$) can be determined simultaneously using the O^{15} inhalation method.

These thresholds play a major role in determining outcome in stroke patients[30] (Fig. 21). Ischemic areas showed depressed metabolic demand with normal or increased blood flow, but perfusion and metabolism differed between the core and borders of the infarct. The halo of glucose hypermetabolism around an infarct[31] indicating increased anaerobic glycolysis was not seen, though uncoupling of aerobic glycolysis was apparent in the dissociation of rCBF from $rCMRO_2$. The behavior of this rim metabolism may hold the key to reversal of ischemia.

PET-scanning stroke patients as early as possible, Wise and coworkers[32] studied only those with initially elevated rOER. When CBF falls, mitochondrial function remains initially intact, rOER is maximal for the trickle of blood available, and $CMRO_2$ remains largely unchanged. Presumably, at this stage the ischemia is reversible. As CBF continues to fall, mitochondrial function begins to fail and rOER and $rCMRO_2$ decrease, even though the CBF is not changed. Infarction is now imminent and soon irreversible (Fig. 22).

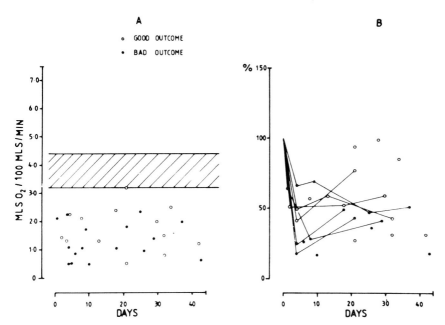

○ GOOD OUTCOME
● BAD OUTCOME

FIGURE 21. Relationship between regional oxygen consumption (rCMRO$_2$) and the core of the infarct. Absolute (A) and relative (B) rCMRO$_2$ in gray matter in the center of the infarct. Shaded area represents normal mean rCMRO$_2$. In the acute phase of the stroke, six of nine patients had rCMRO$_2$ below 1.25 ml O$_2$/100 ml/min. All patients with a poor outcome had rCMRO$_2$ values less than 50 percent of that in the contralateral region. (From Lenzi, et al,[30] with permission.)

TOLERANCE OF THE BRAIN TO ISCHEMIA

Most cells withstand brief anoxia or ischemia to resume normal function, but brain cells tolerate ischemia badly and may be irreversibly damaged even if the organism survives. Their vulnerability is due to the unique metabolism of cerebral tissue, which is totally dependent from moment to moment on its blood supply for its two major substrates, glucose and oxygen. Glucose storage is limited and oxygen storage nonexistent. In addition, anaerobic glycolysis is energy inefficient, and the resulting lactic acidosis damages glia, neurons, and vascular endothelium.[12]

If cerebral circulation stops abruptly, the patient lapses into coma and death within 5 minutes. Animal experiments indicate that death of the organism does not equate with brain death. Even under conditions of total cerebral ischemia, primitive brain function may continue for up to an hour, judging by metabolic and electrical indices (Table 12),[4] although certain factors limit recovery:

1. Integrated brain function—that is, clinical recovery—must be distinguished from simple restoration of neurophysiologic or metabolic status. Mere cellular survival is insufficient.[5]
2. Cerebral anoxia differs from cerebral ischemia. Anoxia alone will not produce cerebral edema,[16] but brain swelling is a major factor in ischemia, especially once necrosis of the blood-brain barrier occurs.[33]

REVERSIBILITY OF
CEREBRAL ISCHEMIA

47

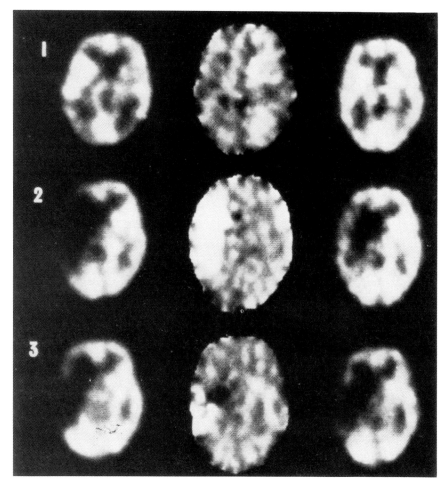

FIGURE 22. Functional images of three studies of the same patient. Cerebral blood flow images are at left, oxygen extraction ratios at center and regional oxygen consumption at right.

Study 1: After a left-hemisphere TIA
Study 2: 7 hours after a major stroke 10 days later
Study 3: 4 days after the stroke

The high regional oxygen extraction ratio within the early infarct (2) fell in association with a decline in cortical regional oxygen consumption (3). (From Wise, et al,[32] with permission.)

TABLE 12. Experimental Studies Reporting Resistance to Cerebral Anoxia-Ischemia

Author	Subject	Duration of Ischemia (min)	Type of Recovery
Kabat et al, 1941	Dog	6.0–8.0	Clinical neurologic
Hirsh et al, 1957[14]	Dog	12.0	Clinical neurologic
Brockman and Jude, 1960	Dog	12.0	Clinical neurologic
Neely and Youmans, 1970	Dog	25.0	Clinical neurologic
Miller and Myers, 1970	Monkey	20.0	Clinical neurologic
Hossmann and Kleihues, 1973[4]	Monkey	60.0	Neurophysiologic, neurochemical

From Plum,[12] with permission.

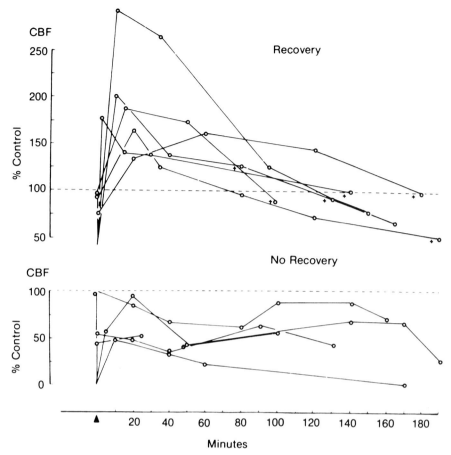

FIGURE 23. Cerebral blood flow in the cat following complete ischemia for 1 hour. Animals in upper diagram recovered spontaneous EEG activity. Note postischemic hyperemia. Animals in lower diagram had no functional recovery. (From Hossmann and Kleihues,[4] with permission.)

3. Complete ischemia is less devastating to the brain than is incomplete ischemia.[4]
4. Postischemic hyperemia is an index of potential recovery, whereas sustained low CBF following ischemia predicts a poor outcome (Fig. 23).[4]
5. Duration of ischemia is as important to cellular survival as its severity (Fig. 24).

THE CEREBRAL ISCHEMIC "CASCADE"

The "cascade" of disordered metabolism triggered by ischemia is partly reversible.[5,9,34] Acute cerebral ischemia swells the glia and shrinks neurons microvacuolated with ballooned mitochondria.[35] Bloating of the astrocytes from glial pump failure distances the neurons from their oxygen supply, increasing the ischemia.[36] As calcium is released from the endoplasmic reticulum and mitochondria, and floods in from the opening of membrane calcium gates, its intracellular concentration rises. The

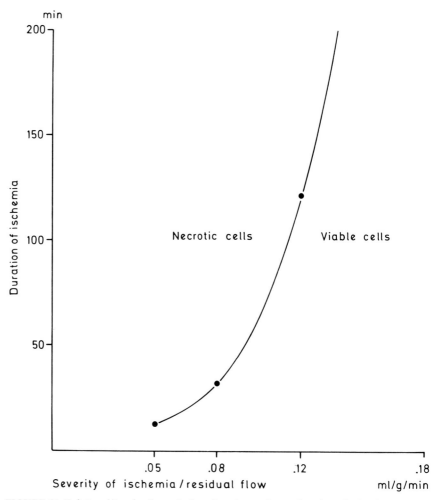

min

FIGURE 24. Relationship of cell survival to duration and severity of cerebral ischemia. (From Heiss, WD, and Rosner, G: *Functional recovery of cortical neurons as related to degree and duration of ischemia.* Ann Neurol 14:294, 1983.)

threshold of membrane failure is about 6 to 8 ml/100 g/min, when there is loss of potassium from cells.[10]

Mitochondrial function is as important a homeostatic defense as is the cell membrane. Brain mitochondria are relatively resistant to ischemia. Mitochondrial respiration, although impaired within a few minutes of complete ischemia, returns to normal 30 minutes after recirculation.[5] This does not occur in incomplete ischemia.

"Free radicals" such as superoxide ($-O_2^-$) are highly toxic products of ischemia, and they destroy lipids and proteins, the major constituents of cell membranes. Certain enzymes, ascorbic acid, other naturally occurring substances, and drugs such as barbiturates may protect the ischemic brain, mainly by scavenging free radicals.[37,38]

If some oxygen is available, free fatty acids accumulate, especially arachidonic acid, producing endoperoxides and leucotrienes. If no oxy-

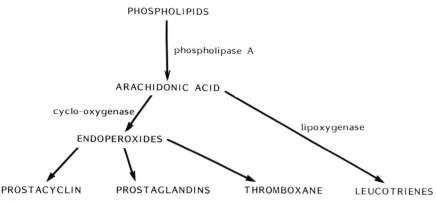

FIGURE 25. Suggested pathways for ischemic cerebral metabolism. (Adapted from Siesjö,[5] and Siesjö and Wieloch,[39] with permission.)

gen is available, this toxic process is arrested, but a surge of damaging endoperoxide reactions occurs on reoxygenation. Endoperoxides injure cells directly as free radicals and indirectly by producing prostaglandins and thromboxane, a vasoconstrictor. Released free radicals also inhibit prostacyclin synthesis, removing the homeostatic vasodilator influence. The excess of leucotrienes may add to neuronal damage, though the metabolic pathway for this has not yet been demonstrated in the brain (Fig. 25).[39]

Siesjö[5] identifies several reversible points along the biochemical cascade pathway of cerebral ischemia at which the whole process could be reversed:

1. Therapeutic use of known free radical scavengers, such as barbiturates or drugs, that block enzymatic degradation of free fatty acid
2. Amelioration of perineuronal glial swelling; that is, intracellular edema
3. Calcium blockers to inhibit the initial rise of cytosolic Ca^{++}

Calcium—The Trigger of the Ischemic Cascade

The viability of cells incubated with different membrane-toxins decreases in the presence of calcium,[40] probably since the influx of calcium through the damaged membrane compounds the damage. In the model proposed by Hass, ischemia releases intracellular calcium, which is normally sequestered within mitochondria or extruded from the cell.[9] This accelerates phospholipid degradation, releasing free fatty acids that act as detergents of the cell membrane, creating a vicious circle by allowing further calcium influx. This chain reaction inhibits mitochondrial respiration, destroying the cell. "The well-contained fire on the hearth thus spreads to involve the entire house."[9] Magnesium also protects against experimental ischemic damage either by reducing cellular calcium influx, by stabilizing plasma membranes, or by reducing ATP requirements.[41]

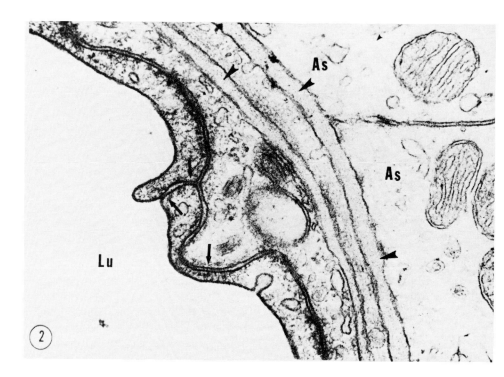

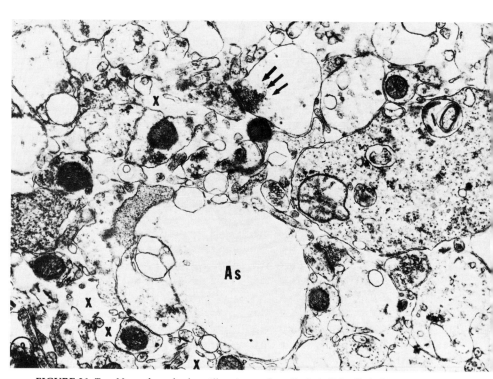

FIGURE 26. *Top,* Normal cerebral capillary in monkey. Endothelial cells held together by tight junctions *(arrows).* Basement membrane *(arrowheads).*

 Bottom, Monkey cortex 5 hours after middle cerebral artery occlusion. Astrocytic process (As) enlarged and extracellular space widened (X). Swollen presynaptic terminal contains vesicles *(arrows).* (From Garcia, et al,[48] p 125, with permission.)

REVERSIBILITY OF CEREBRAL EDEMA

Disordered water balance between cellular, extracellular, and vascular compartments may be as devastating but as reversible as the ionic imbalance following ischemia. Cerebral edema is the commonest cause of death in acute stroke,[42,43] although its role in producing neurologic deficits is disputed.[44] Focal ischemia produces brain swelling by vasoparalysis within minutes, and by metabolic (cytotoxic) edema from ionic shifts within hours, later leaking larger molecules such as proteins and producing vasogenic edema.[45] Rather than cerebral edema, the ionic shifts of the first few hours may represent a totally reversible transfer of water from extracellular to intracellular space.[46] At this stage, electron microscopy shows swelling of the astrocytes with protein-free fluid.

By 6 hours, tissue necrosis and widespread rupture of cell membranes with massive accumulation of fluid begins.[47] Enlargement of the extracellular space is a late event following rupture of the astrocytes.[48] (Fig. 26; Table 13). Glia and neurons succumb to ischemic damage long before the relatively resistant capillary endothelium. During this stage of "vasogenic" edema, the blood-brain barrier becomes permeable to macromolecules, probably by increased pinocytotic activity in the capillary endothelium.[46] Protein extravasation and osmotic extracellular edema flow along the white matter by hydrostatic pressure gradients rather than by diffusion, so producing massive shifts of brain structure. This edema resolves by reaching the CSF and by reabsorption into blood vessels.[49]

Hossmann and Schuier suggest that the best chance of reversal occurs at the stage of metabolic edema by maintaining blood flow above the critical threshold of 15 ml/100 g/min.[45] Controlled hypertension

TABLE 13. Types and Lower Limits of Ischemic Thresholds

Threshold	Lower Limit	Source
Electrical	17 ml/100 g/min, CBF	Trojaborg and Boysen, 1973[16] Sharbrough, Messick, and Sundt, 1973[17]
Evoked response	15 ml/100 g/min, CBF	Branston, Symon, and Crockard, 1976[18]
Lactate damage	16–30 mmol/kg, serum lactate	Rehncrona, Rosen, and Siesjö, 1981[19] Plum, 1982[12]
Metabolic edema	15 ml/100 g/min, CBF	Hossmann and Schuier, 1979[45]
Gray matter damage	10–12 ml/100 g/min, CBF	Marcoux et al, 1982[56]
White matter damage	>14 ml/100 g/min, CBF	Marcoux et al, 1982[56]
Cerebral infarct (core value)	1.5 ml O_2/100 g/min, $CMRO_2$	Lenzi, Frackowiak, and Jones, 1982[30]
Intracellular K^+ release	8 ml/100 g/min, CBF	Astrup, 1982[10]
Duration of ischemia	5 ml/100 g/min for 13 min 8 ml/100 g/min for 30 min 18 ml/100 g/min (? indefinitely)	Heiss and Rosner, 1983 Heiss and Rosner, 1983 Heiss and Rosner, 1983

during metabolic edema could restore CBF without promoting brain swelling but is harmful in the presence of vasogenic edema, which only supervenes after some hours. "Metabolic inhibitors" might retard the cerebral metabolic rate, equilibrating oxygen requirements with reduced oxygen delivery to the brain.[45]

THRESHOLDS OF ISCHEMIC STRUCTURAL DAMAGE

Structural changes occur in neurons within the first few hours (possibly the first few minutes) following ischemia.[35] Neuronal cytoplasmic vacuolation from swollen organelles (mainly mitochondria) is followed by shrinkage of the cell body and nucleus, terminating in their dissolution (Fig. 27).[50] Selective vulnerability occurs in certain areas, determined by differing regional perfusion and metabolism:[50]

1. Cerebral cortex (layers 3, 5, and 6)
2. Hippocampus (Sommer sector and endofolium)
3. Amygdaloid nucleus
4. Cerebellum (Purkinje and basket cells)
5. Certain brainstem nuclei
6. Variable damage occurs to central gray matter such as thalamus and pallidum
7. The spinal cord proves most resistant

The "No-Reflow" Controversy

The concept of selective vulnerability due to regional dependence on vascular supply was supported by the finding of patchy areas of impaired reperfusion following total cerebral ischemia (Fig. 28).[51,52] Swollen perivascular glia and capillary endothelial blebs prevented reperfusion.[53] Ischemia had to be complete and to last longer than 5 minutes to produce this "no-reflow" phenomenon.[54] This endothelial obstruction was later considered artifact, the primary cause of no-reflow being increased blood viscosity from stasis of red blood cells.[55] The role of this phenomenon in the disordered physiology of cerebral ischemia remains controversial and probably minimal.

Thresholds of Tissue Necrosis

When the degree of cerebral tissue damage is correlated with regional CBF values, critical perfusion thresholds are found corresponding to gray and white matter blood flow.[56] Critical gray matter flow is 10 to 12 ml/ 100 g/min but varies for different sites such as caudate, putamen, and

→

FIGURE 27. Monkey cortex. *Top,* 1½ hours following hypotensive episode, ischemic neuron with cytoplasmic microvesicles.

    Middle, Electromicrograph of hippocampal neuron with increased electron density of nucleus, swollen mitochondria, and expanded cisterni. Note expanded astrocyte processes around the neuron and at blood vessel.

    Bottom, 3 hours after status epilepticus. Ischemic cell change with microincrustations. (From Brierley, Meldrum, and Brown,[50] with permission.)

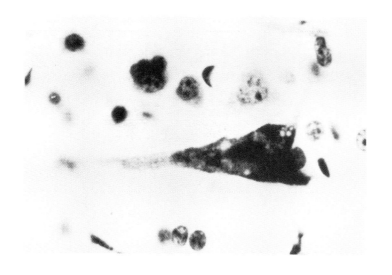

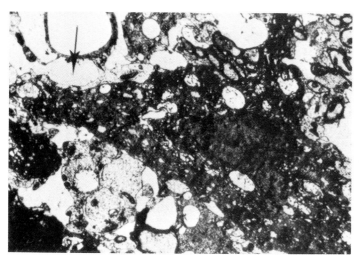

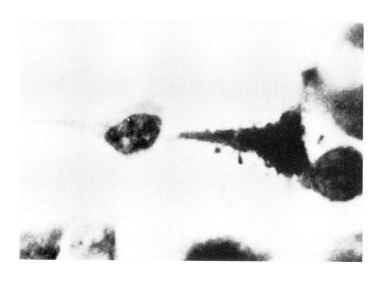

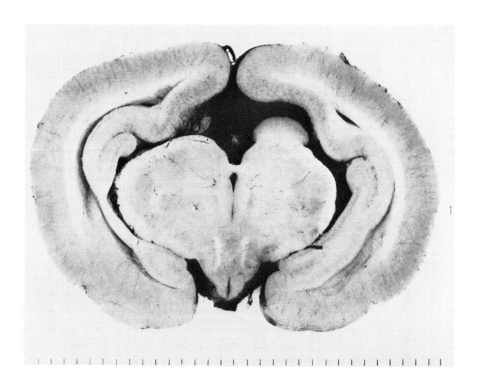

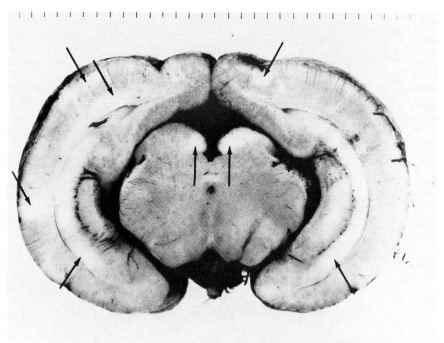

FIGURE 28. *Top,* Normal rabbit brain after carbon black perfusion. *Bottom,* After 5 minutes ischemia, there are areas of impaired carbon perfusion scattered throughout the brain. (From Ames, et al,[52] with permission.)

cortex. Gray matter was more sensitive to reduced perfusion than was white matter, suggesting that greater metabolic activity may require more substrate to maintain functional integrity.

REVERSIBILITY OF HEMATOLOGIC FACTORS IN CEREBRAL ISCHEMIA

Blood Viscosity

Viscosity is the friction between adjacent moving layers of blood and depends upon:[57]

1. Red and white cell concentration of the blood
2. Blood levels of fibrinogen or abnormal immunoglobulins
3. Red cell rigidity
4. Greater flow
5. Diameter of vessel

Low cerebral flow occurs in polycythemia, the paraproteinemias, and sickle cell disease; it may be reversed by appropriate treatment, such as venesection for polycythemia or plasmapheresis for paraproteinemia.

In the Framingham Study, nonpolycythemic people with hemoglobin levels greater than normal had a significantly increased incidence of ischemic stroke.[58] Patients with high-normal hematocrit (0.47 to 0.53)

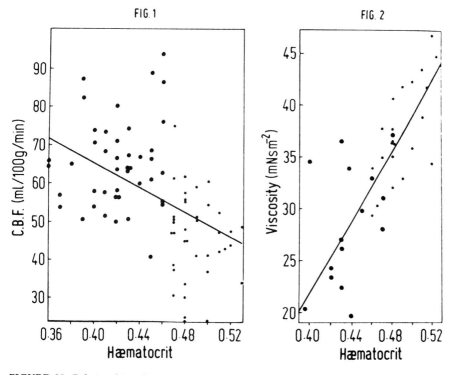

FIG. 1

FIG. 2

FIGURE 29. Relationship of cerebral blood flow and blood viscosity to hematocrit. (From Thomas, DJ, et al: *Effect of haematocrit on cerebral blood-flow in man*. Lancet 2:941, 1977, with permission.)

have significantly lower CBF levels than those with low-normal hematocrit (0.36 to 0.46),[59] and CBF increases dramatically after venesection (Fig. 29).

When regional CBF is already impaired owing to local arterial disease, increased viscosity may lower it to levels below tissue viability. Blood viscosity may also be the primary factor in the no-reflow phenomenon. Red cell clumping by fibrinogen in acute cerebral ischemia causes additional lowering of regional CBF, so that reducing fibrinogen levels could be therapeutic by increasing tissue perfusion.[60]

Platelet Abnormalities

Abnormal platelet behavior may play a primary or secondary role in cerebral ischemia.[61-65] Platelet aggregation is a normal response to vascular endothelial injury, which helps form the initial thrombus. The platelets then release substances such as ADP, serotonin, and catecholamines, producing secondary platelet agglutination,[62] which further obstructs the microcirculation distal to the occluding thrombus.[66]

Platelet aggregation increases significantly within 10 days after ischemic stroke or TIA but then returns to normal,[63] a response unaffected by aspirin or dipyridamole therapy (Fig. 30, *left*). Dougherty and associates[63] reported a patient who, while taking aspirin/dipyridamole following a TIA, had another TIA 19 days later. The percentage of aggregated platelets fell to normal after the first TIA, then rose again during the second event (Fig. 30, *right*) in spite of continuing antiplatelet medication. The data do not allow exact correlation of timing of the platelet change with the clinical event, but the authors indicate that these platelet changes appear to follow and not precede the ischemic events. Abnormal platelet activity may be a precipitating factor for thromboembolism in mitral valve prolapse,[67] explaining the relative infrequency of stroke symptoms in this otherwise common cardiac disorder. The therapeutic potential of platelet inhibiting drugs such as aspirin may lie in disrupting the initial thrombotic process. However, if their only effect is on secondary platelet aggregation occurring distal to the thrombus, they would limit the degree but not the occurrence of ischemia.

THE DAMAGING EFFECT OF INCOMPLETE ISCHEMIA

Brain damage is more severe following incomplete than it is following complete ischemia. Histologically, mitochondrial changes first signal ischemic cell damage,[3] mitochondrial function recovering after complete but not after incomplete cerebral ischemia (Fig. 31).[68]

The continued though reduced supply of glucose during incomplete ischemia promotes pronounced lactic acidosis, a cellular toxin.[19] Oxidative reactions smolder during incomplete ischemia, the tissue losing factors that normally prevent oxidative damage upon recirculation.

Plum elaborated further on the singularly damaging effect of incomplete ischemia.[12] Rats subjected to nearly complete cerebral ischemia produced by four-vessel (cervical) occlusion survived for days even after 30 minutes of total occlusion. Despite severe cerebral ischemia, fast-

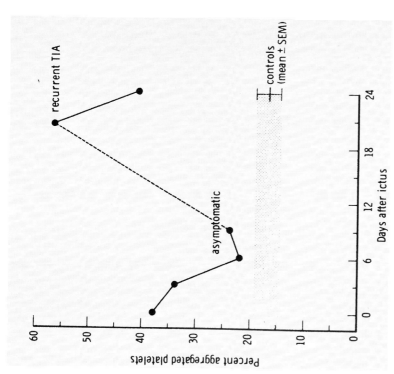

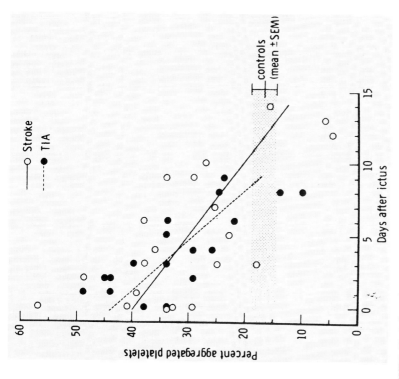

FIGURE 30. *Left,* Relationship of platelet aggregation to days after stroke. *Right,* Pattern of platelet aggregation in patient with recurrent TIAs treated with aspirin/dipyridamole. (From Dougherty, Levy, and Weksler,[63] with permission.)

REVERSIBILITY OF CEREBRAL ISCHEMIA

59

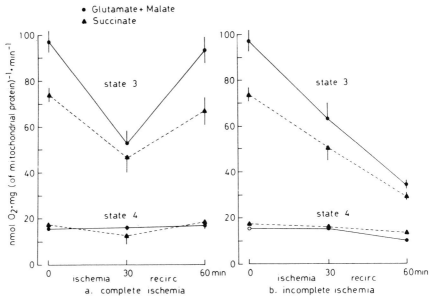

FIGURE 31. Differences in mitochondrial oxygen consumption between animals subjected to (A) complete and (B) incomplete cerebral ischemia. Recirculation restores respiratory activity in the complete ischemia group, but progressive deterioration is irreversible in those with incomplete ischemia. States 3 and 4 relate to substrate activity. (From Rehncrona, Mela, and Siesjö,[68] with permission.)

ing animals showed only selective laminar necrosis rather than infarction. When cerebral blood flow is reduced but not absent, such as in experimental carotid ligation, rapid and dramatic infarction is produced.

The secret of the damaging effect of incomplete ischemia may rest with cellular, especially astrocytic, metabolism. Rats with four-vessel occlusion pretreated with glucose fared so badly that it was difficult for them to survive the length of the experiment.[69] Survivors showed extensive histologic damage with large areas of infarction. With complete ischemia and no available oxygen, the glycogen-rich astrocytes cannot form lactate, remaining unscathed. The brunt of the ischemia then falls upon the neurons. With incomplete ischemia, severe lactic acidosis occurs from continuing anaerobic glycolysis and, once the lactate threshold is exceeded, astrocytes rupture and endothelium necroses. Loss of metabolic and nutritional support from disrupted glia and the microcirculation compound the ischemic damage to neurons (Fig. 32).

CONCLUSION

The concept that ischemic stroke results from "dead brain" betrays a simplistic and unduly pessimistic view. Evidence from clinical observation, neurophysiologic changes, neurochemical studies, and neurohistology indicates a wide spectrum of potentially reversible events preceding brain cell death.

Earlier methods of managing patients with cerebral infarction presupposed that areas of brain deprived of blood simply need reperfusion by vasodilation. Reperfusion may be harmful, making it preferable to

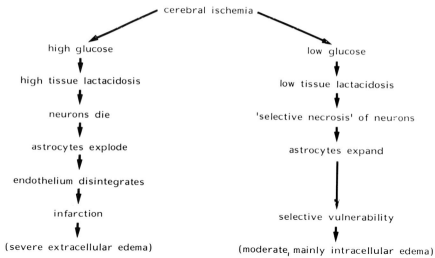

cerebral ischemia

high glucose → high tissue lactacidosis → neurons die → astrocytes explode → endothelium disintegrates → infarction → (severe extracellular edema)

low glucose → low tissue lactacidosis → 'selective necrosis' of neurons → astrocytes expand → selective vulnerability → (moderate, mainly intracellular edema)

FIGURE 32. Adverse effects of hyperglycemia in cerebral ischemia. (Adapted from Plum,[12] with permission.)

arrest or reverse the metabolic and structural changes of the ischemic brain. For instance, deprivation of glucose to prevent damaging lactacidosis during incomplete ischemia may be more therapeutic than reperfusion.

Histochemical techniques, ultramicroscopy, evoked potentials, and brain imaging have defined a wide range of thresholds for tissue viability in ischemia. Determining these outer limits of tolerance to the ischemic insult may be a major factor preceding the discovery of effective therapy.

REFERENCES

1. WHISNANT, JP, ET AL: *Natural history of stroke in Rochester, Minnesota, 1945 through 1954.* Stroke 2:11, 1971.
2. NORRIS, JW, ET AL: *Outcome of brainstem strokes.* In BERGUER, R, AND BAUER, RB (EDS): *Vertebrobasilar Arterial Occlusive Disease.* Raven Press, New York, 1984, p 37.
3. BROWN, AW, AND BRIERLEY, JB: *The nature and time course of anoxic-ischemic cell change in the rat brain—An optical and electron microscopic study.* In BRIERLEY, AW, AND MELDRUM, B (EDS): *Brain Hypoxia.* William Heinemann, London, 1971, p 49.
4. HOSSMANN, K-A, AND KLEIHUES, P: *Reversibility of ischemic brain damage.* Arch Neurol 29:375, 1973.
5. SIESJÖ, BK: *Cell damage in the brain: A speculative synthesis.* J Cereb Blood Flow Metab 1:155, 1981.
6. ASTRUP, J, SIESJÖ, BK, AND SYMON, L: *Thresholds in cerebral ischemia—The ischemic penumbra.* Stroke 12:723, 1981.
7. FRACKOWIAK, RSJ, AND WISE, RJS: *Positron tomography in ischemic cerebrovascular disease.* Neurol Clin 1:183, 1983.
8. MYERS, RE, AND YAMAGUCHI, S: *Nervous system effects of cardiac arrest in monkeys.* Arch Neurol 34:65, 1977.
9. HASS, WK: *The cerebral ischemic cascade.* Neurol Clin 1:345, 1983.
10. ASTRUP, J: *Energy-requiring cell functions in the ischemic brain—Their critical supply and possible inhibition in protective therapy.* J Neurosurg 56:482, 1982.
11. ASTRUP, J, ET AL: *Cortical evoked potential and extracellular K^+ and H^+ at critical levels of brain ischemia.* Stroke 8:51, 1977.
12. PLUM, F: *What causes infarction in ischemic brain? The Robert Wartenberg Lecture.* Neurology 33:222, 1983.
13. SIESJÖ, BK: Personal communication. September, 1983.

14. HIRSCH, H, EULER, KH, AND SCHNEIDER, M: *Ueber die Erholung des Gehirns nach kompletter Ischaemie Hypothermie.* Pflugers Arch 265:314, 1957.

15. NORRIS, JW, AND PAPPIUS, HM: *Cerebral water and electrolytes: Effect of asphyxia, hypoxia and hypercapnia.* Arch Neurol 23:248, 1970.

16. TROJABORG, W, AND BOYSEN, G: *Relation between EEG, regional cerebral blood flow and internal carotid stump pressure during carotid endarterectomy.* Electroencephalogr Clin Neurophysiol 34:61, 1973.

17. SHARBROUGH, FW, MESSICK, JM, AND SUNDT, M, JR: *Correlations of continuous electroencephalograms with cerebral blood flow measurements during carotid endarterectomy.* Stroke 4:674, 1973.

18. BRANSTON, NM, SYMON, L, AND CROCKARD, HA: *Recovery of the cortical evoked response following temporary middle cerebral artery occlusion in baboons: Relation to local blood flow and Po₂.* Stroke 7:151, 1976.

19. REHNCRONA, S, ROSEN, I, AND SIESJÖ, BK: *Brain lactic acidosis and ischemic cell damage: 1. Biochemistry and neurophysiology.* J Cereb Blood Flow Metab 1:297, 1981.

20. KETY, SS, AND SCHMIDT, CF: *Oxide method for the quantitative determination of cerebral blood flow in man. Theory, procedure and normal values.* J Clin Invest 27:476, 1948.

21. LASSEN, NA, AND INGVAR, DH: *The blood flow of the cerebral cortex determined by radioactive 85-Krypton.* Experientia (Basel) 17:42, 1961.

22. OLESEN, J, PAULSON, OB, AND LASSEN, NA: *Regional cerebral blood flow in man determined by the initial slope of the clearance of intraarterially injected 133-Xe.* Stroke 2:519, 1971.

23. OLESEN, J: *Cerebral Blood Flow Methods for Measurement, Regulation, Effects of Drugs and Changes in Disease.* Acta Neurol Scand 50(Suppl 57):1, 1974.

24. HARPER, AM, AND GLASS, HI: *Effect of alterations in the arterial carbon dioxide tension on the blood flow through the cerebral cortex at normal and low arterial blood pressures.* J Neurol Neurosurg Psychiatry 28:449, 1965.

25. BOYSEN, G: *Cerebral blood flow measurement as a safeguard during carotid endarterectomy.* Stroke 2:1, 1971.

26. LASSEN, NA: *The luxury-perfusion syndrome and its possible relation to acute metabolic acidosis localised within the brain.* Lancet 2:1113, 1966.

27. ABDUL-RAHMAN, A, AGARDH, C-D, AND SIESJÖ, BK: *Local cerebral blood flow in the rat during severe hypoglycemia and in the recovery period following glucose injection.* Acta Physiol Scand 109:307, 1980.

28. FIESCHI, C, AND LENZI, GL: *Cerebral blood flow and metabolism in stroke patients.* In ROSS RUSSELL, RW: *Vascular Disease of the Central Nervous System,* ed 2. Churchill-Livingstone, Edinburgh, 1983, p 101.

29. LASSEN, NA, AND PALVOLGYI, R: *Cerebral steal during hypercapnia and the inverse reaction during hypocapnia observed by the 133-Xenon technique in man.* Scand J Clin Lab Invest 22 (Suppl 102):13D, 1968.

30. LENZI, GL, FRACKOWIAK, RSJ, AND JONES, T: *Cerebral oxygen metabolism and blood flow in human cerebral ischemic infarction.* J Cereb Blood Flow Metab 2:321, 1982.

31. GINSBERG, MD, ET AL: *Local glucose utilisation in acute focal cerebral ischemia: Local dysmetabolism and diaschisis.* Neurology 27:1042, 1977.

32. WISE, RJS, ET AL: *Serial observations on the pathophysiology of acute stroke—The transition from ischemia to infarction as reflected in regional oxygen extraction.* Brain 106:197, 1983.

33. PLUM, F, POSNER, J, AND ALVORD, EC: *Edema and necrosis in experimental cerebral infarction* Arch Neurol 9:563, 1963.

34. RAICHLE, ME: *The pathophysiology of brain ischemia.* Ann Neurol 13:2, 1983.

35. BRIERLEY, JB: *Cerebral hypoxia.* In BLACKWOOD, W, AND CORSELLIS, JAN (EDS): *Greenfield's Neuropathology,* ed 2. Edward Arnold, London, 1976, p 43.

36. VAN HARREVELD, A, AND OCHS, S: *Cerebral impedance changes after circulatory arrest.* Am J Physiol 187:180, 1956.

37. FLAMM, ES, ET AL: *Possible molecular mechanisms of barbiturate-mediated protection in regional cerebral ischemia.* Acta Neurol Scand 56(S64):150, 1977.

38. SMITH, DS, REHNCRONA, S, AND SIESJÖ, BK: *Inhibitory effects of different barbiturates on lipid peroxidation in brain tissue in vitro and comparison of the effects of promethazine and chlorpromazine.* Anesthesiology 53:186, 1980.

39. SIESJÖ, BK, AND WIELOCH, T: *Fatty acid metabolism and the mechanism of ischemic brain damage.* In REIVICH, M, AND HURTIG, HI (EDS): *Cerebrovascular Diseases.* Raven Press, New York, 1983, p 251.

40. SCHANNE, FAX, ET AL: *Calcium dependence of toxic cell death: A final common pathway.* Science 206:699, 1979.

41. AMES, A, AND NESBETT, FB: *Pathophysiology of ischemic cell death. ii. Changes in plasma membrane permeability and cell volume.* Stroke 14:227, 1983.

42. BROWN, M, AND GLASSENBERG, M: *Mortality factors in patients with acute stroke.* JAMA 224:1493, 1973.

43. SILVER, FL, ET AL: *Early mortality following stroke: A prospective view.* Stroke 15:492, 1984.

44. BRUCE, DA, AND HURTIG, HI: *Incidence, course, and significance of cerebral edema associated with cerebral infarction.* In PRICE, TR, AND NELSON, E (EDS): *Cerebrovascular Diseases.* Raven Press, New York, 1979, p 191.

45. HOSSMANN, K-A, AND SCHUIER, FJ: *Metabolic (cytotoxic) type of brain edema following middle cerebral artery occlusion in cats.* In PRICE, TR, AND NELSON, E (EDS): *Cerebrovascular Diseases.* Raven Press, New York, 1979, p 141.

46. KATZMAN, R, ET AL: *iv. Brain edema in stroke.* Stroke 8:512, 1977.

47. LITTLE, JR: *Microvascular alterations and edema in focal cerebral ischemia.* In PAPPIUS, HM, AND FEINDEL, W (EDS): *Dynamics of Brain Edema.* Springer-Verlag, Heidelberg, 1976, p 236.

48. GARCIA, JH, ET AL: *Fine structure and biochemistry of brain edema in regional cerebral ischemia.* In PRICE, TR, AND NELSON, E (EDS): *Cerebrovascular Diseases.* Raven Press, New York, 1979, p 169.

49. O'BRIEN, MD: *Ischemic cerebral edema, a review.* Stroke 10:623, 1979.

50. BRIERLEY, JB, MELDRUM, BS, AND BROWN, AW: *The threshold and neuropathology of cerebral 'anoxic-ischemic' cell change.* Arch Neurol 29:367, 1973.

51. AMES, A, III, AND GURIAN, BS: *Effects of glucose deprivation of function of isolated mammalian retina.* J Neurophysiol 26:617, 1963.

52. AMES, A, III, ET AL: *Cerebral ischemia. ii. The no-reflow phenomenon.* Am J Pathol 52:437, 1968.

53. FISCHER, EG: *Impaired perfusion following cerebrovascular stasis.* Arch Neurol 29:361, 1973.

54. KAGSTRÖM, E, SMITH, M-J, AND SIESJÖ, BK: *Recirculation in the rat brain following incomplete ischemia.* J Cereb Blood Flow Metab 3:182, 1983.

55. FISCHER, EG, AMES A, III, AND LORENZO, AV: *Cerebral blood flow immediately following brief circulatory stasis.* Stroke 10:423, 1979.

56. MARCOUX, FW, ET AL: *Differential regional vulnerability in transient focal cerebral ischemia.* Stroke 13:339, 1982.

57. THOMAS, DJ: *Whole blood viscosity and cerebral blood flow.* Stroke 13:285, 1982.

58. KANNEL, WB, ET AL: *Hemoglobin and the risk of cerebral infarction: The Framingham study.* Stroke 3:409, 1972.

59. THOMAS, DJ, ET AL: *Cerebral blood-flow in polycythemia.* Lancet 2:161, 1977.

60. GROTTA, J, ET AL: *Whole blood viscosity parameters and cerebral blood flow.* Stroke 13:296, 1982.

61. KALENDOVSKY, Z, AUSTIN, JH, AND STEELE, P: *Increased platelet aggregability in young patients with stroke.* Arch Neurol 32:13, 1975.

62. WEISS, HJ: *Platelet physiology and abnormalities of platelet function, part 1.* N Engl J Med 293:531, 1975.

63. DOUGHERTY, JH, JR, LEVY, DE, AND WEKSLER, BB: *Platelet activation in acute cerebral ischemia.* Lancet 1:821, 1977.

64. CANADIAN COOPERATIVE STUDY GROUP: *A randomized trial of aspirin and sulfinpyrazone in threatened stroke.* N Engl J Med 299:53, 1978.

65. BARNETT, HJM: *The Canadian cooperative study of platelet-suppressive drugs in transient cerebral ischemia.* In PRICE, TR, AND NELSON, E (EDS): *Cerebrovascular Diseases.* Raven Press, New York, 1979, p 221.

66. BARNETT, HJM: *Platelets, drugs and cerebral ischemia.* In HIRSH, J, ET AL (EDS): *Platelets, Drugs and Thrombosis.* S Karger, Basel, 1975, p 233.

67. SCHARF, RE, ET AL: *Cerebral ischemia in young patients: Is it associated with mitral valve prolapse and abnormal platelet activity in vivo?* Stroke 13:454, 1982.

68. REHNCRONA, S, MELA, L, AND SIESJÖ, BK: *Recovery of brain mitochondrial function in the rat after complete and incomplete cerebral ischemia.* Stroke 10:437, 1979.

69. PULSINELLI, WA, ET AL: *Hyperglycemia converting ischemic neuronal damage into brain infarction.* Neurology 32:1239, 1982.

Chapter 5

DIAGNOSIS OF TRANSIENT ISCHEMIC ATTACKS

Suddenly darkness flooded over him . . .
a numbness and weakness in the left arm and leg?
Why did the muscles on one side of his face
feel as though they were sagging?
. . . He noted that his speech was slurred.
Irving Stone, *The Agony and the Ecstasy*, describing Michelangelo

The hallmark of a cerebrovascular lesion is the sudden onset of a focal neurologic deficit that gradually resolves. The more removed the clinical picture from this pattern, the less likely it is vascular. When other lesions present with a stroke-like onset, the underlying pathogenesis also is often vascular, such as hemorrhage into a tumor, or intracerebral steal.[1] Once a cerebrovascular etiology has been decided, a transient ischemic attack (TIA) must be distinguished from a completed stroke. Even in large metropolitan centers, patients rarely present to a physician sooner than a few hours after onset of the deficit, so the clinical distinction between the two is not usually difficult. Although the duration of TIA is defined as less than 24 hours, patients with minor strokes lasting days or weeks have an identical prognosis.[2,3]

The term "transient ischemic attack" implies more precision than is achieved clinically. Usually the diagnosis rests on the history, since attacks seldom are witnessed by the physician. The history can only establish that an acute, transient focal neurologic deficit has occurred, since physical examination is usually negative. The term "presumed TIA" is preferable, since seizures, migraine, and cerebral tumor are other causes of acute focal neurologic deficits. TIAs of the carotid or vertebro-basilar territory can be differentiated by their characteristic clinical pictures. Hemispheric or brainstem hemorrhages also produce transient neurologic episodes indistinguishable from those of ischemic origin, and lumbar puncture may not indicate the true nature of the lesion; only CT scanning may distinguish them.

The concept of transient stroke developed in parallel with discovery of the etiologic role of carotid bifurcation lesions in stroke. The original criteria for "transience" differed widely. Acheson and Hutchinson[4] decided that episodes longer than 1 hour were "strokes," whereas Ziegler and Hassanein[5] believed that deficits of less than 15 minutes did not qualify as TIAs. It is generally agreed that TIAs last no more than 24 hours. "PRINDs" (presumed resolving ischemic neurologic deficits) are stroke deficits lasting a few days, but this definition is not clinically useful. The likelihood of finding a CT scan lesion increases as the duration of TIAs merges imperceptibly into completed stroke.[6]

TIAs probably last hours, not minutes. In the Toronto series, the duration of TIAs was accurately determined on admission in 66 patients and found to have a mean of 3 hours and 10 minutes (range 1 minute to 24 hours). In the Cooperative Study of TIAs,[7] the median duration of carotid attacks was 14 minutes and of vertebrobasilar events was 8 minutes. Ninety percent of carotid TIAs lasted less than 6 hours, and 90 percent of vertebrobasilar TIAs only 2 hours.

Differences between studies are probably real and represent referral bias. The detection rate may vary with the nature and duration of symptoms. The patient notices every second of transient hemiplegia but dismisses slight residual numbness. Culture, education, and access to medical care may all dictate the patient's response to symptoms. Causes of referral bias vary from physicians' lack of concern to overemphasis by centers with a special interest in patients with TIAs.

The proportion of carotid compared with vertebrobasilar TIAs does not reflect the preponderance of carotid to vertebrobasilar infarction. Infarction in the carotid territory is about six times commoner than vertebrobasilar infarction (Table 14), yet carotid TIAs occur only 1.6 times as frequently as vertebrobasilar TIAs.

This may represent the bias of referral pattern, since patients with carotid TIAs are more commonly surgical candidates than are those with vertebrobasilar TIAs. Carotid territory symptoms are generally distinctive, but syncope and nonspecific dizziness are easily mistaken for vertebrobasilar insufficiency.[8] Also, retrospective diagnosis of carotid TIAs is easier, since infarction follows more commonly than in the vertebrobasilar territory.[9]

TABLE 14. Relative Frequency of TIAs in Carotid and Vertebrobasilar Territory

	Carotid TIAs	Vertebrobasilar TIAs	Frequency
Marshall, 1964[19]	82	76	1.1
Acheson, 1964[4]	38	44	0.86
Friedman, 1969*	47	11	4.3
Dyken, 1977[7]	400	112	3.6
Norris et al, unpublished	110	72	1.6

*From Friedman, GD, et al: *Transient ischemic attacks in a community.* JAMA 210:1428, 1969.

USUAL PRESENTATIONS OF TIAS

Evaluating the nature and outcome of TIAs is complicated by the great variety of symptoms attributed to them. This uncertainty is reflected in drug companies' promises of therapeutic effect in vague or unlikely symptoms such as "forgetfulness" or "dizzy attacks." Whereas some authors strenuously exclude "seizures, syncope and migraine,"[5] others[10] include "complex pleasing hallucinations," periodic stupor, and akinetic mutism. The problem is compounded by reliance on the history, since the physician seldom witnesses the episode (13 percent in the Cooperative Study of TIAs).[11]

In the Cooperative Study of TIAs,[12] the most frequent presentations of carotid TIAs were transient monocular blindness, contralateral weakness or sensory symptoms, and language disturbances, while the com-

TABLE 15. Diagnostic Guidelines Proposed by the Study Group for TIAs

Carotid TIA

1. Motor dysfunction: weakness, paralysis, clumsiness of one limb or both limbs on the same side
2. Sensory alteration: numbness, loss of sensation, paresthesias involving one or both limbs on the same side
3. Speech or language disturbance: difficulty in speaking or writing; incomprehension of language, in reading or in performing calculations
4. Visual disturbances: Loss of vision in one eye or part of one eye in a person with previously intact vision; homonymous hemianopia
5. A combination of any of the above

(When sensory-motor manifestations occur, they usually appear all at one time, i.e., without a "spread" or "march" effect)

Vertebrobasilar TIA

1. Motor dysfunction similar to above but sometimes changing from side to side in different attacks and varying in degree from slight loss of voluntary movement to quadriplegia
2. Sensory alteration: as above but usually involving one or both sides of the face, mouth, or tongue
3. Visual loss: as above but including partial loss of vision in both homonymous fields (bilateral homonymous hemianopia); homonymous hemianopia
4. Disequilibrium of gait or postural disturbance, ataxia, imbalance, or unsteadiness
5. Diplopia, dysphagia, dysarthria, or vertigo: none of these symptoms alone should be considered evidence of a vertebrobasilar TIA
6. Combinations of the above

Symptoms *Not* Considered TIA

1. Altered consciousness or syncope
2. Dizziness, "wooziness," or giddiness
3. Impaired vision associated with alterations of consciousness
4. Amnesia alone, confusion alone, vertigo alone, diplopia alone, dysphagia alone, or dysarthria alone
5. Tonic-clonic motor activity
6. March of motor or sensory deficits
7. Focal symptoms associated with migraine headache
8. Bowel or bladder incontinence

DIAGNOSIS OF
TRANSIENT
ISCHEMIC ATTACKS

Adapted from Study Group on TIA Criteria and Detection (Heyman, A, et al)[13] with permission.

monest symptoms in vertebrobasilar TIAs were bilateral visual blurring, diplopia, atazia, and dizziness. The most frequent symptoms in patients later discovered not to have TIAs were loss of consciousness, confusion, and bilateral leg weakness. These presentations confirmed the diagnostic guidelines proposed in 1974 by the Study Group on TIA Criteria and Detection (Table 15).[13]

UNUSUAL PRESENTATIONS OF TIAS

Headache

Grindal and Toole[14] found an incidence of 25 percent in a retrospective review of TIA patients, a figure identical to our data (Table 16). Headache preceding or accompanying the neurologic symptoms of TIAs is generally attributed to increased flow in collateral channels, normally under low perfusion. Pain due to this rapid opening and stretching of collateral vessels was dubbed "Willis headache," after the first decription in 1667 by Thomas Willis of a patient with carotid artery occlusion.[15]

Seizures

The Study Group on TIA[13] does not include seizures as a feature of TIA. Russell[10] noted that TIAs occasionally present as seizures, and Barnett[16] found no seizures in the vertebrobasilar group but found 1.5 percent in the carotid group among 483 TIA patients. Completed strokes presenting as seizures are easier to distinguish, since permanent deficits remain. TIAs presenting as seizures can only be confidently diagnosed when they occur during the course of multiple systemic embolism.

Loss of Consciousness

Patients with carotid TIAs seldom lose consciousness although they may describe temporary "daze" or "confusion." Loss of consciousness did not occur among patients in the Toronto series. Transient interruption of brainstem arousal mechanisms could theoretically alter consciousness in patients with vertebrobasilar TIAs, though this is undocumented. Vertebrobasilar embolism to the occipital lobe also could cause unconsciousness following a seizure, though it was not reported in the Canadian Cooperative Study.[2] In the Cooperative Study of TIAs, loss of conscious-

TABLE 16. Prospective Evaluation of the Frequency of Headache in 897 Stroke Patients Admitted to the Toronto Unit

	Headache	Total Patients
Cerebral infarction	141 (20%)	692
Cerebral hemorrhage	24 (39%)	62
TIA	32 (24%)	132
Amaurosis fugax	0 (0%)	11

ness occasionally occurred with both carotid and vertebrobasilar TIAs.[11] Our analysis of their original data[17] suggests that other interpretations might explain the episodes of impaired consciousness. Seizures could not always be excluded but, in some of their cases, loss of consciousness accompanied otherwise typical TIAs.

Drop Attacks

In drop attacks the patient, often an elderly woman, suddenly falls to the ground without loss of consciousness and, after a brief delay, scrambles to her feet. Although these episodes are attributed to transient vertebrobasilar ischemia,[18-20] little data support this contention. Transient interruption of descending reticulospinal pathways by momentary brainstem ischemia inhibiting motor power but not consciousness is an attractive but unproven hypothesis.[21] These episodes do not occur with other symptoms of vertebrobasilar ischemia nor in cases of known vertebrobasilar embolism. They may recur alone for years. Sudden head movements, especially looking up, may produce kinking of the arteries in the bony cervical canal, causing hemodynamic rather than thromboembolic TIAs. Occurring alone, they do not warrant further investigation.

Transient Global Amnesia

Transient global amnesia is a symptom, not qualifying as a TIA unless other specific symptoms are also present. Indistinguishable episodes may occur in hysteria, temporal lobe epilepsy, and other conditions. One remarkable patient in our series experienced both a drop attack and transient global amnesia during episodes of vertebrobasilar TIAs.

> **Case History.** A 58-year-old woman who had a pacemaker inserted for sick sinus syndrome had a sudden drop attack several days later, when her legs buckled and she fell without loss of consciousness. A month later, while looking into the refrigerator, she suddenly could not see anything in her right visual field for 5 minutes. Some months after this, she had a "funny feeling," as though her arms were floating above her head, her thoughts seemed scrambled, and her speech garbled for about 10 minutes. While at dinner later, her daughter saw the patient leave the table, wander around the room and ask "What time is it?" and "What are we doing here?" The symptoms cleared in 30 minutes and the patient remembered nothing of the event. Cerebral angiography, CT scan, EEG, and echocardiography were normal.

Similarity to the permanent confabulatory amnesia following bilateral posterior cerebral artery occlusion suggests transient vertebrobasilar ischemia as the cause.[22] Nystagmus noted during transient global amnesia suggests brainstem ischemia in some cases,[23] but Fisher, reviewing his own data, believes that the pathogenesis is epilepsy and argues against any cerebrovascular basis.[24,25]

Amaurosis Fugax

The pathogenesis of carotid TIAs and amaurosis fugax is identical, though transient monocular blindness does not affect the brain. Retinal emboli usually originate from ulceration in the internal carotid artery,[26] sometimes from the external carotid artery when the internal carotid artery is occluded[27] or from the ophthalmic artery.[28] Transient monocular blindness from presumed cardiac emboli was found in one third of patients with chronic rheumatic heart disease examined in an anticoagulant clinic[29] and may occur with mitral valve prolapse.[30]

Few disorders can be confused with amaurosis fugax, in which vision dims suddenly or is like "a shutter coming down," leaving a horizontal lower or upper margin of blindness. There may be photopsias, quickly disappearing stationary flecks of light that do not shimmer or scintillate like the fortification spectra of migraine. Amaurosis fugax may last from seconds to hours[26] but most commonly fades slowly over 5 or 10 minutes. Migraine, with its march of symptoms, cannot be confused with this disorder,[26,29,31] since fortification spectra shimmer distinctively and move across the visual field, producing homonymous hemianopia or temporary blindness. Spasm of the central retinal artery in Raynaud's disease, producing intermittent blindness, is rare.[32] Careful examination will distinguish hemianopia or quadrantanopia from amaurosis fugax.

PHYSICAL EXAMINATION OF PATIENTS WITH TIAS

As in completed stroke, patients sometimes had no visual complaints yet had homonymous hemianopia on examination.[33] Sensory deficits were uncommon and retinal emboli were seen in only 2 (2.5 percent) of 121 patients. Tachycardia was common but cardiac arrhythmias were unusual, although only two patients were actually monitored by ECG during their attacks. Transient increases in pulse rate and blood pressure were considered nonspecific effects of stress.

DIFFERENTIAL DIAGNOSIS OF TRANSIENT ISCHEMIC ATTACKS

Since the diagnosis of TIAs is largely based on the patient's history, few clinical evaluations are more taxing of the examiner's acumen and expertise. Diagnostic accuracy reflects the level of neurologic training.[11] Nonneurologist physicians diagnosed TIAs more readily in patients presenting with vague, nonspecific symptoms such as dizziness or ataxia (Table 17), and they missed minor fixed deficits more frequently. Mistaken diagnoses not only subject the patient to unnecessary investigations but may also delay appropriate treatment.

The condition most commonly mistaken for TIA is ischemic or hemorrhagic *completed stroke*,[11] often only discovered on CT scanning (Fig. 33). Since TIA is a clinical diagnosis, the discovery of cerebral infarction on CT should not alter it.

A variety of *postseizure states* masquerade as stroke or TIAs and present a major problem in diagnosis.[10,11,34] The combination of an old

TABLE 17. Initial Complaint and Final Diagnosis in 123
Patients Found Not to Have TIA (95 Patients With
Completed Stroke Excluded)

Initial Complaint	Final Diagnosis	Number
Fainting	Postural hypotension	18
	Syncope	16
Dizziness	Vertigo	7
	Other (including cardiac arrhythmias)	16
Loss of consciousness	Seizures	18
Anxiety	Neurosis	14
Headache	Migraine and tension	5
Visual symptoms	Papillitis	2
	Retinal artery occlusion	2
Confusion	Other organic confusional states	7
Other	Tumor, iatrogenic, and others	18

From Calanchini, et al,[11] with permission.

stroke with a first seizure is especially confusing and is not clarified by
CT scan. Since both postictal states and TIAs last only hours, they may
be impossible to differentiate, even in retrospect. Postictal states include
hemiparesis (Todd's paralysis), gaze palsy, hemianopia, and hemianesthesia, which may last several days. Postictal confusional states, stupor,
and coma must also be differentiated from TIA (Fig. 34; Table 18).

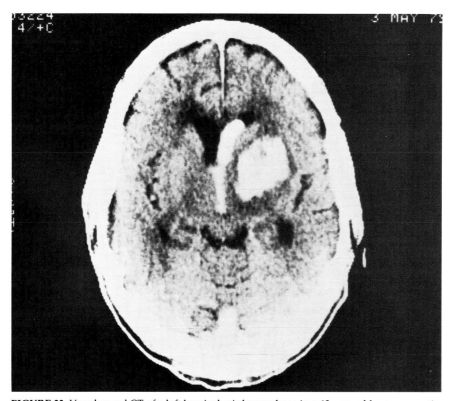

FIGURE 33. Unenhanced CT of a left hemispheric hemorrhage in a 62-year-old man presenting
with a 1-day episode of dysphasia that completely resolved.

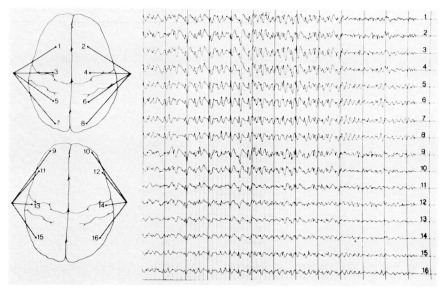

FIGURE 34. An 80-year-old man was admitted with confusion and mild right hemiparesis. EEG showed 3 percent in spike and wave activity. With intravenous diazepam, the EEG instantly reverted to normal, the "stroke" disappeared, and the patient became alert and fully oriented. (From Norris and Hachinski,[34] with permission.)

Complicated *migraine* may also present as TIA or stroke. In classical migraine, transient occipital dysfunction results in flashing or scintillating scotomata. Gradual enlargement of a scintillating scotoma over 5 to 30 minutes ("march") distinguishes the migrainous TIA. Paresthesias of the face, tongue, and limbs on one side often accompany the visual symptoms. In patients over 40, migraine is not suspected as a cause of TIAs and yet such visual accompaniments (excluding the usual scintillating scotomata) occur, sometimes with motor and sensory symptoms.[30] This presentation of migraine in the older patient is particularly deceptive, since only half have headaches. The concept of "migraine without headache" preceded knowledge of more subtle forms of cerebral embolism such as mitral valve prolapse, and the explanation of such silent cerebral ischemic events may need revision. "Basilar migraine" may produce drop attacks, often with loss of consciousness, as well as a variety of ophthalmoplegias, resulting from brainstem ischemia.

The commonest presentation of cerebral *tumor* simulating TIAs is as a postictal state. A less common but more intriguing cause is intrace-

TABLE 18. Clinical Presentation of 81 Patients Misdiagnosed as "Stroke" in the Toronto Unit

Presenting Symptom	Seizure Group	Nonseizure Group	Total
Focal neurologic deficit	19	16	35
Stupor or coma	15	5	20
Acute confusional state	8	18	26
Totals	42 (52%)	39 (48%)	81

rebral steal. The abnormal vasculature of cerebral tumors responds poorly to changes in P_{CO_2}, so that hyperventilation produces shunting of blood from normally vasoconstricting brain to unreacting tumor vessels, thus "stealing" blood from adjacent brain.[1]

Premonitory symptoms prior to rupture of a saccular *aneurysm* may be indistinguishable from TIAs (Fig. 35; Table 19). Severe headache of sudden onset often accompanies subarachnoid hemorrhage[35] but prerupture symptoms may be painless. Aneurysmal leaking, pressure on surrounding structures by the aneurysm, or even prerupture spasm are suggested mechanisms.[36] Subarachnoid hemorrhage with transient neurologic deficits but without headache may be discovered only on CT scanning or lumbar puncture. In rare cases, saccular aneurysm causing the neurologic deficit is only discovered by chance on angiography.

Chronic subdural *hematoma* may present with a variety of fleeting neurologic deficits, including dysphasia. Sometimes, surgical evacuation of the clot completely abolishes the symptoms, indicating causality and not coincidence.[37] Since symptoms from such mass lesions are indistinguishable from "true" TIAs, early CT scanning is imperative.

Transient neurologic symptoms of *hypertensive encephalopathy* are commonly nonspecific, such as headache, confusion, seizures, visual

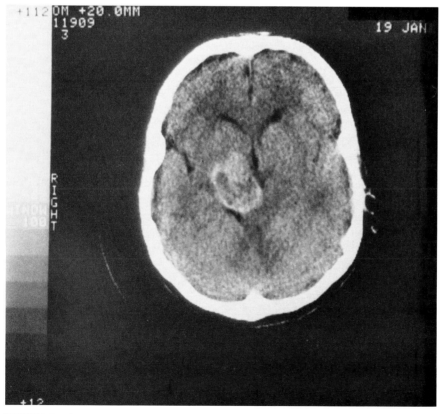

FIGURE 35. A 49-year-old woman had episodic painless diplopia and blurred vision for 2 months, diagnosed as vertebrobasilar ischemia. Examination during an episode revealed a right third nerve palsy. Enhanced CT scan and later angiography showed a giant saccular aneurysm. The episodes resolved when the aneurysm was clipped.

TABLE 19. Presenting Symptoms of Subarachnoid Hemorrhage in 41 Patients

	Number of Patients
Headache	35
Nausea	18
Vomiting	14
Brief loss of consciousness	13
Neck stiffness or pain	6
Hemiparesis	6
Vertigo	6
Faintness	5
Confusion	5
Convulsions	3
Coma	3
Hearing loss	3
Visual loss	2
Diplopia	2
Malaise and diffuse aches	2
Photophobia, back pain, leg pain, ataxia, speech disturbance, chest pain, paraparesis	1 each

From Adams, et al,[36] with permission.

blurring, and, occasionally, focal neurologic deficits. Initially, these symptoms were attributed to vasospasm,[38] but autopsy data indicate that these deficits mostly result from infarction and hemorrhage, and visual blurring is probably due to the retinal changes of malignant hypertension.[39] This entity is rare and overdiagnosed, especially in severely hypertensive patients.[39]

The symptoms of *hypoglycemia* usually consist of nervousness, flushing, sweating, tremor, confusion, ataxia, drowsiness, and stupor. Focal neurologic deficits unaccompanied by these generalized symptoms are rarely due to hypoglycemia. Focal cerebral symptoms are determined by regional variations in cerebral perfusion. The patient is usually diabetic with iatrogenic hypoglycemia. "Reactive hypoglycemia" is a diagnosis and panacea usually offered to anxious, demanding, and otherwise healthy patients. Rarely, hypoglycemia due to an insulinoma is detected by routine administration of glucose to a patient with TIA or stroke in the emergency room.

Patients with *hysterical hemi- or monoparesis* may undergo extensive investigations, including cerebral angiography, unless they are carefully examined in the acute stage. The movements and tone of the affected "paralyzed" limb are inappropriate to the power demonstrated by clinical examination. When testing for limb drift, if the arm or leg is persistently held up, curious jerking or tremulousness may ensue, working to a climax in which the limb jerks wildly in all directions. The patient commonly appears little concerned over these curious effects and may even smile with "la belle indifference." "Signs" such as hemisensory loss may be induced in a suggestible patient by inexperienced medical examiners. Total loss or diminution of all sensory modalities may occur, including loss of vibration sensation to the midline of the forehead or sternum. The gait is often bizarre, without the patient actually falling, and even inexperienced observers may suspect that the patient is play-acting.

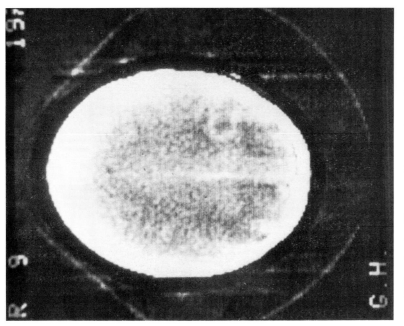

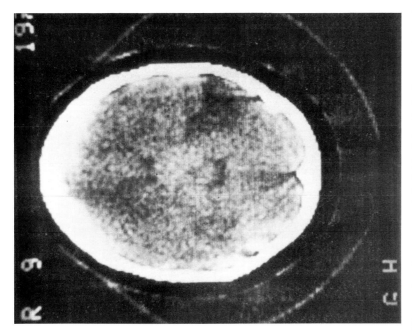

FIGURE 36. CT scan showing an area of diminished density in the posterior parietal region (*left*) and a ring-like area of increased vascularity on enhancement (*right*) in a patient later found to have multiple sclerosis. (From Norris and Hachinski,[34] with permission.)

DIAGNOSIS OF
TRANSIENT
ISCHEMIC ATTACKS

75

Multiple sclerosis may produce transient symptoms and signs often attributed to TIAs in younger patients, especially when they last only hours. The clinical picture often correlates poorly with CT appearances or laboratory data such as brainstem evoked responses, CSF cell, and biochemical analysis.[40] The most sensitive method of imaging plaques is probably magnetic resonance.[41] One patient admitted to the unit with acute hemiplegia was later found to have acute multiple sclerosis (Fig. 36).

CONCLUSION

TIAs are underestimated by patients and physicians alike, since they are brief and rarely disabling. They should be sought assiduously and investigated scrupulously in stroke-prone individuals, since they often signal impending but avoidable disaster.

Transient neurologic focal deficits with an abrupt onset and gradual resolution strongly favor a vascular origin. Diagnosis rests mainly on history, since most TIAs last only a few hours and patients can rarely be examined during attacks. Carotid TIAs must be distinguished from vertebrobasilar TIAs, because their management differs. Clinical acumen is more valuable than a battery of investigations, especially since CT scanning is usually negative and angiographic evidence of cerebrovascular disease may be a chance finding.

The distinction between TIA, completed stroke, and other differential diagnoses becomes important, as the prognosis and management for each are different.

REFERENCES

1. HACHINSKI, VC, ET AL: *Symptomatic intracranial steal.* Arch Neurol 34:149, 1977.
2. CANADIAN COOPERATIVE STUDY GROUP: *A randomized trial of aspirin and sulfinpyrazone in threatened stroke.* N Engl J Med 299:53, 1978.
3. BOUSSER, MG, ET AL: *Essai coopératif contrôlé "AICLA."* Rev Neurol 139:335, 1983.
4. ACHESON, J, AND HUTCHINSON, EC: *Observations on the natural history of transient cerebral ischemia.* Lancet 2:871, 1964.
5. ZIEGLER, DK, AND HASSANEIN, RS: *Prognosis in patients with transient ischemic attacks.* Stroke 4:666, 1973.
6. LADURNER, G, ET AL: *A correlation of clinical findings and CT in ischemic cerebrovascular disease.* Eur Neurol J 18:281, 1979.
7. DYKEN, ML, ET AL: *Cooperative study of hospital frequency and character of transient ischemic attacks. i. Background, organization, and clinical survey.* JAMA 237:882, 1977.
8. BARNETT, HJM: *Progress towards stroke prevention: Robert Wartenberg Lecture.* Neurology 30:1212, 1980.
9. MARSHALL, J: *Summary of the Seventh International Salzburg Conference on Cerebral Vascular Disease. September 25–29, 1974.* Stroke 6:109, 1975.
10. ROSS RUSSELL, RW: *Transient cerebral ischaemia.* In ROSS RUSSELL, RW (ED): *Vascular Disease of the Central Nervous System,* ed 2. Churchill-Livingstone, Edinburgh, 1983, p 204.
11. CALANCHINI, PR, ET AL: *Cooperative study of hospital frequency and character of transient ischemic attacks. iv. The reliability of diagnosis.* JAMA 238:2029, 1977.
12. FUTTY, DE, ET AL: *Cooperative study of hospital frequency and character of transient ischemic attacks. v. Symptom analysis.* JAMA 238:2386, 1977.
13. STUDY GROUP ON TIA CRITERIA AND DETECTION (HEYMAN, A, ET AL): *xi. Transient focal cerebral ischemia: Epidemiological and clinical aspects.* Stroke 5:277, 1974.
14. GRINDAL, AB, AND TOOLE, JF: *Headache and transient ischemic attacks.* Stroke 5:603, 1974.

15. FEINDEL, W (ED): *Willis, Thomas: The anatomy of the brain and nerves, 1667.* McGill University Press, Montreal, 1965.

16. BARNETT, HJM: *The Canadian cooperative study of platelet-suppressive drugs in transient cerebral ischemia.* In PRICE, TR, AND NELSON, E (EDS): *Cerebrovascular Diseases.* Raven Press, New York, 1979, p 221.

17. DYKEN, ML: Personal communication. February, 1983.

18. WILLIAMS, D, AND WILSON, TG: *The diagnosis of the major and minor syndromes of basilar insufficiency.* Brain 85:741, 1962.

19. MARSHALL, J: *The natural history of transient ischaemic cerebrovascular attacks.* Q J Med 33:309, 1964.

20. KUBALA, MJ, AND MILLIKAN, CH: *Diagnosis, pathogenesis, and treatment of "drop attacks."* Arch Neurol 11:107, 1964.

21. MARSHALL, J: *Management of Cerebrovascular Disease,* ed 2. J & A Churchill, London, 1968.

22. VICTOR, M, ET AL: *Memory loss with lesions of hippocampal formation.* Arch Neurol 5:244, 1961.

23. LONGRIDGE, NS, HACHINSKI, V, AND BARBER, HO: *Brain stem dysfunction in transient global amnesia.* Stroke 10:473, 1979.

24. FISHER, CM, AND ADAMS, RD: *Transient global amnesia.* Acta Neurol Scand (Suppl 9) 40:1, 1964.

25. FISHER, CM: *Transient global amnesia—Precipitating activities and other observations.* Arch Neurol 39:605, 1982.

26. MARSHALL, J, AND MEADOWS, S: *The natural history of amaurosis fugax.* Brain 91:419, 1968.

27. BURNBAUM, MD, ET AL: *Amaurosis fugax from disease of the external carotid artery.* Arch Neurol 34:532, 1977.

28. WEINBERGER, J, BENDER, AN, AND YANG, WC: *Amaurosis fugax associated with ophthalmic artery stenosis: clinical simulation of carotid artery disease.* Stroke 11:290, 1980.

29. SWASH, M, AND EARL, CJ: *Transient visual obscurations in chronic rheumatic heart-disease.* Lancet 2:323, 1970.

30. BARNETT, HJM, ET AL: *Further evidence relating mitral-valve prolapse to cerebral ischemic events.* N Engl J Med 302:139, 1980.

31. FISHER, CM: *Late-life migraine accompaniments as a cause of unexplained transient ischemic attacks.* Can J Neurol Sci 7:9, 1980.

32. WALSH, FB, AND HOYT, WF: *Clinical neuro-ophthalmology, vol 3.* Williams & Wilkins, Baltimore, 1969, p 1806, 1914.

33. PRICE, TR, ET AL: *Cooperative study of hospital frequency and character of transient ischemic attacks, vi. Patients examined during an attack.* JAMA 238:2512, 1977.

34. NORRIS, JW, AND HACHINSKI, VC: *Misdiagnosis of stroke.* Lancet 1:328, 1982.

35. FISHER, CM: *Headache in cerebrovascular disease.* In VINKEN, PJ, AND BRUYN, GW (EDS): *Handbook of Neurology, Vol 5: Headaches and Cranial Neuralgias.* North-Holland, Amsterdam, 1968, p 124.

36. ADAMS, HP, ET AL: *Pitfalls in the recognition of subarachnoid hemorrhage.* JAMA 244:794, 1980.

37. WELSH, JE, ET AL: *Chronic subdural hematoma presenting as transient neurologic deficits.* Stroke 10:564, 1979.

38. BYROM, FB: *The pathogenesis of hypertensive encephalopathy and its relation to the malignant phase of hypertension: Experimental evidence from the hypertensive rat.* Lancet 2:201, 1954.

39. CHESTER, EM, ET AL: *Hypertensive encephalopathy: A clinicopathologic study of 20 cases.* Neurology 28:928, 1978.

40. POSER, CM: *Exacerbations, activity and progression in multiple sclerosis.* Arch Neurol 37:471, 1980.

41. YOUNG, IR: *Nuclear magnetic resonance imaging of the brain in multiple sclerosis.* Lancet 2:1063, 1981.

Chapter 6

DIAGNOSIS OF STROKE

More puzzles are solved by taking a second history
than by doing all the tests.
Gordon Holmes

Diagnosis underlies rational management, yet stroke is often diagnosed when absent or missed when present. Making the diagnosis of stroke is easier than deciding its type.[1,2] History and examination still remain the most reliable, repeatable, and cost-effective ways of evaluating stroke. Deciding its location is easier than determining its etiology. The highly organized CNS is clinically eloquent when injured, but the cause of the injury carries no such clues, and laboratory investigations are often necessary for further management. CT scanning helps to identify the site and type of pathology, to distinguish nonvascular from vascular lesions, and to identify vascular subtypes, but it remains a complement of and not a substitute for clinical evaluation.[3]

The diagnosis of stroke depends essentially upon the interpretation of the history and examination, first localizing the lesion and then characterizing its type and cause.

HISTORY

The time profile characterizes a stroke, although the physician usually sees the patient hours later, making an accurate history critical to diagnosis. It is important to inquire in detail about the very first symptom and to overcome the tendency of patients to relate the most dramatic or the most recent events. The primacy of the initial symptom cannot be overemphasized, since it often offers the best clues to localization and etiology.

In unsophisticated patients, it may be necessary to review their daily activities to establish whether a neurologic event has affected them. Although many stroke patients are unable to give a history because of aphasia or unconsciousness, those who can often describe paralysis of the affected limbs as "heavy" or dragging, and it may be impossible to differentiate paresis from anesthesia. Patients may say that they "fell to one side" or could not get out of bed. They rarely describe hemianopia but they may bruise the side of their body in the absent visual field. In unraveling the patient's history, descriptive rather than categorical language is preferable; "unsteadiness" may not be "ataxia," and "speech difficulty" not necessarily "aphasia."

The clinical picture will usually decide the cerebral location. Weakness more in the arm than in the leg suggests carotid stroke, whereas

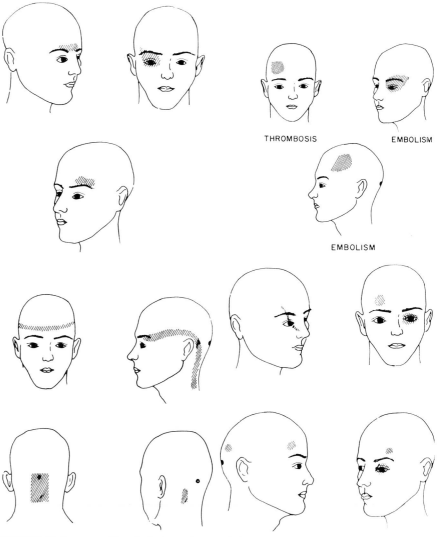

THROMBOSIS   EMBOLISM

EMBOLISM

ACUTE STROKE

80

FIGURE 37. Patterns of headache in occlusion of the internal carotid artery *(top, left)*, middle cerebral artery *(top, right)*, basilar artery *(bottom, left)*, and posterior cerebral artery *(bottom, right)*. (From Fisher,[8] with permission.)

TABLE 20. Headache at Onset in 964 Consecutive Admissions to the Toronto Unit

	Yes	No	Unknown	Total
Infarct	141 (20%)	351	50	742
Hemorrhage	24 (39%)	38	16	78
TIA	32 (24%)	100	1	133
Amaurosis fugax	0	11	0	11

equal involvement suggests a capsular or brainstem lesion. Unawareness that a stroke has occurred suggests the nondominant hemisphere. It is difficult to differentiate dysphasia from dysarthria by history alone. Vertigo, ataxia, diplopia, or dysphagia suggest a vertebrobasilar site, although swallowing difficulties occur with both carotid and vertebrobasilar stroke.

An abrupt onset, with rapidly intervening stupor or coma, may occur in cerebral hemorrhage or a brainstem stroke. Patients with hemispheric emboli may initially lose consciousness, possibly due to unwitnessed seizures. More commonly, patients with carotid stroke are aware of spreading hemiweakness and numbness over several minutes and remain conscious, at least until the onset of cerebral edema several days later. There is no evidence that cerebral embolism occurs with more frequency at any time during the diurnal cycle.

About 50 percent of patients with ischemic stroke have prior TIAs.[4-6] Past history of hypertension, cardiac disease, peripheral vascular disease, diabetes, and peripheral or pulmonary embolism may all be relevant to the recent illness.

Stroke patients often have a positive family history for diabetes, hypertension, stroke, and myocardial infarction, compared with the family history of their spouses.[7] A family history of vascular disease becomes more relevant the earlier it occurs. Smoking, drinking, drug addiction, and the contraceptive pill are risk factors for stroke. A history of migraine should be considered in the differential diagnosis of stroke.

Headache is unusual with cerebral infarction and, if severe and sudden, suggests subarachnoid hemorrhage or migraine. Headache preceding the "stroke" by weeks or months suggests cerebral tumor. Carotid strokes are more likely to produce frontoparietal headache and vertebrobasilar stroke frontal or occipital headache[8] (Fig. 37). Headache in cerebral hemorrhage is more abrupt, severe, and dramatic, twice as common as in cerebral infarction (Table 20), and often followed by loss of consciousness. Vomiting at onset is very suggestive of intracranial hemorrhage. Seizures at onset occur in about 5 percent of patients, suggesting cerebral embolism or cerebral hemorrhage.[9]

EXAMINATION

Almost a thousand years ago, Ibn Ridwan of Cairo[10] tested his patients' acuity of hearing and vision, their muscle power by having them lift weights and grasp objects, and their gait by observing them walk forward and back. We should be no less thorough, especially in observing stroke patients.

General Appearance

An inquiring glance yields more information than any other part of the examination. The approximate age, sex, ethnic origin, habitus, alertness, responsiveness, language, and attitude become immediately evident to the discerning eye.

In an aphasic or unresponsive patient, handedness can be determined with 90 percent accuracy by observing that the thumb nailbed of the dominant hand is broader and has a less rounded contour than that of the other thumb.[11] Onset of the stroke can be estimated from a man's beard growth and the freshness of a woman's make-up.

The body build may suggest a systemic condition. Hypertension often accompanies obesity. Women obese in the upper body are eight times as likely to develop diabetes as other women.[12] A marfanoid habitus (tallness with long slender limbs) may be associated with mitral valve prolapse.[13] In blacks, sickle cell trait may precipitate stroke.

Smoking leaves its stain on the fingers and its smell on breath and clothes. Alcoholism may be suspected from a pleasing, evasive demeanor or from the trail of enlarged venules or capillaries on the face, particularly on the nose. Chronic alcoholic smokers have a characteristic tremulousness of limb and hoarseness of voice. Subdural hematoma, common among alcoholics, may present as "stroke."

Corneal arcus occurs more frequently with increasing age and in men. It is an independent risk factor for coronary heart disease in men under 50 years, their chance of myocardial infarction being almost twice as great.[14] Xanthelasma, lipid deposits around the eyes, may be innocent or suggest type II hyperlipidemia.

The general physical examination may yield other relevant signs such as valvular heart disease, petechial hemorrhages, or infection relating to etiology. The neurovascular examination identifies arterial disease and suggests the presence of stenoses and occlusions, whereas the standard neurologic examination provides the most information on cerebral localization.

NEUROVASCULAR EXAMINATION

Ophthalmoscopy

The retinal vessels mirror the brain vasculature, allowing direct observation of arterial narrowing secondary to hypertension, diabetic retinopathy, and retinal artery or branch occlusions with secondary retinal infarction. Although increased intracranial pressure is common in stroke, papilledema only occurs with cerebral hemorrhage, or when a mass lesion mimics stroke. Birefringent cholesterol emboli in the retina usually indicate the presence of carotid stenoses and ulceration. Their significance may be exaggerated, since they are sought most avidly in symp-

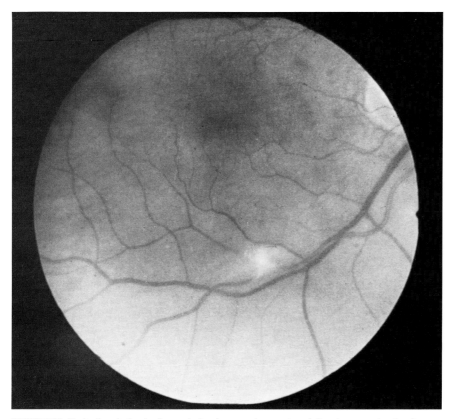

FIGURE 38. Retinal embolus in the optic fundus seen in a patient following an episode of amaurosis fugax.

tomatic patients but go undetected in asymptomatic patients (Fig. 38). Subhyaloid hemorrhage indicates subarachnoid blood.

Palpation

Palpation of the carotid arteries is an unreliable measure of their patency and risks bradycardia or dislodgment of atheroma or thrombus. Palpation of the branches of the external carotid arteries proves more useful and less risky. An absent temporal artery pulse suggests common carotid artery occlusion, and a tender, tortuous, and enlarged temporal artery suggests arteritis. Blood pressure asymmetries may not be reflected in inequalities of pulse, and measurements in both arms are required to detect significant subclavian or brachial artery obstruction or subclavian "steal."

Auscultation

Cranial bruits arise from arteriovenous malformation, aneurysms, neoplasms, hemodynamic states, and ectopically located vessels.[15]
Bruits from carotid stenosis occur near the angle of the jaw (Fig. 39), and neither loudness nor pitch are reliable indicators of stenosis.[16] Dis-

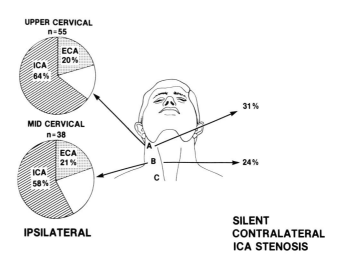

UPPER CERVICAL
n=55

ECA 20%
ICA 64%

MID CERVICAL
n=38

ECA 21%
ICA 58%

IPSILATERAL

31%

24%

A
B
C

SILENT
CONTRALATERAL
ICA STENOSIS

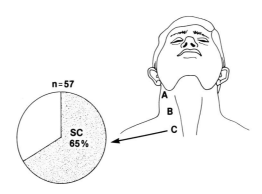

n=57

SC 65%

A
B
C

SILENT
IPSILATERAL
ICA STENOSIS
11%

SILENT
CONTRALATERAL
ICA STENOSIS
4%

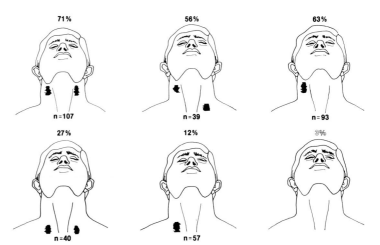

71%
n=107

56%
n=39

63%
n=93

27%
n=40

12%
n=57

3%

covery of carotid stenosis makes demands on clinical judgment in deciding whether it is relevant to the patient's symptoms, since up to 10 percent of routine postmortem examinations demonstrate carotid lesions that were asymptomatic in life.[17]

NEUROLOGIC EXAMINATION

The neurologic examination is most helpful in localization, which narrows the diagnostic possibilities. Higher cortical dysfunction suggests a hemispheric lesion and cranial nerve impairment brainstem involvement. Unilateral motor or sensory deficits of the face, arm, and leg characterize hemispheric lesions, whereas bilateral signs suggest brainstem involvement.

Carotid stroke is distinguished from vertebrobasilar stroke by the characteristic pattern of symptoms and signs. In carotid stroke there are hemiplegia, hemianesthesia, and hemianopia, and cortical deficits such as aphasia. The motor deficit is maximal in the arm, except in anterior cerebral artery territory lesions when the leg is affected most. In vertebrobasilar strokes, brainstem or cerebellar signs such as diplopia or ataxia are prominent, and hemiparesis or hyperreflexia are commonly bilateral.

Vascular lesions may deviate from their anatomically dictated arterial territories,[18–20] because of individual variations in blood supply, or when emboli lodge only in some arterial branches. Even when totally occluded, the vascular territory may be salvaged by collateral circulation, but occlusion of an artery that supplies more than its own vascular territory causes a larger infarction. The duration of ischemia may vary, and the handedness and perhaps the gender[21] of the patient may influence the resulting clinical picture. Acute occlusion causes more extensive damage than does slow stenosis, which allows development of collateral circulation.

Approach to the Conscious Patient

Hemiparesis

A hemispheric lesion is probable in patients who are awake and gazing away from their inert limbs. In uncooperative or aphasic patients, the paralyzed limb flops uselessly by their side. The downward drift against gravity of an arm or leg (Fig. 40) compared with its fellow denotes less

---

FIGURE 39. *Top,* Doppler findings in 93 patients wtih unilateral carotid bruits. When carotid and subclavian bruits were heard on the same side of the neck, the carotid bruit was regarded as the most relevant. ICA = Internal carotid artery or carotid bifurcation stenosis of at least 35 percent. ECA = External carotid artery stenosis.

Middle, Doppler findings in 57 patients with unilateral subclavian bruits. SC = Subclavian stenosis.

Bottom, Prevalence of ICA stenosis, by Doppler, of at least 35 percent on either or both sides of the neck in 336 patients divided among five auscultatory categories. Shading represents the bruit location. The bottom right diagram illustrates the prevalence of ICA stenosis in persons without cervical bruits (derived from published data). (From Chambers and Norris,[16] with permission.)

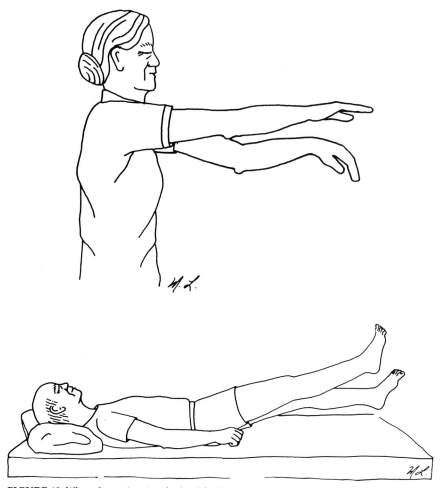

FIGURE 40. When the patient is asked to lift a limb against gravity, the weak limb tends to drift downward.

severe weakness. More subtle signs of minimal weakness may be the abductor digiti quinti sign[22] or the abducted thumb sign (Fig. 41). The "tramp sign," with the leg "down and out" (externally rotated with plantar flexion), suggests weakness of the leg (Fig. 42).

Distal weakness suggests a cortical lesion, and uniform weakness of a limb suggests a deep brain lesion. Commonly the arm is more affected than the leg in lesions of the middle cerebral artery territory, since few collaterals protect the centrosylvian area. Leg weakness greater than arm weakness suggests a lesion in the anterior cerebral artery territory. Rarely, weak limbs with sparing of the face reflect a spinal cord lesion such as infarction. Occasionally, a weak face, arm, or leg occurs with lacunar infarcts[23] of the internal capsule or the basis pontis.

Abnormalities appear as the patient gets out of bed, dresses, and walks. A stiff limb, a fumbling hand, and tilting posture all suggest unilateral weakness. Decreased arm swing, circumduction of the leg, and a syncopated footfall denote a hemiplegic gait.

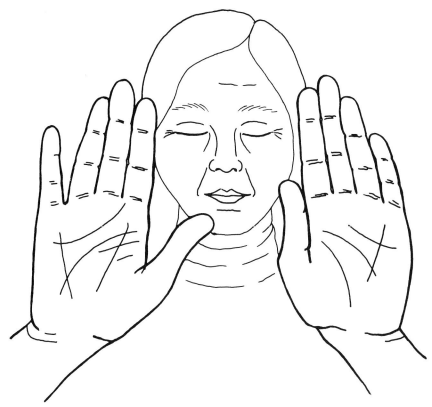

FIGURE 41. With minor corticospinal impairment, the thumb may assume an abducted position when the arms are outstretched. At times the little finger will also be abducted.

Tone. In acute stroke, the hemiparetic limb is initially flaccid, becoming hypertonic within days, and later hyperreflexia and "clasp knife" spasticity supervene. Flaccidity of a limb for days suggests a poor prognosis.

Reflex hyperactivity may be subtle, and only appreciated by greater deflection and decreased latency between the hammer blow and the response. When testing for slight differences one may tap very gently with the middle finger on each side until a response is obtained; the affected side usually will require fewer taps. Tapping vigorously may mask and lose the differences between the two sides; an affected leg may be displaced from the bed. Differences magnify further by reinforcing reflexes (for example, having the patient make a fist just before the examiner taps the patellar tendon).

The Babinski sign may be equivocal at first, with only a qualitative difference between the two sides. It later becomes frankly extensor.

Incoordination

Impaired position sense, weakness, and cerebellar or basal ganglia disturbances all cause truncal or limb incoordination. Cerebellar lesions are commonest, producing limb ataxia and sometimes truncal ataxia when the vermis is involved.

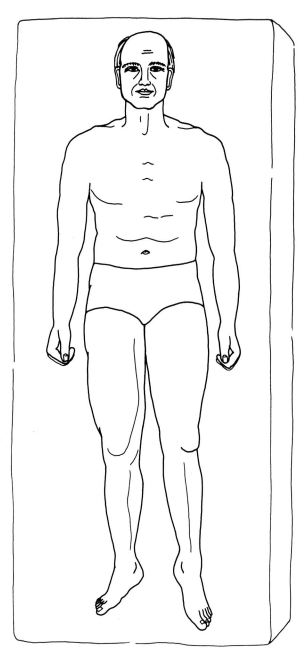

FIGURE 42. With corticospinal weakness, the foot often assumes a position of plantar flexion with eversion at the ankle.

Hemisensory Impairment

Sensation is often impaired but seldom lost on the contralateral side in hemispheric stroke. Pain and temperature sensation are affected more than proprioception. Patients with cortical lesions have touch and pain sensation largely intact but may complain of a limb "feeling funny." Examination may demonstrate impaired two-point discrimination, proprioception, and graphesthesia. Sometimes no sensory impairment can be demonstrated except inattention to simultaneous stimuli of both sides, touch on the impaired side going unreported.

Patchy abnormalities of the face or individual fingers suggest cortical localization, whereas involvement of the whole head, the trunk or abdomen, or extension of impairment to the midline suggest a deep lesion, usually encompassing the thalamus or surrounding area.[24]

Crossed anesthesia is often present in brainstem lesions, with ipsilateral facial impairment of pain or touch and contralateral body and limb abnormalities.

Gaze Deviation

Forced deviation of the eyes and often the head is an important localizing sign of stroke. Damage to a frontal eyefield results in unopposed action of the intact contralateral side, so that the eyes are forced to look toward the affected hemisphere (away from the hemiplegic side) (Fig. 43, *top*). The patient with brainstem stroke looks away from the affected side,

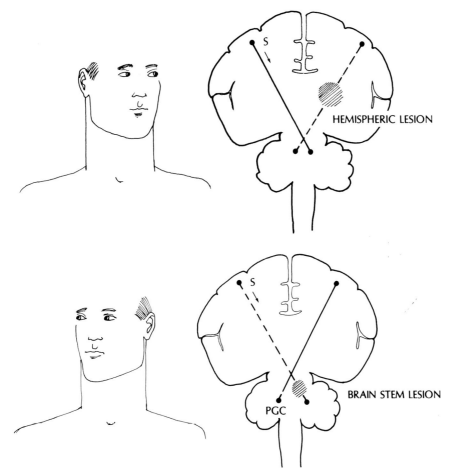

HEMISPHERIC LESION

PGC   BRAIN STEM LESION

FIGURE 43. Forced deviation of the head and eyes toward the side of the hemispheric lesion (*top*) and away from the side of the brainstem lesion (*bottom*).

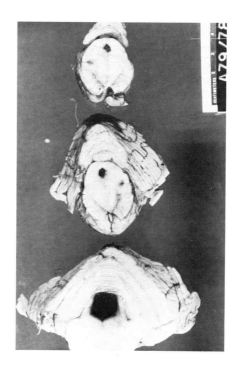

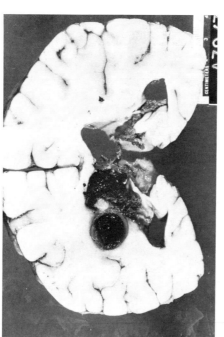

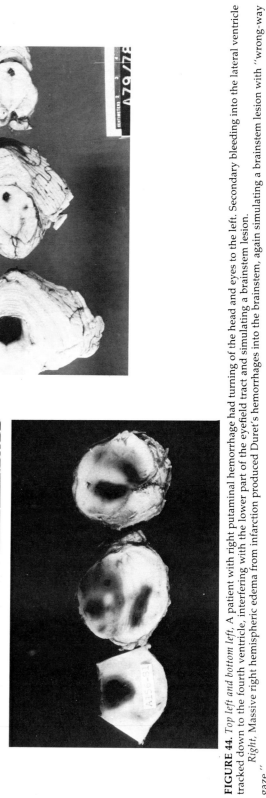

FIGURE 44. *Top left and bottom left,* A patient with right putaminal hemorrhage had turning of the head and eyes to the left. Secondary bleeding into the lateral ventricle tracked down to the fourth ventricle, interfering with the lower part of the eyefield tract and simulating a brainstem lesion.

Right, Massive right hemispheric edema from infarction produced Duret's hemorrhages into the brainstem, again simulating a brainstem lesion with "wrong-way gaze."

toward the hemiplegic side (Fig. 43, *bottom*), since descending tracts to the lateral gaze centers in the pons decussate in the upper midbrain. Rarely, infarction or hemorrhage in the rostral midbrain above the decussation mimic hemispheric lesions.

"Wrong-way" gaze,[25] though very unusual, may cause diagnostic confusion when, for instance, a patient with right hemiplegia has forced gaze to the right. In cerebral hemorrhage, it may result from blood tracking down to the ipsilateral brainstem (Fig. 44, *top left, bottom left*); and in cerebral infarction, from Duret's hemorrhages (Fig. 44, *right*).

Cranial Nerve Impairment

Hemianopia alone usually indicates a lesion in the vertebrobasilar system but may occur in carotid strokes when the posterior cerebral artery arises from the carotid artery or when the anterior choroidal artery supplies the optic radiation exclusively (15 to 20 percent of patients).[19] Hemianopia suggests an intrinsic cerebral lesion, seldom occurring with compressive lesions such as subdural hematoma, except when the patient nears coma.[26]

Facial weakness that disappears with emotional expression suggests a cortical lesion. If it persists, a deep lesion involving the thalamus, globus pallidus, or upper midbrain becomes likely. Lesions of the facial nucleus or its outflow tract produce weakness of the upper and lower face, inability to close the eye or furrow the brow, and drooping of the mouth on the affected side. Minimal facial weakness is suggested by a wider palpebral fissure and flattened nasolabial fold on the hemiparetic side with hemispheric lesions (Fig. 45). The *corneal reflex* may be depressed on the hemiparetic side.[27,28] Transient asymmetric *tongue deviation* to the hemiparetic side often occurs despite bilateral innervation.

Dysarthria

Dysarthria most frequently arises from brainstem lesions, from interference with medullary nuclei, tracts, or cerebellar connections. It also occurs with left hemispheric and more often with right hemispheric lesions.[29]

Dysphagia

Persistent dysphagia commonly results from a brainstem stroke, especially medullary infarction; but acute hemispheric lesions also produce transient dysphagia.

Higher Cortical Dysfunction

The term "dominant hemisphere" betrays an unjustified assumption of a natural hierarchy. The cerebral hemispheres are more alike than different, and the differences are complementary rather than subordinate.

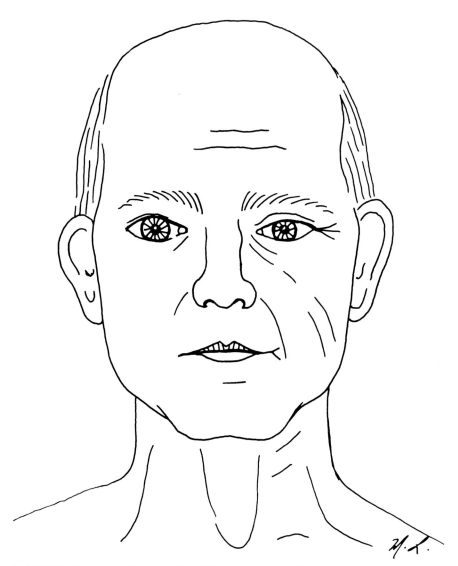

FIGURE 45. Flattening of the nasolabial fold and asymmetry of the mouth characteristic of facial weakness.

The brain works as an integrated and harmonious whole, both structurally and functionally. It is best to refer the lesion to the right or left hemisphere and to state the patient's handedness.

Re-evaluation of brain function emphasizes the importance of cerebral network disruption as opposed to single-locus lesions[30] and recognizes that deep lesions can produce cortical syndromes.[31] Nevertheless, the recognition of specific clinical entities retains localizing value.

Aphasia is a disorder of written and spoken language characterized by anomia (word-finding difficulty), paraphasias (roundabout speech), and comprehension deficits of varying degrees. Initially, a stroke patient may be mute or may express only inappropriate, stereotypical words such as "yes." Over the ensuing weeks, this deficit may recede into a more specific expressive or receptive language disorder.

Unless a clear account of "wrong words" emerges, only examination, and not history alone, distinguishes dysphasia from dysarthria (difficulty articulating). Aphasia is invariably associated with dysgraphia, although writing aphasia can occur without speaking aphasia.[32] A patient writing correct sentences usually suffers from dysarthria, not aphasia, however distorted the speech.[32] Aphasic syndromes result from left-hemisphere injuries almost always in dextrals and in two thirds of sinistrals.

Broca's nonfluent aphasia is characterized by few words, often fragments of nouns or verbs uttered with difficulty and expressed in frustration. Comprehension may be unaffected but repetition is always impaired. Lesions restricted to the posterior third frontal convolution (Broca's area) usually produce mild or transient expressive aphasia. When persistent, the underlying lesion frequently involves Broca's area, the anterior rolandic region area, and, to a variable extent, the anterior parietal and temporal areas.[33,34]

Patients with *Wernicke's fluent aphasia* are loquacious and circumlocutory. What they say sounds sensible but is meaningless ("politician's speech"), often consisting of neologistic paraphasias (jargon). Patients can neither understand nor repeat the examiner's words.[32] Comprehension and repetition difficulty occurring without paraphasias is termed "pure word deafness."

Involvement of Wernicke's area alone produces mild, transient, fluent aphasia. In persistent or severe jargon aphasia, the inferior parietal and supramarginal areas are also involved.[34]

In *conduction aphasia*, comprehension usually remains normal and spontaneous speech is nearly fluent. Difficulties arise in repetition, especially of short words, "no ifs, ands, or buts."[32] Conduction aphasia arises from deep parietal lesions, just above the sylvian fissure, often involving the arcuate fasciculus, insula, or both.[35]

Transcortical motor aphasia produces poor speech output but good repetition and comprehension, resulting from injury to the supplementary motor area, near Broca's area or the basal ganglia. *Transcortical sensory aphasia* consists of fluent, often meaningless speech with good repetition but poor comprehension. Temporo-occipital and basal ganglia lesions are usually responsible. In *anomic aphasia*, occurring during recovery from other aphasias and in metabolic disorders, comprehension and repetition remain intact. It lacks localizing value, since it may result not only from lesions in the angular gyrus or adjacent lower temporal lobe but also from frontal and subcortical lesions.

Pure aphasic syndromes may help pinpoint the lesion (Fig. 46). However, mixed aphasias outnumber pure types, and the characteristics of a patient's aphasia may change with time.[34,36]

Apraxia is a disturbance of purposeful movement in the absence of paralysis or a comprehension deficit.[37] Patients are unable to act on command but can act automatically, so they will not wave when asked but will wave when the examiner departs.[34]

Ideomotor apraxia is the inability to connect the idea of an act with the action. It commonly occurs with aphasia. The patient cannot protrude the tongue on command or on imitation but will later do so while licking

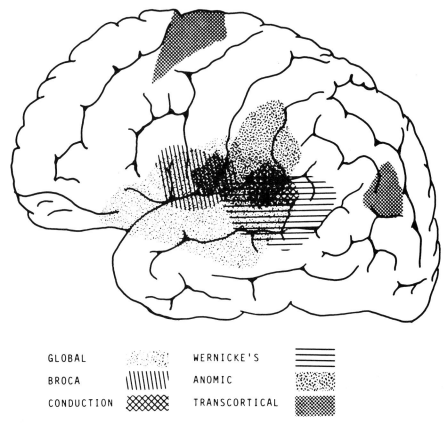

GLOBAL		WERNICKE'S	
BROCA		ANOMIC	
CONDUCTION		TRANSCORTICAL	

FIGURE 46. Usual sites of lesions producing the different aphasias. (From Kertesz,[34] with permission.)

the lips. Ideational apraxia usually involves difficulty in carrying out complex, sequenced commands, such as pretending to butter toast. Unlike the patient with ideomotor apraxia, this patient cannot perform these actions even when served toast. Dressing apraxia probably represents not an apraxia but a disorder of visuospatial orientation.[38] Buccofacial or oral apraxia may occur independently from limb apraxia and is seen most often with anterior insular lesions. Other apraxias follow left frontal or parietal lesions, disconnecting lesions of the corpus callosum, and the superior longitudinal fasciculus.[39]

Gerstmann's syndrome is characterized by impairment in the handling of symbols (agraphia and dyscalculia) and by somesthetic deficits (right-left disorientation and finger agnosia), sometimes with coexisting hemianopia or quadrantanopia and a hemisensory defect. The syndrome seldom occurs alone, most often accompanying anomic aphasia. It is seen in lesions of the left parietal lobe, sometimes limited to the angular gyrus.

Right-Hemisphere Syndromes

ACUTE STROKE

94

Predominantly frontal lesions cause motor inattention, cingulate-gyrus lesions cause motivational impairment, and parietal lesions cause visuospatial difficulties. Lesions of the right hemisphere tend to cause hemineglect syndromes such as left-sided sensory and motor neglect, and

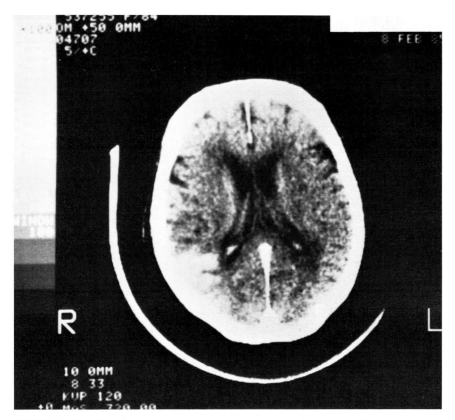

FIGURE 47. This 69-year-old previously well woman, vacationing alone in Florida, was found wandering around the pool in a dazed and confused state. Neurologic examination 5 days later showed only a left visual and sensory inattention. There were no motor signs. Her agitated and confused state resolved in a week. CT scan showed a superficial right-sided cortical infarct.

anosognosia (denial of illness).[34] Right parietal lesions also cause unilateral neglect in drawing and constructional apraxia.[31] Right middle cerebral artery infarction may cause acute confusion,[40] probably due to injury to the association cortex (Fig. 47).

The emotional components of speech (for example, prosody and emotional gesturing) are controlled from the right hemisphere. Damage to areas in the right hemisphere that are homologous to left hemispheric speech centers produce motor, sensory, global, transcortical, and other "aprosodias."[41] Inappropriate jocularity suggests right-sided frontal lesions, and undue emotionality (usually bursts of crying), bilateral lesions.

Memory Impairment

Left hippocampal lesions cause temporary amnesia, while bilateral hippocampal damage causes persistent "amnestic stroke."[42]

Approach to the Unconscious Patient

Patients with hemispheric infarcts are initially alert even with large lesions but, as ischemic edema evolves over several days, they become drowsy or stuporous, or comatose. Brainstem lesions produce rapid unconsciousness, since the reticular activating system is vulnerable throughout its length. Infarcts or hemorrhages in the cerebellum act like brainstem lesions due to direct compression of the brainstem or by acute hydrocephalus. Cerebral hemorrhage more commonly impairs consciousness than cerebral infarction since it is more likely to produce hydrocephalus or rapid distortion of brain parenchyma. Impairment of consciousness in excess of the neurologic deficit suggests subarachnoid hemorrhage, meningoencephalitis, or a metabolic encephalopathy.

Hemispheric Lesions

The infarcted swollen hemisphere acts like a deep midline mass, pushing the diencephalon through the tentorial notch, first compressing the midbrain and then the pons and medulla (rostral caudal deterioration).[43] At the diencephalic stage, pupils are small (1 to 3 mm) and react to light (central Horner's syndrome). There may be bilateral corticospinal signs, decorticate posturing, paratonic rigidity, grasp reflexes, and periodic breathing.[44] The coma is still reversible, but patients succumbing to later stages die.[45] Midpoint fixed pupils herald pontine compression and cardiac and respiration irregularities indicate medullary involvement and pending death.

With more lateral downward herniation, the swollen hemisphere pushes the ipsilateral temporal uncus over the edge of the tentorial incisura, compressing the third nerve, midbrain, and posterior cerebal artery.[46] The ipsilateral pupil initially is dilated and reacts sluggishly, if at all, to light, progressing to a full third nerve palsy. Contralateral decerebrate posturing becomes bilateral as herniation compresses the contralateral peduncle against the tentorial edge. Further deterioration occurs as in the more common central herniation syndrome.[45,47]

Brainstem Lesions

Midbrain lesions produce coma and dilated, irregular, and unresponsive pupils. Pontine lesions cause small reactive pupils, impaired lateral reflex eye movements,[48] and often hemiplegia or quadriplegia. Interruption of the median longitudinal fasciculus may cause dysconjugate eye movements. A "locked-in" syndrome results from a lesion of the ventral pons or midbrain.[43] These patients are conscious, quadriplegic, and capable only of voluntary vertical eye movements and eye closing. Rhythmic vertical eye movements used by patients to signal alertness may be mistaken for the ocular bobbing of pontine coma. Continuous EEG recordings may not show sleep patterns for days, implying patients' loss not only of the ability to move and communicate but also to rest and sleep.[49]

Cerebellar Lesions

A cerebellar mass may compress the pons and midbrain directly against the clivus, causing hydrocephalus. Severe compression and distortion may produce a brainstem infarct or hemorrhage.

Downward protrusion of the cerebellar tonsils compresses the medulla oblongata and seals off the inferior outlet of the posterior fossa, producing hydrocephalus and medullary impaction, and often results in sudden apnea and circulatory collapse.[44] Upward transtentorial herniation occurs when drainage of the lateral ventricles creates a pressure gradient and pushes an infarcted or hemorrhagic mass through the incisura. Herniation of the vermis may compress the vein of Galen against the splenium and the free edge of the falx, producing hemorrhagic infarction of the diencephalon and surrounding white matter.[50]

INTERPRETATION

A practical approach consists of interpreting the most unequivocal "hard" parts of the history and examination first, remembering that common things occur commonly, and rare causes of stroke are best diagnosed by exclusion. The less-definite aspects can buttress or qualify a working diagnosis, whereas their overemphasis may mislead into a diagnostic quagmire. Laboratory investigations should only be ordered when a clinical diagnosis with a list of differential options has been decided.

Etiologic information is derived from the location and history. Location suggests etiology and investigations must complement the clinical evaluation (Fig. 48). The history provides information about the type and cause of the lesion, an abrupt onset typifying a vascular etiology and impairment of consciousness being commoner with cerebral hemorrhage than infarction. Rapidly increasing intracranial pressure from intracerebral hemorrhage or acute hydrocephalus due to subarachnoid bleeding may produce rapid deterioration. Headache, vomiting, papilledema, and coma soon supervene. Neck stiffness and other meningitic signs due to cervical subarachnoid irritation by fresh blood commonly occur.

Although this dramatic picture is distinctive in patients with serious intracerebral hematomas, less serious lesions are commonly missed. Autopsy series give undue weight to hemorrhagic stroke, which is more commonly fatal than is ischemic stroke. The introduction of CT scanning redressed the imbalance between the underestimate of hemorrhagic stroke by clinicians and its overestimate by pathologists.

Cerebral infarcts should be characterized further as thromboembolic or hemodynamic. Hemodynamic infarctions are uncommon, usually resulting from profound hypotension or hypotension in the presence of multiple occlusions or stenoses of cervical arteries. These infarcts tend to occur in watershed areas, where the end-territories of cerebral arteries converge.

DIFFERENTIAL DIAGNOSIS

Thirteen percent of 821 consecutive patients admitted to the Toronto Unit were misdiagnosed (Table 21).[3] Unwitnessed or unrecognized *seizures* were the commonest mimic (39 percent). Twenty-three patients were admitted with postictal confusion, stupor, or coma; and 19 with focal neurologic deficits, including hemiparesis, monoparesis, gaze palsies, or hemisensory deficits. Thirteen patients had had a previous stroke,

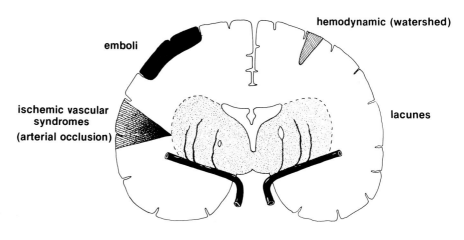

ISCHEMIC

hemodynamic (watershed)

emboli

ischemic vascular
syndromes
(arterial occlusion)

lacunes

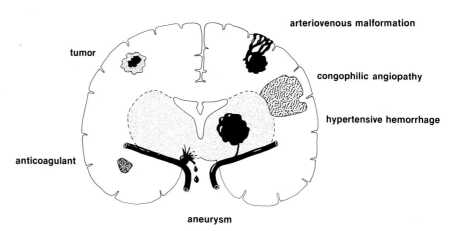

HEMORRHAGE

arteriovenous malformation

tumor

congophilic angiopathy

hypertensive hemorrhage

anticoagulant

aneurysm

FIGURE 48. Typical locations of cerebral infarction *(top)* and hemorrhage *(bottom).*

posing the problem of distinguishing a first seizure from a second stroke. Seizures were generalized or focal. When focal, they did not always manifest with shaking, the perceived hallmark of epilepsy, and were missed. Persistent neurologic deficits occurred not only with motor seizures (Todd's paralysis) but also with seizures that aggravated visual and sensory symptoms, sometimes for days.

Confusion and *impaired consciousness* comprised the second largest group of misdiagnoses, including acute confusion, syncope, drug, or alcohol intoxication and metabolic encephalopathy. Although cerebral infarction may cause confusion,[40] the confusion more often lies with the physician than with the patient. *Coma* due to nonvascular causes may simulate stroke and is overdiagnosed as such,[51] but systematic examination easily establishes whether the cause of the coma is structural.[43]

Cerebral tumor was rarely mistaken for stroke in the Toronto Unit (1 percent). All patients had progressive hemiparesis for weeks or months, and five had papilledema, which is not seen in cerebral infarc-

TABLE 21. Presenting Clinical Picture in 108 Patients Misdiagnosed as Having "Stroke"

Major Presenting Symptom	Seizure Group	Nonseizure Group	Total
Focal neurologic deficit	19	16	35
Acute confusional state	8	18	26
Stupor or coma	15	5	20
Vertigo or syncope	0	19	19
Other	0	8	8
Total	42	66	108

From Norris and Hachinski,[3] with permission.

tion. *Subdural hematoma* was found in three patients presenting with confusion and minimal neurologic signs. Only one had a preceding and uncertain history of trauma.

Miscellaneous diagnoses included vertigo, encephalitis, acute cardiac failure, multiple sclerosis, and psychogenic deficits. Migraine, brain abscesses, cysticercosis, acute meningitis, and hypoglycemia may occasionally also mimic stroke. Although mass lesions of the brain comprise the classic differential diagnosis of stroke, CT scanning easily identifies these, leaving to the physician the purely clinical differential diagnoses of seizures, confusion, and TIA. While technologic advances simplify some diagnoses, they leave a residue of difficult ones to the clinician, confirming the need for better tests as well as better physicians.

CONCLUSION

History and examination remain the standard of the diagnosis of stroke, guiding rational selection and interpretation of laboratory and radiologic investigation. The examination localizes the lesion, the history implies its etiology, and investigations confirm both. A precise diagnosis precedes treatment and helps prognosis.

Brief but close attention to speech, posture, movement, and a few simple maneuvers yields the essentials of the neurologic examination. Undue reassurance can be derived from a lack of arterial bruits and overt cardiac abnormalities, since most arterial disease is silent and cardiac disease is often unapparent.

The differential diagnosis must distinguish between a suddenly discovered deficit and a neurologic deficit of sudden onset, characteristic of all vascular syndromes. Disturbed anatomy can now be imaged but functional disorders can only be identified clinically. No more cost-effective method of diagnosis has yet been found than the knowledgeable physician.

REFERENCES

1. CORWIN, LI, ET AL: *Accuracy of death certification of stroke: The Framingham study.* Stroke 13:125, 1982.
2. HATANO, S: *Experience from a multicentre stroke register: A preliminary report.* Bull WHO 54:541, 1976.
3. NORRIS, JW, AND HACHINSKI, VC: *Misdiagnosis of stroke.* Lancet 1:328, 1982.
4. PESSIN, MS, ET AL: *Mechanisms of acute carotid stroke.* Ann Neurol 6:245, 1979.

5. MOHR, JP, ET AL: *The Harvard Cooperative Stroke Registry: A prospective registry.* Neurology 28:754, 1978.

7. ALTER, M, ET AL: *Cerebral infarction, clinical and angiographic correlations.* Neurology 22:590, 1972.

8. FISHER, CM: *Headache in cerebrovascular disease.* In VINKEN, PJ, AND BRUYN, GW (EDS): *Handbook of Clinical Neurology, Vol 5: Headaches and Cranial Neuralgias.* North-Holland, Amsterdam, 1968, p 124.

9. BLACK, SE, HACHINSKI, VC, AND NORRIS, JW: *Seizures after stroke* (abstr). Can J Neurol Sci 9:291, 1982.

10. ARNALDEZ, R: *Ibn Ridwan.* In GILLISPIE, CC (ED): *Dictionary of Scientific Bibliography,* Vol 11. Charles Scribner's Sons, New York, 1975, p 444.

11. BLOCK, JE: *Letter to the Editor: Thumbs down on left-handedness.* N Engl J Med 291:307, 1974.

12. KISSEBAH, AH, ET AL: *Relation of body fat distribution to metabolic complications of obesity.* J Clin Endocrinol Metab 54:254, 1981.

13. BROWN, OR, ET AL: *Aortic root dilatation and mitral valve prolapse in Marfan's syndrome: An echocardiographic study.* Circulation 52:651, 1975.

14. ROSENMAN, RH, ET AL: *Relation of corneal arcus to cardiovascular risk factors and the incidence of coronary disease.* N Engl J Med 291:1322, 1974.

15. CHAMBERS, BR: *Stroke risk determinants in patients with asymptomatic neck bruits.* M.D. thesis, University of Melbourne, 1984.

16. CHAMBERS, BR, AND NORRIS, JW: *Clinical significance of asymptomatic neck bruits.* Neurology (in press).

17. FISHER, CM: *Occlusion of the carotid arteries—further experiences.* Arch Neurol Psychiatry 72:187, 1954.

18. BEEVOR, C: *The cerebral arterial supply.* Brain 30:403, 1907.

19. LAZORTHES, G, GOUAZE, A, AND SALAMON, G: *Vascularisation et circulation de l'encéphale,* vol 1. Masson, Paris, 1976.

20. SALAMON, G: *Atlas de la vascularisation arterielle du cerveau chez l'homme,* ed 2. Sandoz Editions, Paris, 1973.

21. MCGLONE, J: *Sex differences in human brain asymmetry: A critical survey.* Behav Brain Sci Res 3:215, 1980.

22. ALTER, M: *The digiti quinti sign of mild hemiparesis.* Neurology 23:503, 1973.

23. FISHER, CM: *Lacunar strokes and infarctions: A review.* Neurology 32:871, 1982.

24. FISHER, CM: *Pure sensory stroke and allied conditions.* Stroke 13:434, 1982.

25. FISHER, CM: *Some neuro-ophthalmological observations.* J Neurol Neurosurg Psychiatry 30:383, 1967.

26. LUXON, LM, AND HARRISON, MJG: *Chronic subdural hematoma.* QJ Med 48:43, 1979.

27. LANCE, JW, AND MCLEOD, JG: *A Physiological Approach to Clinical Neurology,* ed 2. Butterworth's, London, 1975.

28. ROSS, RT, AND JOHNSTON, JA: *Corneal reflex in hemisphere disease II.* Can J Neurol Sci 1:196, 1974.

29. BRODAL, A: *Self-observations and neuro-anatomical considerations after a stroke.* Brain 96:675, 1973.

30. MESULAM, M-M: *A cortical network for directed attention and unilateral neglect.* Ann Neurol 10:309, 1981.

31. HIER, DB, MONDLOCK, J, AND CAPLAN, LR: *Behavioral abnormalities after right hemisphere stroke.* Neurology 33:337, 1983.

32. GESCHWIND, N: *Aphasia.* N Engl J Med 285:654, 1971.

33. MOHR, JP: *The evaluation of aphasia.* Stroke 13:399, 1982.

34. KERTESZ, A: *Aphasia and Associated Disorders.* Grune & Stratton, New York, 1979, pp 161, 181.

35. BENSON, DF, ET AL: *Conduction aphasia.* Arch Neurol 28:339, 1973.

36. BRUST, JCM, AND RICHTER, RW: *Stroke associated with addiction to heroin.* J Neurol Neurosurg Psychiatry 39:194, 1976.

37. LIEPMANN, H: *Das Krankheitsbild der Apraxie.* Monatsschr Psychiatr Neurol 17:289, 1905.

38. BRAIN, LORD: *Speech Disorders: Aphasia, Apraxia and Agnosia,* ed 2. Butterworth & Co, 1965.

39. HEILMAN, KM, ROTHI, LJ, AND VALENSTEIN, E: *Two forms of ideomotor apraxia.* Neurology 32:342, 1982.

40. SCHMIDLEY, JW, AND MESSING, RO: *Agitated confusional states in patients with right hemisphere infarctions.* Stroke 15:883, 1984.

41. ROSS, ED: *The aprosodias, functional-anatomic organization of the affective components of language in the right hemisphere.* Arch Neurol 38:561, 1981.

42. BENSON, DF, MARSDEN, CD, AND MEADOWS, JC: *The amnesic syndrome of posterior cerebral artery occlusion.* Acta Neurol Scand 50:133, 1974.

43. PLUM, F, AND POSNER, JB: *Approach to the unconscious patient.* In *The Diagnosis of Stupor and Coma,* ed 3. FA Davis, Philadelphia, 1980, p 345.

44. CARONNA, JJ: *Coma in ischemic cerebral vascular disease.* In ROSS RUSSELL, RW (ED): *Vascular Disease of the Central Nervous System,* ed 2. Churchill-Livingstone, Edinburgh, 1983, p 139.

45. PLUM, F: *Brain swelling and edema in cerebral vascular disease.* In *Cerebrovascular Disease.* (Proc Assoc Res Nerv Ment Dis 41.) Williams & Wilkins, Baltimore, 1966, p 318.

46. JEFFERSON, G: *The tentorial pressure cone.* Arch Neurol Psychiatry 40:857, 1938.

47. NG, LKY, AND NIMMANNITYA, J: *Massive cerebral infarction with severe brain swelling.* Stroke 1:158, 1970.

48. KUBIK, CS, AND ADAMS, RD: *Occlusion of the basilar artery—A clinical and pathologic study.* Brain 69:73, 1946.

49. MARKAND, ON, AND DYKEN, ML: *Sleep abnormalities in patients with brain stem lesions.* Neurology 26:769, 1976.

50. CUNEO, RA, ET AL: *Upward transtentorial herniation—7 cases and a literature review.* Arch Neurol 36:618, 1979.

51. WHISNANT, JP: *The decline of stroke.* Stroke 15:160, 1984.

Chapter 7

VASCULAR SYNDROMES

As the types of the Palsy are manyfold, and its causes divers . . .
Thomas Willis

The accurate localization of a cerebral lesion, the definition of its pathology, and the inability to alter its course have long been the hallmark of neurology. A profusion of stroke syndromes allowed the neurologist to dazzle colleagues with eponyms, without affecting the fate of the patient. This lack of practical application, and the infinite variation of vascular syndromes arising from the vagaries of vascular supply, led to attempts to find ways of classifying acute cerebrovascular disease that are based on advancing diagnostic and therapeutic technology.

Advances in diagnosis and treatment have also cast doubt upon the usefulness of these syndromes. The temporal description of vascular lesions such as TIAs proves more valuable in management than their eponyms. CT can localize and characterize lesions in the carotid territory with greater accuracy than the best clinician, although its visualization of the brainstem and cerebellum remains poor. Cerebral angiography demonstrates that the same syndrome may follow occlusion of different vessels. Vascular syndromes are usually considered from the perspective of ischemic stroke, but CT scanning has taught us that small hemorrhages in any cerebral location are indistinguishable from infarction (Table 22). It is more important to know whether a causal carotid lesion is surgically accessible than to know the exact site of the hemispheric infarction. Diagnosing a cardiac embolic source is more important than deciding the site of the infarct, since diagnosis determines treatment.

TABLE 22. Classification of Vascular Syndromes

Ischemic stroke	Thrombosis
Carotid stroke	Subclavian steal
Internal carotid artery occlusion	Vertebral occlusion
Middle cerebral artery syndromes	Cerebellar infarction
Anterior cerebral artery syndromes	Basilar occlusion
Ocular stroke	"Locked-in" syndrome
Ophthalmic artery occlusion	Lacunar stroke
Central retinal artery occlusion	Hemorrhagic stroke
Retinal artery branch occlusion	Supratentorial
Vertebrobasilar stroke	Centrencephalic
Brainstem centrencephalic stroke	Lobar
Vertebrobasilar embolism	Infratentorial
"Top of the basilar" syndrome	Cerebellar hemorrhage
Posterior cerebral artery occlusion	Pontine hemorrhage
Thalamic stroke	

The differing pathogenesis in vertebrobasilar and carotid stroke is a major factor in outcome. For instance, benign lesions of the penetrating arterioles are commoner in the brainstem, and emboli produce differing effects in the vertebrobasilar and carotid circulation owing to the different vascular anatomy.

ISCHEMIC STROKE

Carotid Stroke

The commonest type of carotid ischemic stroke is wedge-shaped, the base involving the cortex and the apex extending down to the basal ganglia (Fig. 49). This results from occlusion of the middle cerebral artery extending or embolizing from the ipsilateral carotid artery. In situ thrombosis of the middle cerebral artery is rare, and the term "cerebral thrombosis" is inappropriate.[1]

In cerebral embolism, the thrombus fragments to involve smaller arterial branches, limiting the lesion to cortical areas. The initially severe hemiplegia rapidly resolves, leaving residual cortical signs such as aphasia, often with only a minor degree of hemiparesis. This rapid resolution depends on healthy collaterals in the otherwise normal cerebral vascular tree. Cerebral angiography, unless performed within the first few days, is normal.[2]

Internal Carotid Artery Occlusion

Occlusion of the internal carotid artery may be asymptomatic or produce massive infarction in the middle and anterior cerebral arterial territories (Fig. 50). Between these extremes, a spectrum of clinical syndromes is produced from a mixture of middle and anterior cerebral arterial lesions. The closer the lesion to the circle of Willis, the less the chance of collateral circulation and the larger the infarction.

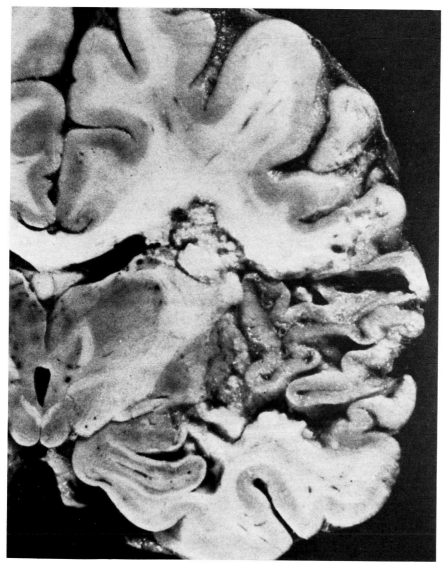

FIGURE 49. Coronal section of brain showing large, wedge-shaped infarct with the apex extending into the internal capsule. (From Fisher, CM: *The anatomy and pathology of the cerebral vasculature.* In Meyer, JS (ed): *Modern Concepts of Cerebrovascular Disease.* Spectrum Publications, New York, 1975, p 1.)

The clinical effects of internal carotid artery stenosis are indistinguishable from occlusion, though neurologic deficits are more severe with occlusion.[3] The final clinical picture depends upon the richness of collaterals, the speed of occlusion, and the individual vascular anatomy.

The *carotid stump syndrome* occurs rarely when an occluded internal carotid artery produces further TIAs or stroke through extension or detachment of a thrombus or embolization through the external carotid artery collateral.[4] Patients with *bilateral internal carotid occlusion* may be asymptomatic but, when symptomatic, often feature dementia and seizures in addition to focal neurologic signs.[5]

VASCULAR
SYNDROMES

105

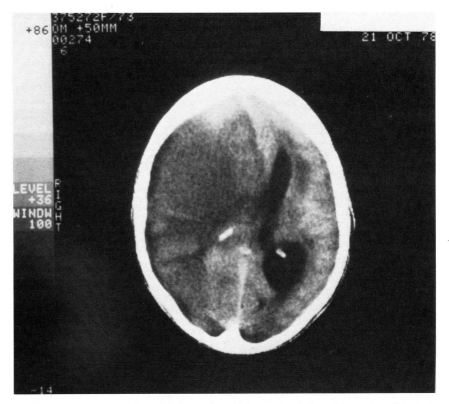

FIGURE 50. CT scan of patient with internal carotid artery occlusion with sparing of posterior cerebral artery territory. Note massive midline shift due to combined middle cerebral artery and anterior cerebral artery territory infarction.

Middle Cerebral Artery Territory Syndromes

Middle cerebral artery territory occlusion rapidly causes drowsiness, hemiplegia of the face, arm and leg, hemisensory loss, homonymous hemianopia, and deviation of the eyes away from the hemiplegic side. Since the arm is always more affected than the leg and weakness is mainly distal, the patient usually retains some proximal leg power, even in dense hemiplegia. The patient with less severe stroke soon regains a functioning though limping "hemiplegic gait," using proximal leg power to swing the weaker distal limb circumductively. If the lenticulostriate arteries are not involved, the resulting infarct is mainly cortical, with relative sparing of the leg and visual pathways. Left-hemisphere infarction also produces various aphasias. Right-hemisphere infarction commonly produces unilateral neglect with anosognosia (unawareness of the hemiplegia); visual, sensory, and auditory inattention; and spatial disorientation.

Less devastating lesions and disabilities are produced by branch occlusions by embolic fragments. For instance, there may be paralysis of the arm and face with Broca's aphasia, or an isolated Wernicke's aphasia with no other neurologic signs. The anterior branches of the middle cerebral artery produce more consistent clinical syndromes than the posterior branches[6] (Fig. 51).

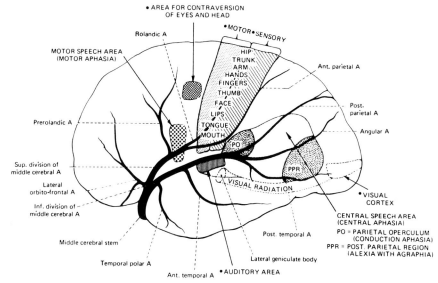

FIGURE 51. Lateral view of the cerebral hemisphere, showing the middle cerebral artery distribution with its corresponding areas of functional localization. (From Petersdorf, RG, et al,[56] with permission.)

Anterior Cerebral Artery Territory Syndromes

Occlusion of the anterior cerebral artery produces hemiparesis, minimal in the face and maximal in the leg, with loss of sensation in the leg. When occlusion of the common stem of both arteries causes bilateral frontal infarction, the patient is indifferent to his urinary incontinence and may have memory impairment[7] (Fig. 52).

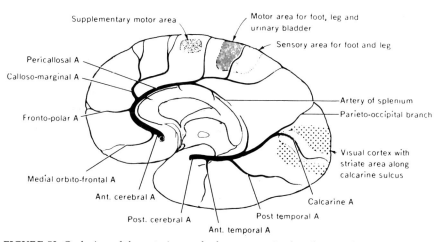

FIGURE 52. Occlusion of the anterior cerebral artery proximal to the anterior communicating artery is usually asymptomatic but, if distal, causes loss of power and sensation in the contralateral leg. Partial weakness of the arm may also occur. The classical anterior cerebral artery triad of leg weakness, urinary incontinence, and mental changes only occurs with bilateral anterior cerebral artery ischemia due to occlusion of a common proximal trunk. (From Petersdorf, RG, et al,[56] with permission.)

Ocular Stroke

Ophthalmic artery occlusion rarely leads to blindness because of its profuse collaterals, but occlusion of the central retinal artery or its branches results in retinal infarction. Retinal artery branch occlusions are usually due to microemboli, which may be white, suggesting a cardiac source, or birefringent, suggesting cholesterol from the carotid artery or the aortic arch (Hollenhorst plaque) or rarely platelet emboli. These emboli may be silent or produce amaurosis fugax or retinal infarction. In situ thrombosis seldom occurs, and embolism remains the leading cause.

Amaurosis fugax and retinal infarction rank among the commonest forms of "threatened stroke." They may produce little or no disability but indicate probable ulceration or stenosis of the internal carotid artery. Too often they are dismissed as insignificant by both patients and physicians. The next embolic episode may be massive cerebral embolism, and all patients with these symptoms should have cerebral angiography, unless contraindicated because of age or systemic illness.

Vertebrobasilar Stroke

A profusion of eponymous brainstem vascular syndromes has taxed the memories of medical students for years, without adding to management. Caplan[8-13] has suggested a management-oriented reclassification based on pathogenesis and on data from cerebral angiography and CT scanning.

Although there are as many varieties of vertebrobasilar stroke as carotid stroke, it is still investigated as a single entity, since it is less easily visualized by angiography and CT scanning and is less amenable to surgery. The pathogenesis may be qualitatively different[8] than in the carotid system, since emboli behave differently and hemodynamic strokes are probably commoner.[14,15]

The pattern of parenchymal damage in stroke reflects the organization of the vertebrobasilar vasculature (Fig. 53). Segmental arteries emerging at right angles from the basilar trunk perforate the pons directly, while larger circumferential vessels wind around the brainstem to supply more distal areas such as the cerebellum. Hypertension affects mainly the small pontine perforators, causing small or lacunar infarcts in the pontine centrencephalon. Emboli traverse the vertebral arteries, pass into the basilar trunk, and only impact at its bifurcation. Thromboemboli arising from ulcerated plaques are rarer than in the carotid territory and may plug medium-sized vessels such as the vertebral artery, or produce in situ thrombosis as in the main basilar trunk.

Brainstem "Centrencephalic" Stroke

Occlusion of a basilar branch or perforating arteriole produces a limited medial or lateral pontine infarct (Fig. 54), or a deeper lacuna. The primary arterial lesion is hypertensive arteriolar necrosis or lipohyalinosis.[16] These are relatively common lesions, since 20 percent of ischemic strokes in the Harvard Stroke Registry were lacunar.[17]

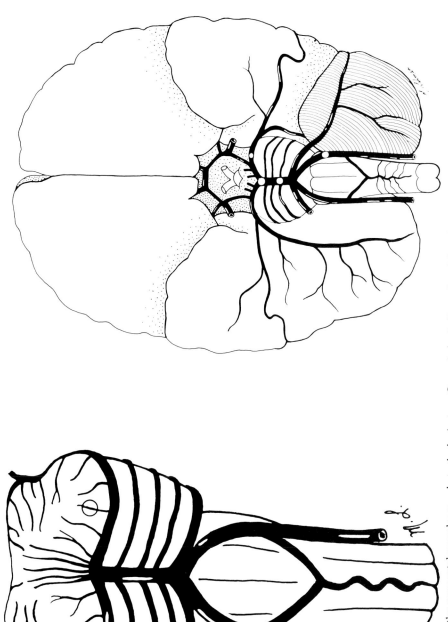

FIGURE 53. Illustration of the segmental vascular supply to the brainstem. Open circles indicate site of thromboembolism in the vertebrobasilar system.

VASCULAR
SYNDROMES

109

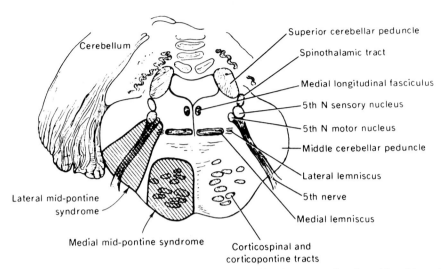

FIGURE 54. Medial midpontine infarction (occlusion of basilar paramedian branch) and lateral midpontine syndrome (occlusion of short circumferential). (From Petersdorf, RG, et al,[56] with permission).

The clinical manifestations are usually benign, reflecting the limited size of the lesion. Headache is absent, since no significant collateral flow occurs. Occlusion of the thalamogeniculate perforators at the basilar bifurcation causes paresthesias of the contralateral limbs, with hemichorea or hemiataxia of ipsilateral limbs. A variety of lacunar syndromes has been described, including pure motor and pure sensory stroke, sensorimotor stroke, dysarthria/clumsy-hand syndrome, homolateral ataxia with crural paresis, and others.[18-20] These strokes occur mainly in elderly or hypertensive patients. They are minor and self-limiting, and anticoagulants are useless and dangerous.

Vertebrobasilar Embolism

Emboli pass through the vertebral artery into the basilar artery, and only impact at the narrower, rostral end where it bifurcates. Hence, vertebrobasilar emboli produce either rostral brainstem damage ("top-of-the-basilar" syndrome) or, if they fragment and pass distally, infarct the medial temporal lobe or occipital pole (Fig. 55).

"Top-of-the-basilar" syndrome[10,13] consists of:

1. Disordered vertical gaze or skew deviation of the eyes
2. "Pseudo–sixth" nerve palsy (impaired ocular abduction without sixth nerve damage)
3. Large, unreactive (sometimes tiny) pupils
4. Behavior changes due to a rostral brainstem lesion, amnestic features of temporal lobe ischemia, and cortical blindness
5. Absence of hemiplegia due to sparing of long tracts

Posterior cerebral artery occlusion occurs when the embolus fragments and is carried distally, with the sudden onset of homonymous hemianopia, without other clinical signs. Visual neglect, as in hemiano-

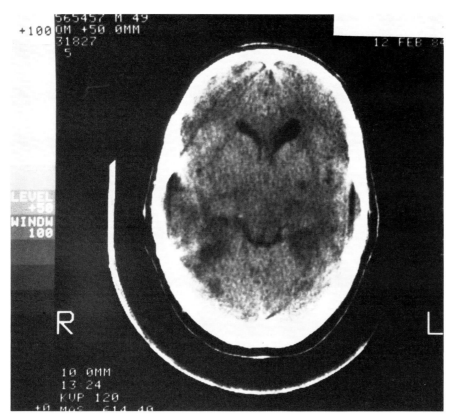

FIGURE 55. This 52-year-old man suddenly collapsed unconscious at home. No seizure movements were seen. On arrival in the hospital several hours later, he was fully awake and oriented but had no memory of the incident and little of the preceding days. He was cheerfully unaware of his total blindness, claiming that objects were too far away to be seen or "things seem a little hazy." The optic fundi were normal but both pupils were dilated and fixed. There was a left third nerve palsy and bilateral brisk hyperreflexia with bilateral Babinski signs.

Three months earlier, he had had a severe myocardial infarction. ECG on this admission suggested a cardiac aneurysm, which was confirmed by x-ray screening. The admission CT scan was normal, but CT on day 3 showed extensive infarction of both medial temporal lobes and both occipital lobes. The cerebral angiogram showed occlusion of the distal branch of the left PCA, compatible with embolism.

During the next 2 weeks, the third nerve palsy and cortical blindness partly resolved, leaving a patchy right homonymous hemianopia and extremely impaired vision in the left homonymous fields. Anticoagulant therapy was given on the assumption that a cardiogenic embolus had impacted at the basilar bifurcation, causing brainstem ischemia and temporo-occipital infarction.

pia from middle cerebral artery occlusion, is absent. The patient may see multiples of the same object on the hemianopic side (visual perseveration)[10] (Fig. 56). Left occipital infarction may also cause anomic aphasia, alexia without agraphia, visual agnosia, or an amnestic syndrome. Right occipital infarction may be associated with the absence of visual dreaming and prosopagnosia (inability to recognize faces).[21] If the embolus divides into two, the resulting bilateral posterior cerebral artery infarction produces cortical blindness and, sometimes, an amnestic state due to bilateral temporal lobe ischemia.[22]

More proximal posterior cerebral artery occlusion may infarct the posteroventral thalamic nuclei, producing hemianesthesia without other

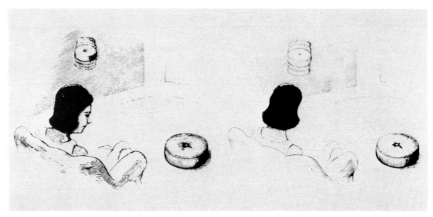

FIGURE 56. *Left,* The cushion viewed in the right homonymous visual field suddenly appears in the left (defective) homonymous fields as well, resulting in diplopia as long as the actual object remains in view. *Right,* Illusory image is palinoptic, persisting 15 minutes after the patient has turned her head to the left and the real cushion is no longer in view. The illusory image is smaller than the real one and appears to be oscillating; otherwise it is an exact replica of the original. (From Jacobs, L: *Visual allesthesia.* Neurology 30:1059, 1980, with permission.)

deficits (*"thalamic stroke"*). The sensory loss may fade, to be replaced after some months by a continuous unpleasant hemibody sensation, "thalamic pain." This may occur after lacunar infarction ("sensory stroke") of the thalamus. If the adjacent midbrain is also involved, there may be superimposed ocular signs such as skew-deviation or forced downward conjugate gaze.

Thrombosis in the Vertebrobasilar System

The more proximal the arterial occlusion, the less the clinical effect. Proximal vertebral artery occlusion may be found by chance during angiography, most lesions being asymptomatic, probably due to rich collateral supply from the thyrocervical trunk.[23] Suboccipital vertebral artery lesions result mainly from trauma such as chiropractic manipulation, sometimes infarcting the lower brainstem and cerebellum.[24,25] Bilateral distal vertebral occlusion is rare, usually fatal, and functionally equivalent to proximal basilar occlusion.[12]

Occlusion or stenosis of the subclavian artery proximal to the vertebral artery origin causes "subclavian steal." Brainstem TIAs result from diversion of blood from the vertebrobasilar system into the subclavian artery during arm exercise but subclavian steal rarely causes infarction.[8]

Unilateral vertebral artery occlusion may produce medial or lateral medullary infarction (Wallenberg's syndrome) (Fig. 57).[26]

Cerebellar infarction produces a clinical picture indistinguishable from cerebellar hemorrhage. Ischemic edema balloons the cerebellar hemisphere and may fatally compress the adjacent brainstem or kink the aqueduct to produce severe acute hydrocephalus.[27,28] There is sudden vascular headache from dilated collateral flow, vertigo, vomiting, and cerebellar ataxia. The eyes show skew-deviation and occasional sixth

ACUTE STROKE

112

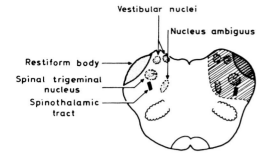

Vestibular nuclei

Nucleus ambiguus

Restiform body

Spinal trigeminal
nucleus

Spinothalamic
tract

LATERAL MEDULLARY SYNDROME

1. Loss of pain and temperature
   sensations over the ipsilateral
   face and contralateral half of
   the body
2. Ataxia (loss of coordination)
3. Vertigo
4. Loss of gag reflex, difficulty in
   swallowing and difficulty in
   articulation
5. Ipsilateral Horner's syndrome
6. Vomiting

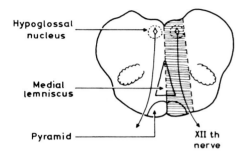

Hypoglossal
nucleus

Medial
lemniscus

Pyramid

XII th
nerve

MEDIAL MEDULLARY SYNDROME

1. Paralysis of homolateral half
   of tongue
2. Contralateral paralysis
3. Contralateral loss of
   kinesthesia and discriminative
   touch

FIGURE 57. Lateral *(top)* and medial *(bottom)* medullary syndromes. (From Afifi, AK, and Berg-man, RA: *Basic Neurosience.* Urban & Schwarzenberg, Baltimore, 1980, pp 133–134, with permission.)

nerve palsy and the pupils are pinpoint but reactive due to sympathetic outflow compression with intact midbrain pupilloconstrictors. Motor signs are minimal since the pyramidal tracts are compressed rather than damaged, so decompression by ventricular drainage or removal of infarcted tissue leaves the patient with minimal sequelae.

Basilar artery occlusion is often fatal.[29] Three of Drake's five cases of basilar artery ligation for cerebral aneurysm ended in death or disaster.[30] Basilar occlusions probably start as in situ thrombosis of the proximal or mid-trunk, while distal occlusions are mainly due to emboli, though there are exceptions.[31] As the thrombus enlarges over several days, the patient's clinical state worsens.[13] Early signs are occipital headache, transient dizziness, and diplopia, followed by progressive hemi- or quadriparesis, bulbar paralysis, and impaired conjugate gaze. Anticoagulant therapy has been advocated at the first signs, though there is no convincing evidence of its effectiveness.[13] If the long circumferential cerebellar collaterals can bridge the gap between the distal and proximal basilar trunk, the patient may escape with only minor disability.[9]

The *"locked-in" syndrome*[32] is the most devastating form of basilar stroke where total quadriparesis, including the face, follows ventral pontine infarction, usually from basilar occlusion[33,34] (Fig. 58). The tegmentum is spared, so the patient stays alert and oriented, the only remaining movement being vertical gaze. Moving the eyes frantically up and down are the patient's only means of signaling distress and the comprehension of bedside discussions of the prognosis. Survival, though rare, usually leaves the patient severely crippled with brainstem impairment.[35]

VASCULAR
SYNDROMES

113

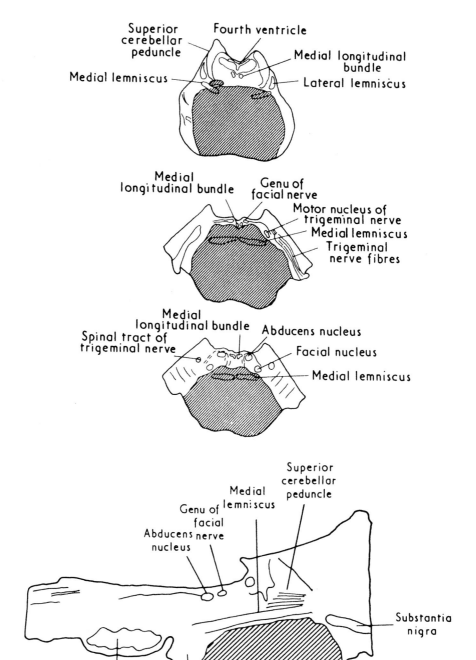

FIGURE 58. Distribution of lesions in a patient with ventral pontine infarction producing the "locked-in syndrome." (From Hawkes,[34] with permission.)

TABLE 23. Frequency of Lacunar Compared with Other Ischemic Strokes in the Toronto Unit, 1983

Site of Infarction	Lacunar	Other	Total
Hemispheric	17	145	162 (10%)
Vertebrobasilar	4	26	30 (13%)

Lacunar Stroke

Lacunae are tiny infarcts (rarely larger than 15 mm) located deeply within the brain, mainly in the basal ganglia, internal capsule, and pons. Although lacunae were first described in 1901,[36] their relevance to other stroke syndromes did not emerge until their clinical spectrum was delineated by Fisher.[37-42] They are relatively common, 10 to 20 percent in most stroke registries[17] (Table 23), although they may become less frequent with the decline of hypertension.[43] Since lacunae usually result from arteriolar lipohyalinosis, angiography is negative. Their clinical course is benign and self-limiting, and anticoagulants are not indicated. In "état lacunaire" the brain is riddled with lacunae, causing spastic ataxia, pseudobulbar palsy, and end-stage dementia.

Clinicopathologic correlation indicates at least four clearly defined syndromes (Table 24). Lacunar syndromes are distinct from other types of stroke since they are not associated with seizures, hemianopia, or cortical deficits such as aphasia. Other varieties have been described, such as sensorimotor stroke, hemichorea, hemiballismus, and other varieties of basilar branch occlusion,[19] but their place in the hierarchy of lacunar syndromes is uncertain since they often lack pathologic correlation.[20] Some lacunar syndromes initially attributed to specific locations are produced by lesions at various sites; for example, pure motor hemiplegia can result from an internal capsule lesion,[37] a pontine infarct,[19] or even medullary damage.[44] Additional features often help localize the lesion. Ataxic hemiparesis due to a supratentorial lesion often has sensory involvement, but when the brainstem is involved, nystagmus, dysarthria, and cranial nerve abnormalities also occur.[45]

Lacunae are sometimes found by chance on CT scans performed for other reasons. The CT appearance of a lacuna is deceptive. Part of the confusion results from misinterpretation of the CT scan. The early stages

TABLE 24. Lacunar Syndromes

	Symptoms	Location
Pure motor hemiparesis	Weakness of face, arm, leg	Internal capsule, basis pontis
Pure sensory stroke	Paresthesias of face, arm, leg	Thalamus
Motor-sensory stroke	Weakness and paresthesias of face, arm, leg	Internal capsule
Ataxic hemiparesis	Hemiparesis, ipsilateral ataxia	Internal capsule, basis pontis
Dysarthria, clumsy hand	Dysarthria, clumsy hand	Internal capsule, basis pontis

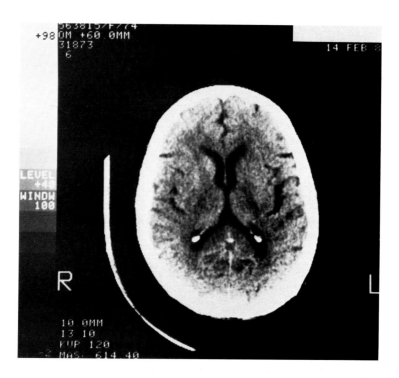

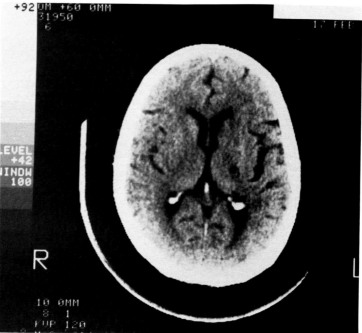

FIGURE 59. A 75-year-old housewife had several episodes of weakness of the right arm lasting a few minutes, 1 month prior to admission for carotid surgery. On awakening from the anesthetic following a left carotid endarterectomy, she was alert but had a mild right sensorimotor hemiparesis. On hospital discharge 3 weeks later, she had a residual limp and weakness of the right hand. Although the CT scan on admission was normal (top), a second CT scan 3 days after surgery (bottom) showed a "lacunar" infarction in the left internal capsule.

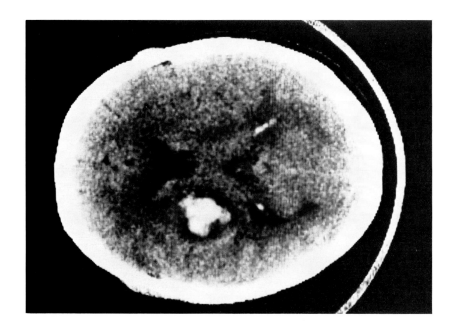

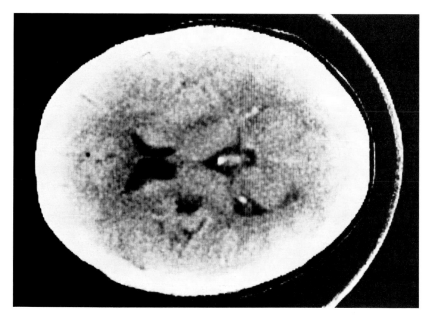

FIGURE 60. Traumatic intracerebral hemorrhage (*top*) that preceded "lacuna" (*below*) 6 months earlier.

of a large, wedge-shaped infarct may initially show only the tip of the wedge, simulating a lacuna. A "lacuna" may also appear after cerebral embolism (Fig. 59) or a small capsular hemorrhage[46] (Fig. 60). Lacunae may be missed if they are tiny or if the CT is performed too early to visualize the lesion.[47] Sequential CT scans over several months will demonstrate the lesions in 69 percent of cases.[48]

Since lacunae are small and deep, the EEG should be unaffected,[49] and this is our experience, although changes have been reported.[46]

HEMORRHAGIC STROKE

Superimposed on focal neurologic deficits are signs of raised intracranial pressure and evidence of meningeal irritation due to blood[26] (Table 25). Papilledema is rarely (if ever) seen in cerebral infarction but occasionally occurs within the first few days of cerebral hemorrhage from the tamponade effect of the hematoma, progressive cerebral edema, and acute hydrocephalus. Headache, vomiting, and rapid lapse into unconsciousness are often seen in cerebral hemorrhage, combined with neck stiffness and other meningitic signs, as blood tracks through the ventricular system into the spinal subarachnoid space.

Although this dramatic picture is distinctive of serious intracerebral hematomas, lesser lesions are commonly missed. Autopsy series give undue weight to hemorrhagic strokes, which are more commonly fatal than ischemic strokes. Only since the introduction of CT scanning has the imbalance been redressed between clinicians' underestimation and pathologists' overestimation of the frequency of hemorrhagic stroke.

Unfortunately, cerebral hemorrhage is commonly so catastrophic that distinguishing between hypertensive hemorrhage, ruptured berry aneurysm, or arteriovenous malformation is academic. In the Toronto Unit, 80 percent of patients died within the first week. Arteriovenous malformation may be suspected but not found, suggesting autodestruction, especially in hemorrhages at atypical locations. In milder hemorrhages, it is mandatory to search for underlying vascular lesions, anticoagulant complications, and systemic disorders such as blood dyscrasia.

Supratentorial Hemorrhage

Most intracerebral hemorrhages occur in the *vascular centrencephalon* (Table 26) in the region of the putamen and thalamus.[50] If the patient stays conscious long enough to be examined, hemiplegia, hemianes-

TABLE 25. Neurologic Features of Cerebral Hemorrhage

	Motor Deficit	Eye Deviation	Pupils
Supratentorial			
Putaminal	Dense hemiplegia	Opposite to hemiplegia	Ipsilateral, dilated, fixed
Thalamic	Dense hemiplegia	Down	Small, unreactive
Lobar	Depends on site	None	Normal
Infratentorial			
Pontine	Dense quadriplegia	Neutral position or "bobbing"	Pinpoint, reactive
Cerebellar	Quadriparetic but moves all limbs	Skew	Pinpoint, reactive

TABLE 26. Site of Intracerebral Hemorrhage at Autopsy in 393 Cases

Corpus striatum	42%
Pons	16%
Thalamus	15%
Cerebellum	12%
White matter	10%
Other	5%

From Freytag,[50] with permission.

thesia, and hemianopia are found, with forced conjugate gaze away from the hemiplegic side in putaminal hemorrhage and forced downward gaze in thalamic hemorrhage. Commonly, the patient lapses into coma with decerebrate rigidity and dies from coning within 2 or 3 days. If the shift of brain resulting from raised intracranial pressure is lateral rather than downward, arteries may be trapped and occluded, causing cerebral infarcts at remote locations (Fig. 61).

Small hemorrhages may mimic cerebral infarction and were often treated as ischemic strokes prior to CT scanning.[51] Intracerebral hemorrhages may even by asymptomatic.[52]

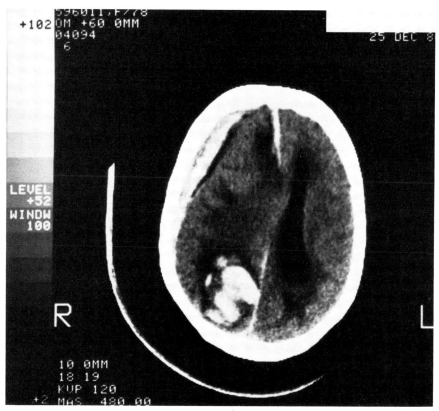

FIGURE 61. This 77-year old woman complained of headache and collapsed unconscious 15 minutes later. CT showed a large right frontal subdural hematoma (SDH) causing lateral cerebral shift. This temporarily occluded the right posterior cerebral artery (PCA) resulting in an occipital infarction. When the shift reversed following mannitol infusion, reperfusion of the PCA territory converted the ischemic area into a hemorrhagic infarct.

Lobar intracerebral hemorrhages usually produce milder deficits. They occur in subcortical white matter, often arise from underlying treatable lesions such as tiny angiomas or other arteriovenous malformations, and are much more accessible surgically than centrencephalic hemorrhages. Occipital hemorrhage presents with severe pain around the ipsilateral eye and dense hemianopia. Parietal hemorrhage produces an anterior temporal headache and a hemisensory deficit. Left temporal hemorrhage causes pain around the ear, fluent aphasia with good repetition and poor comprehension, and incomplete hemianopia. Frontal hemorrhage causes frontal headache and severe contralateral arm weakness with minimal face and leg involvement.[53]

Infratentorial Hemorrhage

Cerebellar hemorrhage usually presents with sudden frontal or occipital headache, vertigo, vomiting, and a staggering cerebellar ataxia,[54] rapidly progressing to coma in severe cases. An alert patient has striking cerebellar ataxia of all limbs and may be unable to stand or walk. There may be bilateral hyperreflexia and Babinski signs, but there is no hemiparesis. There may be lateral gaze nystagmus, with either skew-deviation of the eyes or forced conjugate gaze in the direction opposite the lesion. A sixth nerve palsy resulting from raised intracranial pressure may be a false localizing sign. The pupils are small, equal, and reactive. Decreasing consciousness from cerebellar edema or acute hydrocephalus compressing the brainstem[55] indicates a poor outcome and a need for emergency surgical decompression.

Pontine hemorrhage is usually more devastating, producing coma and decerebrate quadriplegia, distinct from cerebellar hemorrhage. The pupils are also pinpoint and reactive, but conjugate gaze is in the neutral position and unaffected by ice-cold irrigation of the ears. If the patient is not comatose, lateral gaze nystagmus is sometimes seen. "Ocular bobbing," a slow rhythmic conjugate vertical movement of the eyes, may be seen in both conditions but is commoner in cerebellar lesions. CT scan may be the only certain way of differentiating pontine from cerebellar hemorrhage.

CONCLUSION

Eponymous syndromes are being abandoned as progress in diagnostic techniques such as CT scanning and angiography emphasize their lack of application. Single artery syndromes are found more commonly in textbooks than in neurologic practice. New classifications of stroke syndromes are being proposed, to reflect the location and etiology of the lesion and to relate them to management.

Current stroke classifications emphasize etiology rather than specific arterial anatomy. Cerebral embolism and lacunar stroke together constitute a large and important minority of ischemic strokes. Control of hypertension is producing a striking decline in the incidence of hemorrhagic stroke and is changing the proportion of ischemic stroke.

Vascular syndromes are determined by their vascular supply, carotid or vertebrobasilar; by their location vis-à-vis the vascular centrencephalon; and by their temporal profile. Rational management can only be based on such a taxonomy.

REFERENCES

1. McCall, AJ, and Fletcher, PJH: *Pathology*. In Hutchinson, EC, and Acheson, EJ: *Strokes*. WB Saunders, London, 1975, p 36.
2. Dalal, PM, Shah, PM, and Aiyar, RR: *Arteriographic study of cerebral embolism*. Lancet 2:358, 1965.
3. Dyken, ML, et al: *Complete occlusion of common or internal carotid arteries*. Arch Neurol 30:343, 1974.
4. Barnett, HJM, Peerless, SJ, and Kaufman, JCE: *"Stump" of internal carotid artery—A source for further cerebral embolic ischemia*. Stroke 9:448, 1978.
5. Wortzman, G, Barnett, HJM, and Lougheed, WM: *Bilateral internal carotid occlusion: A clinical and radiological study*. Can Med Assoc J 99:1186, 1968.
6. Waddington, MM, and Ring, BA: *Syndromes of occlusions of middle cerebral artery branches—angiographic and clinical correlation*. Brain 44:685, 1968.
7. Meadows, JC: *Clinical features of focal cerebral hemisphere infarction*. In Ross Russell, RW (ed): *Vascular Disease of the Central Nervous System*, ed 2. Churchill-Livingstone, Edinburgh, 1983, p 169.
8. Caplan, LR, and Rosenbaum, AE: *Role of cerebral angiography in vertebrobasilar occlusive disease*. J Neurol Neurosurg Psychiatry 38:601, 1975.
9. Caplan, LR: *Occlusion of the vertebral or basilar artery. Follow up analysis of some patients with benign outcome*. Stroke 10:277, 1979.
10. Caplan, LR: *"Top of the basilar" syndrome*. Neurology 30:72, 1980.
11. Caplan, LR: *Vertebrobasilar disease—Time for a new strategy*. Stroke 12:111, 1981.
12. Caplan, LR: *Bilateral distal vertebral artery occlusion*. Neurology 33:552, 1983.
13. Caplan, LR: *Patterns of posterior circulation infarctions: Correlation with vascular pathology*. In Berguer, R, and Bauer, RB (eds): *Vertebrobasilar Arterial Occlusive Disease*. Raven Press, New York, 1984, p. 15.
14. Moossy, J: *Anatomy and pathology of the vertebrobasilar system*. In Berguer, R, and Bauer, RB (eds): *Vertebrobasilar Arterial Occlusive Disease*. Raven Press, New York, 1984, p 1.
15. Bauer, RB: *Mechanical compression of the vertebral arteries*. In Berguer, R, and Bauer, RB (eds): *Vertebrobasilar Arterial Occlusive Disease*. Raven Press, New York, 1984, p 45.
16. Fisher, CM: *The arterial lesions underlying lacunes*. Acta Neuropathol (Berlin) 12:1, 1969.
17. Mohr, JP, et al: *The Harvard Cooperative Stroke Registry: A prospective registry*. Neurology 28:754, 1978.
18. Fisher, CM, and Caplan, LR: *Basilar artery branch occlusion: A cause of pontine infarction*. Neurology 21:900, 1971.
19. Mohr, JP: *Lacunes*. Stroke 13:3, 1982.
20. Miller, VT: *Lacunar stroke, a reassessment*. Arch Neurol 40:129, 1983.
21. Cohn, R, Neumann, MA, and Wood, DH: *Prosopagnosia: A clinicopathological study*. Ann Neurol 1:177, 1977.
22. Benson, DF, Marsden, CD, and Meadhows, JC: *The amnesic syndrome of posterior cerebral artery occlusion*. Acta Neurol Scand 50:133, 1974.
23. Fisher, CM: *Occlusion of the vertebral arteries, causing transient basilar symptoms*. Arch Neurol 22:13, 1970.
24. Easton, JD, and Sherman, DG: *Cervicalmanipulation and stroke*. Stroke 8:594, 1977.
25. Krueger, BR, and Okazaki, H: *Vertebral-basilar distribution infarction following chiropractic manipulation*. Mayo Clin Proc 55:322, 1980.
26. Fisher, CM, Karnes, WE, and Kubik, CS: *Lateral medullary infarction—The pattern of vascular occlusion*. J Neuropathol Exper Neurol 20:323, 1961.
27. Sypert, G, and Alvord, EC: *Cerebellarinfarction, a clinicopathological study*. Arch Neurol 32:357, 1975.
28. Khan, M, et al: *Massive cerebellar infarction: "Conservative" management*. Stroke 14:745, 1983.
29. Kubik, CS, and Adams, RD: *Occlusion of the basilar artery—A clinical and pathological study*. Brain 69:73, 1946.
30. Drake, CG: *Ligation of the vertebral (unilateral or bilateral) or basilar artery in the treatment of large intracranial aneurysms*. J Neurosurg 43:255, 1975.

31. GROTTA, JC: *Letter to the Editor: Distal basilar artery occlusion syndrome.* Neurology 32:456, 1982.

32. PLUM, F: *Brain swelling and edema in cerebral vascular disease.* In *Cerebrovascular Disease* (Proc Assoc Res Nerv Ment Dis 41). Williams & Wilkins, Baltimore, 1966, p 318.

33. GILROY, J: *The "locked in" syndrome.* In BERGUER, R, AND BAUER, RB (EDS): *Vertebrobasilar Arterial Occlusive Disease.* Raven Press, New York, 1984, p 73.

34. HAWKES, CH: *"Locked-in" syndrome: Report of seven cases.* Br Med J 4:379, 1974.

35. KHURANA, RK, GENUT, AA, AND YANNAKAKIS, GD: *Locked-in syndrome with recovery.* Ann Neurol 8:439, 1980.

36. MARIE, P: *Des foyers lacunaire de désintégration et de différents autres états cavitaires du cerveau.* Rev Med 21:281, 1901.

37. FISHER, CM: *Lacunes: Small deep cerebral infarcts.* Neurology 15:774, 1965.

38. FISHER, CM, AND COLE, M: *Homolateral ataxia and crural paresis, a vascular syndrome.* J Neurol Neurosurg Psychiatry 28:48, 1965.

39. FISHER, CM, AND CURRY, HB: *Pure motor hemiplegia of vascular origin.* Arch Neurol 13:30, 1965.

40. FISHER, CM: *A lacunar stroke, the dysarthria–clumsy hand syndrome.* Neurology 17:614, 1967.

41. FISHER, CM: *The arterial lesions underlying lacunes.* Acta Neuropathol 12:1, 1969.

42. FISHER, CM: *Thalamic pure sensory stroke: A pathologic study.* Neurology 28:1141, 1978.

43. WHISNANT, JP: *The decline of stroke.* Stroke 15:160, 1984.

44. ROPPER, AH, FISHER, CM, AND KLEINMAN, GM: *Pyramidal infarction in the medulla: A cause of pure motor hemiplegia sparing the face.* Neurology 29:91, 1979.

45. FISHER, CM: *Ataxic hemiparesis.* Arch Neurol 351:126, 1978.

46. RASCOL, A, ET AL: *Pure motor hemiplegia: CT study of 30 cases.* Stroke 13:11, 1982.

47. WEISBERG, LA: *Computed tomography and pure motor hemiparesis.* Neurology 29:490, 1979.

48. DONNAN, GA, TRESS, BM, AND BLADIN, PF: *A prospective study of lacunar infarction using computerized tomography.* Neurology 32:49, 1982.

49. CAPLAN, LR, AND YOUNG, RR: *EEG findings in certain lacunar stroke syndromes.* Neurology 22:403, 1972.

50. FREYTAG, E: *Fatal hypertensive intracerebral haematomas: A survey of the pathological anatomy of 393 cases.* J Neurol Neurosurg Psychiatry 31:616, 1968.

51. KINKEL, W: *Computerized tomography in clinical neurology.* In BAKER, AB (ED): *Clinical Neurology,* Vol 4. Harper & Row, Philadelphia, 1983.

52. RUDICK, RA: *Asymptomatic intracerebral hematoma as an incidental finding.* Arch Neurol 38:396, 1981.

53. ROPPER, AH, AND DAVIS, KR: *Lobar cerebral hemorrhages: Acute clinical syndromes in 26 cases.* Ann Neurol 8:141, 1980.

54. FISHER, CM, ET AL: *Acute hypertensive cerebellar hemorrhage: Diagnosis and surgical treatment.* J Nerv Ment Dis 140:38, 1965.

55. SHENKIN, HA, AND ZAVALA, M: *Cerebellar strokes: Mortality, surgical indications, and results of ventricular drainage.* Lancet 2:429, 1982.

56. PETERSDORF, RG, ET AL (EDS): *Harrison's Principles of Internal Medicine* (ed 10). McGraw-Hill, New York, 1983, pp 2028–2060.

Chapter 8

THE DETERIORATING STROKE

Healing is a matter of time, but it is sometimes a matter of opportunity.
Hippocrates

The onset of stroke is usually sudden, dramatic, and complete, but its course commonly fluctuates, tending usually to improve—but sometimes to deteriorate.

DEFINITION OF "DETERIORATING STROKE"

The term "deteriorating stroke" was coined to include not only "stroke-in-evolution" but also other strokes that deteriorate during the first week from either cerebral (69 percent) or systemic causes (31 percent).[1] The "deteriorating stroke" has multiple etiologies, including propagation of thrombus in a critical cerebral blood vessel, which is cited as the usual cause of "stroke-in-evolution."[2]

"Stroke-in-evolution" ("progressing stroke") occurs when the stroke progresses stepwise or smoothly over several hours.[3] In the Toronto Unit (Table 27), a stepwise onset was as common in ischemic as in hemorrhagic completed strokes. An abrupt onset is commoner in cerebral hemorrhage than in cerebral infarction, reflecting the more dramatic and devastating pathology.

"Recurrent stroke" from further cardiac embolism or continuing carotid thromboembolism may occur within minutes, days, weeks, or longer after onset of the original event and so may contribute to all of the above profiles of clinical evolution. These terms merge into one another and their frequency of occurrence depends largely on definition and timing of deficits, and the method of data collection. For instance, in a retrospective review of 298 cases, Carter[4] reported that 38 percent of

TABLE 27. Type of Onset in 820 Consecutive Patients with Completed Stroke Admitted to the Unit

Stroke Type	Abrupt	Gradual	Stepwise	Unknown	Total
Infarction	431 (58%)	84 (11%)	120 (16%)	107 (14%)	742
Hemorrhage	55 (70%)	10 (13%)	5 (6%)	8 (11%)	78

TABLE 28. Incidence of Deteriorating Stroke Related to Stroke Type in 300 Consecutive Admissions to the Unit

Stroke Type		Total	Deteriorating
Cerebral infarction	Hemispheric	235	81 (34%)
(n = 268)	Brainstem	33	9 (27%)
Cerebral hemorrhage	Hemispheric	27	19 (70%)
(n = 32)	Brainstem	5	3 (60%)

ischemic strokes were "ingravescent" (progressive) during 2 hours. In a similar review, neurologic rating at 7 days was unchanged in 39 percent, improved in 35 percent, and worse in 26 percent.[5] The deteriorated group comprised 19 percent who stabilized within 48 hours, 3 percent who continued to remit and relapse, and 4 percent who worsened only at the end of the observation period. In the Toronto Unit, 30 percent of 300 stroke patients deteriorated, 40 percent remained "stable," and 30 percent improved, as assessed prospectively by their Toronto Stroke Score during the first week (Table 28; Fig. 62).[1]

The frequency with which deterioration is documented depends largely on the quality of observation, which initially often relies on the

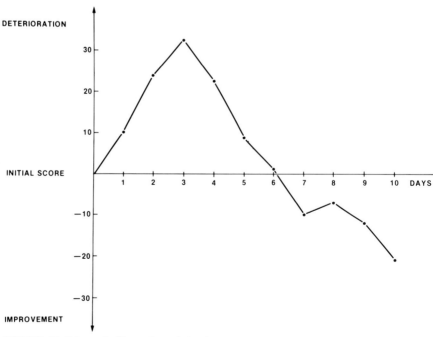

FIGURE 62. Schematic illustration of the deteriorating stroke, based on the Toronto Stroke Scoring System. This patient with ischemic stroke became drowsy and more hemiplegic over the first 3 days, but subsequently improved. This pattern is common in cerebral infarction and presumably indicates ischemic cerebral edema.

TABLE 29. Causes of Deterioration in Stroke

Cerebral factors	Systemic factors
Infarction	Cardiac
Cerebral edema	Heart failure
Hemorrhagic infarction	Cardiac arrhythmias
Recurrent embolism	Pulmonary
Progressive thrombosis	Pneumonia
(Postictal states)	Pulmonary embolism
Hemorrhage	Metabolic
Cerebral edema	Renal/hepatic failure
Rebleeding	Syndrome of inappropriate ADH
Acute hydrocephalus	Septicemia
(Postictal states)	Psychologic
	Drugs

patient's or relatives' recollections. In at least one third of patients stroke occurs when the patient is asleep,[6] making it difficult to ascertain the time and mode of onset. Detection of deterioration is unlikely in patients dismissed as "CVA" and kept at home or admitted to chronic care without further examination. In acute care units with frequent observation, the number of deteriorating patients may seem surprisingly high. In the patient with "deteriorating stroke" the first essential is a careful clinical examination to determine whether further laboratory investigations are appropriate. Knowledge of likely causes of deterioration, such as extension of the original stroke, systemic complications, and side effects of drugs, is essential to proper management (Table 29).

CEREBRAL CAUSES OF DETERIORATING ISCHEMIC STROKE

Clinical progression of ischemic stroke is generally assumed due to evolving thrombus,[7] but progressive cerebral edema, an equally plausible mechanism, is usually maximal by the third day, a peak time for deterioration in these patients.[8] Recurrent embolism or secondary bleeding into hemorrhagic infarction may also produce deterioration.

The Concept of Progressive Thrombosis

The pathogenesis of stroke evolving over hours ("stroke-in-evolution," "progressing stroke") may be progressive thrombosis of the major arterial supply, but convincing pathologic, angiographic, and clinical evidence is lacking and remains largely uncorrelated.[7] In an autopsy study of 50 patients with ICA occlusion, thrombosis occurred most commonly (73 percent) in association with tight (greater than 75 percent) stenoses and was invariably (98 percent) found at the carotid sinus. Angiographic/autopsy correlations in five patients suggest that, after establishment of the "white thrombus" in situ, anterograde red thrombosis propagates downstream within hours (Fig. 63). This process, spreading as far as the turbulent junction of the distal internal carotid artery, probably stops when it meets retrograde flow from the ophthalmic artery. If this long thrombus reaches beyond the internal carotid bifurcation, invading the circle of Willis, massive ipsilateral hemispheric infarction could rapidly occur.[9] It could propagate into the middle cerebral artery or break

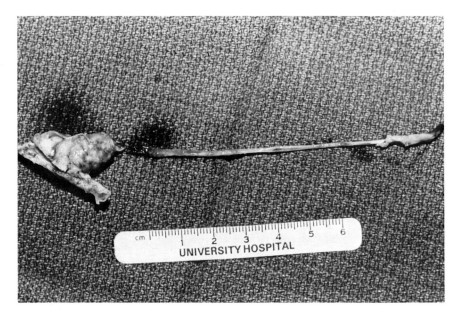

FIGURE 63. Long "red" anterograde clot attached to original white thrombus and extending up the internal carotid artery.

off and embolize into it. This extension might be arrested by anticoagulant treatment, especially since the anterograde clot is composed of "red cells loosely packed in a bag of platelets."[10] Unfortunately no methodologically sound clinical trial exists that tests this promising hypothesis. Surgical intervention might be a feasible alternative, since anterograde extension of clot takes about 3 to 6 hours.[10]

The Role of Cerebral Edema

Experimental arterial occlusion produces "cytotoxic" edema within 1½ hours of focal CBF falling below 20 ml/100 g/min, which then advances through the hemisphere.[11] Restoration of the circulation following removal of the occlusion increases, rather than decreases, the edema, and the clinical deficit worsens. Reactive hyperemia may act similarly so that, paradoxically, patients with good collateral circulation may experience more cerebral edema than those whose collaterals are diffusely impaired by atherosclerosis.[12] In more prolonged ischemia, "vasogenic" edema follows breakdown of the blood-brain barrier, with extravasation of large molecules such as protein. In experimental regional ischemia, O'Brien and colleagues[13] found that radioactive markers extravasated within a few days and remained high for 20 days, though the cerebral water content did not exactly follow the same temporal or spatial distribution (Fig. 64).

The relationship between clinical deterioration and progressive brain swelling is controversial. CT scan results did not correlate retrospectively with clinical evaluation in the study of Bruce and Hertig,[14] although large infarctions with midline displacement were related to higher mortality. They concluded that ischemic damage, and not secondary edema, was the major factor determining outcome.

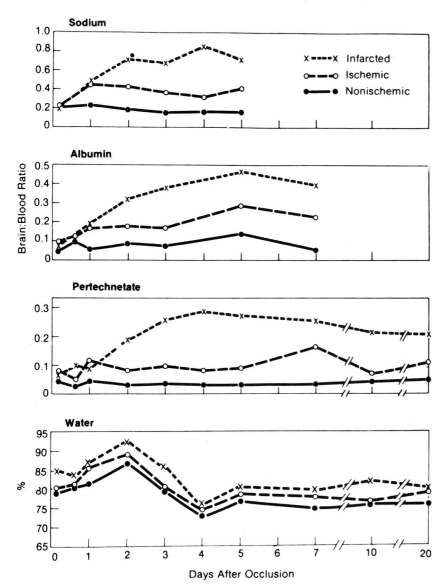

FIGURE 64. Mean values of brain:blood ratios for three radioactive substances compared with mean values for water content of nonischemic, ischemic, and infarcted tissue of brains of cats at different times after MCA occlusion. (From O'Brien, Jordan, and Waltz,[13] with permission.)

Hemorrhagic Infarction

Bleeding into cerebral infarction may be microscopic or catastrophic. It is more frequent in cerebral embolism when dissolution of the embolus leaves a necrotic and leaking arterial tree. Hemorrhagic infarcts expand more rapidly than do "pale" infarcts in the same territory and therefore are more frequently devastating or fatal.[15] The clinical picture of embolic occlusion with widespread extravasation of blood merges imperceptibly into intracerebral hemorrhage, the only clue to the pathogenesis being the CT appearance (Fig. 65). Hemorrhagic ischemic stroke is commonest in embolic infarction, yet these are the very patients in whom anticoag-

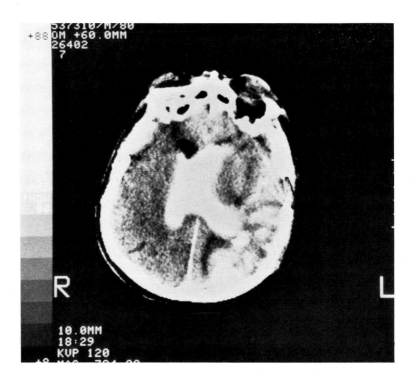

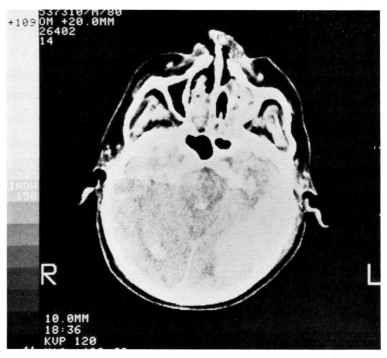

FIGURE 65. This 82-year-old man felt dizzy in the sauna, staggered out, and collapsed, stuporous. He soon lapsed into coma with decerebration of the right limbs and small reacting pupils. *Top,* CT scan showed the classical wedge appearance of a left middle cerebral artery infarction totally suffused with blood. *Bottom,* Duret hemorrhages in the brainstem indicate terminally raised intracranial pressure and transtentorial herniation.

ulants are most indicated. Available retrospective data indicate that secondary hemorrhage into embolic infarction is rare, and should not deter early intervention with anticoagulant therapy.[16]

DETERIORATION OF THE PATIENT WITH HEMORRHAGIC STROKE

In hemorrhagic stroke, deterioration is usually attributed to rebleeding, though progressive cerebral edema is probably more common, sometimes with acute hydrocephalus.[17] Unsuspected causes of rebleeding include subdural hematoma (Fig. 66), undiagnosed berry aneurysm, arteriovenous malformation, or coagulation disorders.

Hemispheric Hemorrhage

Deterioration in intracerebral hemorrhage occurs from cerebral edema, acute hydrocephalus or rebleeding.[17-19] Distinguishing these early is important since the mass effect of hematoma determines survival within the first 2 days.[20] CT scanning is a valuable diagnostic aid. Cerebral edema following cerebral hemorrhage is maximal by the fifth day, producing obstruction or loculation of the ventricular system, especially with lesions near the aqueduct. Rapid filling of the ventricular system with blood may also cause acutely fatal hydrocephalus.

Rebleeding is commonest with saccular aneurysms and arteriovenous malformations.[17] Simultaneous bleeding or rebleeding at different sites in the brain, often superficially, may indicate amyloid angiopathy (Fig. 67)[21,22] Hypertensive hemorrhages usually bleed once—and catastrophically—but these patients sometimes deteriorate from rebleeding as much as 1 week later.[23]

Early detection of deterioration in patients with cerebral hemispheric hemorrhage is mandatory before progressive brain edema prohibits evacuation of the hematoma.[24]

Cerebellar Hemorrhage

Ten percent of all intracerebral hemorrhages were cerebellar in the Boston City Hospital autopsy series, yet, prior to CT scanning, the clinical diagnosis was rarely made.[25]

Clinical diagnosis is notoriously difficult, but, before the advent of CT, posterior fossa craniectomy was often performed on clinical criteria alone.[26] Lumbar puncture is dangerous since it may induce transtentorial herniation and, if performed early, may not even be bloodstained.[25] These problems do not arise when CT scanning is available.

Sudden, devastating deterioration is the rule in patients with cerebellar hemorrhage, and early detection is more important in this than in any other location since it is often totally reversible.[27-29] Many untreated patients, especially if comatose, will die, whereas limited resection of the cerebellum often leaves no residual clinical deficit.[28,30-32]

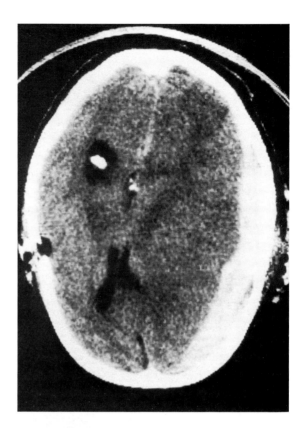

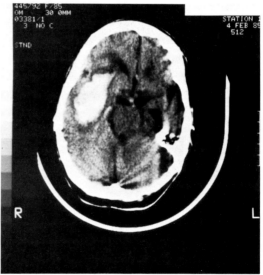

FIGURE 66. *Top,* This 66-year-old alcoholic, with no recent history of head injury, was admitted to the hospital drowsy, with a 1-day history of right hemiparesis. He became comatose 1 day later, and CT showed a left subdural hemorrhage.

Bottom, This 67-year-old woman with idiopathic thrombocytopenic purpura suddenly became comatose with a left hemiplegia. CT showed the typical appearance of cerebral hemorrhage secondary to a blood dyscrasia. There is layering of clot, indicating serial hemorrhage, and a fluid level frontally, indicating an abnormal coagulable state.

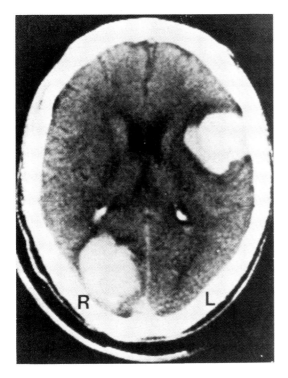

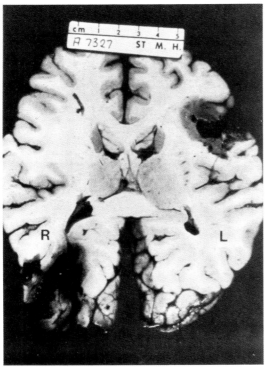

FIGURE 67. CT scan appearance and pathologic correlation in a patient with two simultaneous intercerebral hematomas of atypical location, shown on biopsy to be due to amyloid angiopathy. (From Tucker, Bilbao, and Klodawsky,[21] with permission.)

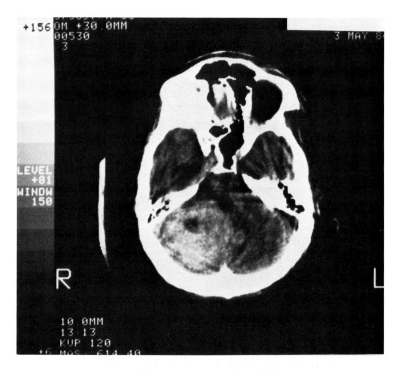

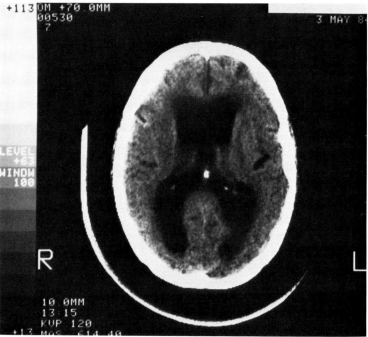

FIGURE 68. Right cerebellar hemorrhage *(top)* with secondary acute hydrocephalus *(bottom).*

Case History. A 65-year-old hypertensive woman collapsed, awake but dysarthric with left sixth nerve palsy, left facial weakness, truncal ataxia, left-beating nystagmus, and left gaze palsy. She had no limb weakness. She remained alert and resting in bed after lumbar puncture, which showed an opening pressure of 230 mm water with bloody fluid, but next day was found dead. Autopsy showed a fresh left cerebellar hemorrhage.[28]

Acute hydrocephalus, from mechanical distortion or engorgement with blood of the ventricular system, may cause upward or downward tonsillar herniation and medullary compression. The outcome may depend on the size of the hemorrhage; in those with a progressive course and brainstem compression, cerebellar hematomas were greater than 3 cm on CT, and there was acute ventricular dilation (Fig. 68). The outcome was benign where the hematoma was less than 3 cm and without ventricular dilation.[33] Alert patients with minimal signs and CT confirmation of the lesion can be observed in an intensive care unit, facilitating emergency craniotomy if they deteriorate.[29]

In cerebellar infarction, deterioration is also due to either direct brainstem compression or involvement by the edematous infarct or secondary to hydrocephalus from aqueduct obstruction. Deterioration may be just as dramatic, and, before CT scanning, cerebellar infarction could not readily be distinguished from cerebellar hemorrhage.[27] The outcome is probably more favorable than in cerebellar hemorrhage, though sufficient cases are not available to confirm this. Prompt surgical treatment for the hydrocephalus may obviate posterior fossa decompression.[34]

Brainstem Hemorrhage

Hypertension-induced hematomas of the brainstem are pontine in location and usually fatal. Survivors of the initial onslaught are usually comatose, quadriplegic, bilaterally decerebrate, and have pinpoint pupils. However, this now may need revising, since CT scanning indicates that smaller hemorrhages were probably mistaken for infarcts, especially when they ran a benign course (Fig. 69). Brainstem hemorrhage is now commonly found in patients with arteriovenous malformations that are less catastrophic and have a greater chance for successful surgical evacuation.[35] Once CT confirms the brainstem location of the hemorrhage, the patient's course should be monitored closely. Sudden deterioration by the fourth or fifth day is common and, though it is more likely due to edema than to rebleeding, urgent evacuation of the hematoma may allow recovery with little or no residual deficit.

Case History. An alert 71-year-old man was admitted with ataxia and eye signs of a midbrain lesion, with CT evidence of a 1-cm mesencephalic tegmental hemorrhage. He began to recover, but on the fifth day he suddenly became drowsy, with loss of all eye movements and progressive brainstem signs. Although the presumptive diagnosis was rebleeding, CT indicated resolution of the hematoma, the deterioration being due to periventricular edema.[36]

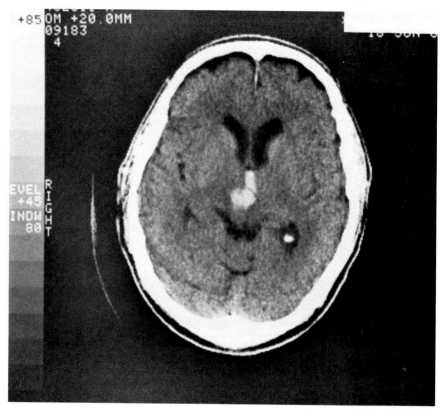

FIGURE 69. Midbrain hematoma presenting as TIA. This 64-year-old man suddenly fell off his chair and lay unconscious for 15 minutes. When he awoke he had left hemiplegia, diplopia, nystagmus, and right palatal palsy. The initial clinical diagnosis on admission was Wallenberg's syndrome, but CT scanning showed a pontine hemorrhage extending into the medulla. The patient was ambulant by 7 days and discharged on the ninth hospital day with very minimal ataxia and nystagmus.

The indications for surgical evacuation of brainstem hemorrhage are controversial.[29] Although there are numerous reports of beneficial surgical results,[35,36] the natural history of brainstem hemorrhage is uncertain and the hematoma may resolve uneventfully.

SYSTEMIC CAUSES OF DETERIORATING STROKE

Cardiac Factors

Cardiovascular disease and hypertension are the commonest disorders associated with stroke, but it is difficult to distinguish a causal from a chance relationship. In the Toronto Unit, serious cardiac arrhythmias, cardiogenic embolism, and other conditions such as heart failure were the commonest systemic disorders associated with deteriorating stroke patients (Table 30).

Post-Stroke Depression

Patients with stroke have mood disorders, especially depression, more often those with comparable disabilities.[37] Depression during acute

TABLE 30. Systemic Disorders (28 Patients, 25 Percent) Associated with Stroke Deterioration in 112 Patients

Cardiac disorders		15
Serious cardiac arrhythmias	7	
Recurrent cardiac emboli	3	
Acute myocardial infarction	2	
Heart failure	3	
Respiratory disorders		6
Metabolic disorders		3
Other		4

stroke occasionally progresses to stupor or psychomotor retardation and must be distinguished from further neurologic damage. Post-stroke depression occurred in 30 percent of 103 stroke patients evaluated by psychiatric questionnaire and examination.[38] The peak incidence of depression was between 6 months and 2 years and was unrelated to age, sex, neurologic impairment, or alteration in lifestyle. It was commonest in patients with left-hemisphere lesions, which may represent the special vulnerability of the left hemisphere to injury of catecholamine pathways.[39-42]

The Syndrome of Inappropriate Antidiuretic Hormone

In the syndrome of inappropriate antidiuretic hormone (SIADH), excessive water retention produces reduced plasma osmolality, yet the urine remains less than maximally dilute in the presence of normal renal and adrenal function.[43] Hyponatremia soon induces cerebral edema[44] with a significant reduction in brain sodium, potassium, and chloride content,[45] which may affect brain energy metabolism[46] and interfere with neurotransmitter amino acid uptake.[47] Symptoms develop as serum sodium levels fall[44] (Fig. 70): confusion occurs at about 120 mEq/L, stupor at 115 mEq/L, and coma supervenes at about 110 mEq/L, often accompanied by seizures.

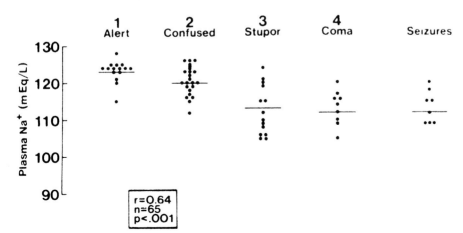

FIGURE 70. Neurologic effects of falling plasma sodium. (From Arieff,[44] with permission.)

TABLE 31. SIADH in 138 Consecutive Patients Admitted to the Toronto Unit

	Definite SIADH*	Possible SIADH†	Total
Hemispheric infarction	5	4	44
Hemispheric hemorrhage	2	3	14
Brainstem infarction	0	0	8
TIA	0	0	50
Nonstroke controls	0	0	22

*Definite SIADH: Na <125 mEq/L, plasma osmolality <270 mOsm/kg, simultaneous urine osmolality > plasma osmolality, no medication known to produce SIADH.
†Possible SIADH: Did not satisfy all "definite" criteria, but patient continued to produce concentrated urine despite hyponatremia and hypo-osmolality.

In patients with SIADH complicating acute stroke, metabolic edema augments the ischemic edema, producing a secondary mass effect, in addition to the biochemical dysfunction. Arginine-vasopressin (antidiuretic hormone) levels may be raised in the absence of clinical symptoms and, in the study of Joynt and associates,[48] none of their stroke patients developing hyponatremia and hypo-osmolality became symptomatic.

This syndrome is infrequent in acute stroke[48,49] and, of 138 consecutive patients evaluated in the Toronto Unit, only 5 (11 percent) of 44 with cerebral hemisphere infarction met the biochemical diagnostic criteria of SIADH[50] (Table 31). Two of 14 patients with hemispheric hemorrhage also qualified biochemically, but none of the remaining patients with either brainstem infarction or TIA were affected. Of the seven patients meeting the biochemical criteria of SIADH, three had seizures, six deteriorated, and four died. In deteriorating patients, hyponatremia worsened progressively over the first 4 days, was maximal at 7 to 9 days, and spontaneously resolved in survivors (Fig. 71).

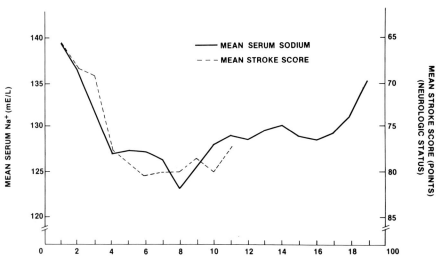

FIGURE 71. Relationship of serum sodium levels to neurologic score in seven patients with SIADH and deteriorating stroke.

Drug Effects

The commonest effect of deterioration from drugs is impairment of consciousness, usually from tranquilizers or sedatives, since neurologic deficits appear to worsen as alertness is impaired. Because sedation may impair accurate neurologic evaluation in patients who may deteriorate from more serious causes, these drugs should be avoided.

Metabolic effects of drugs include inadvertent insulin-induced hypoglycemia in diabetic stroke patients in whom the superimposed neurologic deficit is indistinguishable from a further cerebrovascular episode. Secondary SIADH induced by chlorpropamide and other drugs may be difficult to detect when it occurs days after the drug is stopped. Postural hypotension caused by antihypertensives and other drugs may induce serious secondary infarction or increase the existing area of ischemia, especially when intravenous infusions of nitroprusside or diazoxide are used to treat hypertensive encephalopathy.

The risk of exacerbating a pre-existing cerebral hemorrhage with administration of anticoagulants for "completed stroke" has been considerably reduced since CT scanning made the distinction between cerebral infarction and hemorrhage so clear. The danger of secondary hemorrhage into an area of infarction following anticoagulation for embolic stroke has probably been exaggerated.[16,51]

Other Systemic Factors

The incidence of deterioration does not appear to differ between the sexes, but advancing age is a critical factor. Infections (especially septicemia), pneumonia, pulmonary embolism, and metabolic disorders such as renal and hepatic failure produce deterioration or obtundation in the stroke patient.

INVESTIGATING THE PATIENT WITH DETERIORATING STROKE

Clinical Examination

Successful therapeutic intervention in deterioration depends on early recognition of changing neurologic signs and their accurate interpretation. No amount of laboratory data will substitute. For instance, if acute stupor is an isolated finding unaccompanied by a worsening focal deficit, an acute metabolic or drug-induced cause is most likely. New neurologic deficits in other locations, such as the contralateral hemisphere, suggest continuing embolism. There may be other evidence of systemic emboli, such as acute ischemia in a limb or signs of bacterial endocarditis. Neurologic deterioration from an unwitnessed or unrecognized seizure may remain indistinguishable from a fresh embolic event, even after thorough investigation. Postictal neurologic deficits may last for hours to days and range from hemiparesis (Todd's paralysis) to homonymous hemianopia and even global aphasia.

Patients with a recurrence of intracranial bleeding may be indistinguishable clinically from those with rapidly progressive cerebral edema.

Both may develop neck stiffness, stupor, and other signs of increasing intracranial pressure, and only CT scanning can differentiate.

In the absence of cerebral causes of deterioration, examination should focus on signs of cardiopulmonary failure, systemic infection, drug complications, and SIADH.

Laboratory Investigation

Laboratory tests should always be appropriate to the suspected clinical disorder. Random laboratory screening is generally unrewarding, wasteful of time and resources, and is no substitute for careful clinical examination.

Urgent CT or magnetic resonance scanning will identify cerebral causes such as massive edema or bleeding. Isotope brain scan, skull x-ray (for pineal shift), and lumbar puncture should be performed urgently if CT is not available. Angiography is preferable to lumbar puncture in drowsy patients who may have raised intracranial pressure. Before CT became available, deterioration a few hours after lumbar puncture was occasionally observed in patients with intracranial hemorrhage (Fig. 72).

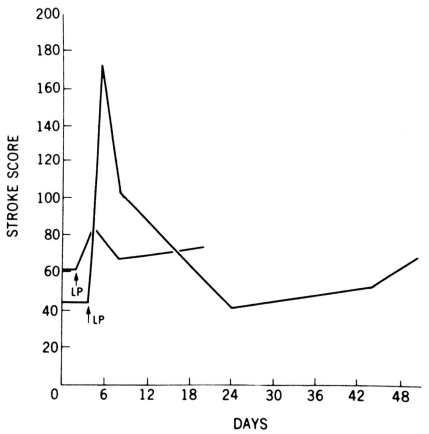

FIGURE 72. Changes in stroke scores in individual patients with cerebral hemorrhage. Lumbar puncture (LP) in two patients with cerebral hemorrhage. Lumbar puncture (LP) caused abrupt deterioration and increase in stroke score. (From Norris, JW, and Hachinski, VC: *Intensive care management of stroke patients.* Stroke 7:573, 1976.)

This was an unavoidable complication, since the diagnosis rested largely on lumbar puncture findings.

CONCLUSION

Approximately one third of stroke patients suffer clinical deterioration in the first week, which threatens their ultimate recovery by potentially increasing the extent of neurologic damage and by limiting or delaying rehabilitation.

New cerebral events such as edema, secondary hemorrhage, and recurrent embolism cause deterioration in 70 percent of cases. Systemic causes, including cardiopulmonary effects, metabolic disorders, and drug complications, are responsible in the remainder.

Vigilant clinical assessment and judicious laboratory confirmation to detect deterioration and discover its cause can realize the patient's full potential for recovery.

REFERENCES

1. HACHINSKI, VC, AND NORRIS, JW: *The deteriorating stroke.* In MEYER, JS, ET AL (EDS): *Cerebral Vascular Disease 3.* Excerpta Medica, Amsterdam, 1980, p 315.
2. CARTER, AB: *Ingravescent cerebral infarction.* QJ Med 29:611, 1960.
3. MARSHALL, J: *The Management of Cerebrovascular Disease.* J & A Churchill, London, 1968, p 113.
4. CARTER, AB: *Ingravescent cerebral infarction.* QJ Med 29:611, 1960.
5. JONES, HR, AND MILLIKAN, CH: *Temporal profile (clinical course) of acute carotid system cerebral infarction.* Stroke 7:64, 1976.
6. MARSHALL, J: *Diurnal variation in occurrence of strokes.* Stroke 8:230, 1977.
7. MILLIKAN, CH, AND McDOWELL, FH: *Treatment of progressing stroke.* Stroke 12:397, 1981.
8. NORRIS, JW, AND LASSEN, NA: *Letter to the Editor: Important points in treatment of progressing stroke.* Stroke 13:403, 1982.
9. CASTAIGNE, P, ET AL: *Internal carotid artery occlusion. A study of 61 instances in 50 patients with post-mortem data.* Brain 93:231, 1970.
10. GAUTIER, JC: *Arterial pathology in cerebral ischemia and infarction.* In GREENHALGH, RM, AND ROSE, FC (EDS): *Progress in Stroke Research.* Pitman, London, 1979, p 28.
11. SYMON, L: *Experimental cerebral infarction.* In GREENHALGH, RM, AND ROSE, FC (EDS): *Progress in Stroke Research 1.* Pitman, Bath, 1979, p 79.
12. BLACKWOOD, W: Personal communication, 1982.
13. O'BRIEN, MD, JORDAN, MM, AND WALTZ, AG: *Ischemic cerebral edema and the blood-brain barrier.* Arch Neurol 30:461, 1974.
14. BRUCE, DA, AND HERTIG, HI: *Incidence, course, and significance of cerebral edema associated with cerebral infarction.* In PRICE, TR, AND NELSON, E (EDS): *Cerebrovascular Diseases.* Raven Press, New York, 1979, p 191.
15. McCALL, AJ, AND FLETCHER, PJH: *Pathology.* In HUTCHINSON, EC, AND ACHESON, EJ: *Strokes.* WB Saunders, London, 1975, p 36.
16. FURLAN, AJ, ET AL: *Hemorrhage and anticoagulation after nonseptic embolic brain infarction.* Neurology 32:280, 1982.
17. RANSOHOFF, J, DERBY, B, AND KRICHEFF, I: *Spontaneous intracerebral hemorrhage.* Clin Neurosurg 18:247, 1971.
18. McKISSOCK, W: *Primary intracerebral hemorrhage.* Lancet 2:221, 1961.
19. GREENBERG, J, SKUBICK, D, AND SHENKIN, H: *Acute hydrocephalus in cerebellar infarct and hemorrhage.* Neurology 29:409, 1979.
20. SILVER, FL, ET AL: *Early mortality following stroke: A prospective view.* Stroke 15:492, 1984.
21. TUCKER, WS, BILBAO, JM, AND KLODAWSKY, H: *Cerebral amyloid angiopathy and multiple intracerebral hematomas.* Neurosurgery 7:611, 1980.

22. WHITE, OB, ET AL: *Letter to the Editor: Death in early stroke, causes and mechanisms.* Stroke 10:743, 1979.

23. KANEKO, M, KOBA, T, AND YOKOKAMA,T: *Early surgical treatment for hypertensive intracerebral hemorrhage.* J Neurosurg 46:579, 1977.

24. FISHER, CM, ET AL: *Acute hypertensive cerebellar hemorrhage: Diagnosis and surgical treatment.* J Nerv Ment Dis 140:38, 1965.

25. ROSENBERG, GA, AND KAUFMAN, DM: *Cerebellar hemorrhage: Reliability of clinical evaluation.* Stroke 7:332, 1976.

26. NORRIS, JW, EISEN, AA, AND BRANCH, CL: *Problems in cerebellar hemorrhage and infarction.* Neurology 19:1043, 1969.

27. OTT, KH, ET AL: *Cerebellar hemorrhage: diagnosis and treatment, review of 56 cases.* Arch Neurol 31:160, 1974.

28. OJEMANN, RG, AND HEROS, RC: *Spontaneous brain hemorrhage.* Stroke 14:468, 1983.

29. HEROS, RC: *Cerebellar hemorrhage and infarction.* Stroke 13:106, 1982.

30. MCKISSOCK, W, RICHARDSON, A, AND WALSH, L: *Spontaneous cerebellar hemorrhage: A study of 34 consecutive cases treated surgically.* Brain 83:1, 1960.

31. SHENKIN, HA, AND ZAVALA, M: *Cerebellar strokes: Mortality, surgical indications, and results of ventricular drainage.* Lancet 2:429, 1982.

32. LITTLE, JR, TUBMAN, DE, AND ETHIER, R: *Cerebellar hemorrhage in adults—diagnosis by computerized tomography.* J Neurosurg 48:575, 1978.

33. KHAN, M, ET AL: *Massive cerebellar infarction: "Conservative" management.* Stroke 14:745, 1983.

34. O'LAOIRE, SA, ET AL: *Brain-stem hematoma, a report of six surgically treated cases.* J Neurosurg 56:222, 1982.

35. DURWARD, QJ, BARNETT, HJM, AND BARR, HWK: *Presentation and management of mesencephalic hematoma.* J Neurosurg 56:123, 1982.

36. SANO, K, AND OCHIAI, C: *Brain stem hematomas: Clinical aspects with reference to indications for treatment.* In PIA, HW, LANGMAID, C, AND ZIERSKI, J (EDS): *Spontaneous Intracerebral Hematomas.* Springer-Verlag, New York, 1980, p 366.

37. FOLSTEIN, MF, MAIBERGER, R, AND MCHUGH, TR: *Mood disorder as a specific complication of stroke.* J Neurol Neurosurg Psychiatry 40:1018, 1977.

38. ROBINSON, RG, AND PRICE, TR: *Post-stroke depressive disorders: A follow-up study of 103 patients.* Stroke 13:635, 1982.

39. ROBINSON, RG, ET AL: *A two-year longitudinal study of post-stroke mood disorders: Findings during the initial evaluation.* Stroke 14:736, 1983.

40. ROBINSON, RG, ET AL: *Post-stroke affective disorders.* In REIVICH, M, AND HURTIG, HI (EDS): *Cerebrovascular Diseases* (ED 13). Raven Press, New York, 1983, p 137.

41. ROBINSON, RG, AND SZETELA, B: *Mood change following left hemispheric brain injury.* Ann Neurol 9:447, 1981.

42. SCHILDKRAUT, JJ: *The catecholamine hypothesis of affective disorders: A review of supporting evidence.* Am J Psychiatry 122:509, 1965.

43. BARTTER, FC, AND SCHWARTZ, WB: *The syndrome of inappropriate secretion of antidiuretic hormone.* Am J Med 42:790, 1967.

44. ARIEFF, AI, ET AL: *Neurological manifestations and morbidity of hyponatremia: Correlation with brain water and electrolytes.* Medicine 55:121, 1976.

45. HOLLIDAY, MA, ET AL: *Factors that limit brain volume changes in response to acute and sustained hyper- and hyponatremia.* J Clin Invest 47:1916, 1968.

46. FISHMAN, RA: *Cell volume, pumps and neurological function: Brain's adaptation to osmotic stress.* In PLUM, F (ED): *Brain Dysfunction in Metabolic Disorders.* New York, 1974, p 159.

47. GAGE, PW, AND QUASTEL, D: *Influence of sodium ions on transmitter release.* Nature 106:1047, 1965.

48. JOYNT, RJ, ET AL: *Hyponatremia in subarachnoid hemorrhage.* Arch Neurol 13:633, 1965.

49. GOLDBERG, M, AND HANLER, J: *Hyponatremia and renal wasting of sodium in a patient with malfunction of the CNS.* N Engl J Med 263:1037, 1960.

50. MAZUREK, MF, AND NORRIS, JW: *Vasopressin and inappropriate antidiuresis in acute neurovascular illness.* Can J Neurol Sci 9:297, 1982.

51. YATSU, FM, AND MOHR, JP: *Anticoagulation therapy for cardiogenic emboli to the brain.* Neurology 32:274, 1982.

Chapter 9

THE YOUNG STROKE

When you have eliminated the possible, whatever remains,
however improbably, must be the truth.
Sherlock Holmes

Stroke in the young looms urgent and compelling to physicians and relatives alike, particularly when dealing with the devastating risk of chronic disability. Young stroke patients have remediable lesions more commonly than do elder stroke patients, and investigation should be full in all cases. Cerebral angiography is mandatory in all cases unless the etiology is unequivocal or the deficit is severe and irreversible.

Since the behavior of the infant and neonatal brain differs so much from that of the child and adult, discussion is limited to stroke occurring in patients between 16 and 45 years of age. These patients represent only 3 to 4 percent of the stroke population, but they encompass the majority of etiologies.

INCIDENCE

No good comparative studies exist of the relative incidence of TIA in young and older stroke patients. Fifty-four of 1278 consecutive patients admitted to the Toronto Unit were between the ages of 16 and 45 years (4.2 percent) (Table 32), similar to the American National Stroke Survey figure of 3.7 percent.[1]

Strokes in young adults are commoner in India, where 30 percent of 850 stroke patients are under the age of 40.[2] This probably reflects a population structure in which young adults predominate: 50 percent of the population is under the age of 20, and life expectancy is 52 years. As

TABLE 32. Cause of Stroke or TIA in 54 Consecutive Patients Under 45 Years of Age Admitted to the Toronto Unit*

ISCHEMIC		
Cardiac		17
MCA trunk or branch occlusions (presumptive cardiac source)	7	
Rheumatic heart disease	4	
Mitral prosthesis	2	
Myocardial infarction with mural thrombosis	1	
Paroxysmal atrial fibrillation	1	
Atrial myxoma	1	
Mitral valve prolapse	1	
Unknown (normal angiograms in 8)		12
Migraine		8
Presumed carotid atherosclerosis		6
Diabetes	5	
Hypercholesterolemia	1	
Trauma		3
Accidents	2	
Chiropractic manipulation	1	
Hypertensive encephalopathy		3
Arteritis		1
Cerebral venous thrombosis		1
HEMORRHAGIC		3
Hypertension	2	
Arteriovenous malformation	1	

*Subarachnoid hemorrhage not included.

lifespan approaches the age at which strokes are commoner, the incidence of stroke in India may rise.[3]

ETIOLOGY

A scheme of the diagnostic possibilities in young patients (Fig. 73) can be used to generate a practical list from local experience. For example, consider moyamoya disease, seldom found in North America but often in Japan.

ISCHEMIC STROKE

Cardiac Causes

The commonest cause of stroke in the young is cardiac embolism, usually to the middle cerebral artery trunk or branches. A normal angiographic appearance suggests a cardiac embolic source, although a cardiac source is not always identified. Two-dimensional (2-D) echocardiography is particularly valuable in these cases, with the growing recognition of nonarteriosclerotic causes of stroke.[4]

    Deaths under the age of 50 from *rheumatic heart disease* have declined 75 percent in Canada in the past 25 years,[5,6] but rheumatic fever remains a significant problem, particularly in the Third World. Mitral stenosis (with or without atrial fibrillation) is the commonest lesion causing neurologic sequelae (Fig. 74).[4] Atrial fibrillation without a cardiac valvular lesion is also a potent cause of stroke.[7]

    While rheumatic heart disease declines, *mitral valve prolapse* (MVP) is apparently rising as a cause of stroke. About 6 percent of the popula-

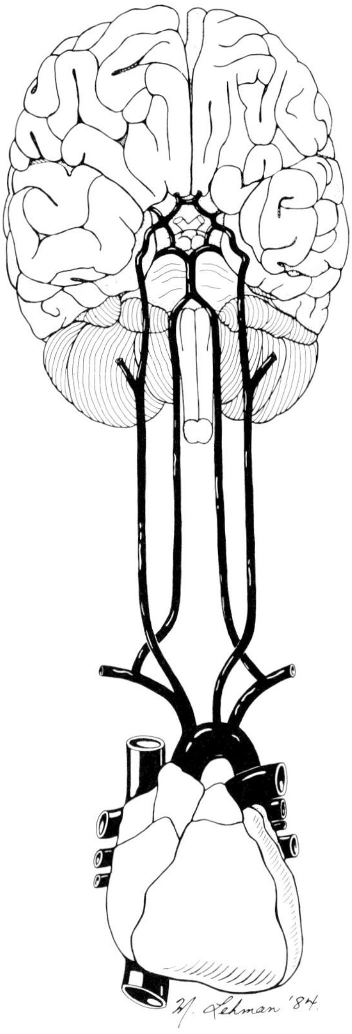

HEAD

MIGRAINE

HEMORRHAGES
Aneurysms
Arteriovenous malformations
Hypertensive hemorrhage

HYPERTENSIVE
ENCEPHALOPATHY

NECK

ATHEROSCLEROSIS
Hypertension
Diabetes
Hyperlipidemia

FIBROUS DYSPLASIA

CHEST

TAKAYASU DISEASE

ARRHYTHMIAS
Atrial fibrillation

MYOCARDIAL INFARCTION
Mural thrombus
Akinetic segments

CARDIOMYOPATHY
Infectious
Chagas' disease
Alcoholism
Idiopathic

BLOOD

HEMOGLOBINOPATHIES
Sickle cell disease

COAGULOPATHIES
Oral contraceptives
Acute alcohol intoxication
Disseminated intravascular
  coagulopathy
Hypercoagulable states
Inflammatory bowel disease
Lupus anticoagulant

ARTERITIS
Infection
 -syphilis
 -tuberculosis
 -virus
Collagen vascular disease
Giant cell disease
Drug abuse
Moyamoya disease
Nishimoto disease

VENOUS INFARCTION

ARTERIAL DISSECTION
Trauma
Spontaneous
Atherosclerosis

TRAUMA
Accidents
? Acute alcohol intoxication
Chiropractic manipulation

PULMONARY VENOUS DISEASE
Pulmonary venous thrombosis
Paradoxical embolus

VALVULAR HEART DISEASE
Mitral valve stenosis
Mitral valve prolapse
Bicuspid aortic valve
Endocarditis
 -infective
 -non-infective
Valvular prostheses

CARDIAC TUMORS
Atrial myxoma

BLOOD DYSCRASIAS
Thrombocytic thrombocytopenic
  purpura
Leukemia
Falciparum malaria

DEFICIENCY DISEASES
C_2 deficiency
Homocystinuria

M. Lehman '84

FIGURE 73. Causes of stroke in the young.

tion has mitral valve prolapse,[8,9] but only a minority suffer symptoms or harm from it, such as TIAs or cerebral infarction. Among 60 patients under the age of 45 years with TIAs or cerebral infarction without demonstrable cause, 40 percent had MVP compared with 6.6 percent of subjects matched for age and sex.[10] The role of MVP in patients over the age of 45 years is obscured by the predominance of other causes of stroke and the frequent presence of arterial lesions, and its role may remain underestimated unless 2-D echocardiography is performed in all patients (Fig. 75). Mitral valve prolapse may be associated with other conditions, such as Marfan's syndrome and mesenchymal disorders.[11–13]

Clinical signs of the syndrome are inconsistent and 2-D echocardiography provides a new standard of diagnosis, although no consistent

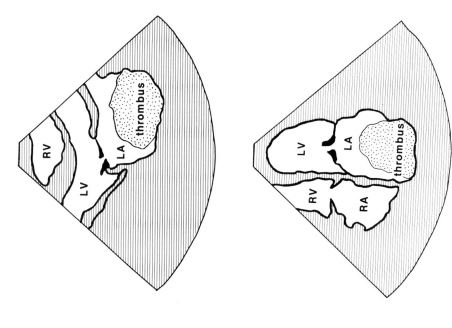

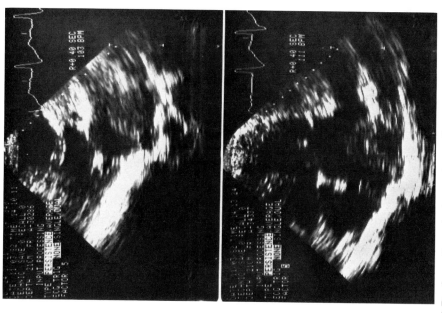

FIGURE 74. 2-D echocardiography in a patient with severe mitral stenosis due to rheumatic heart disease, also showing a major thrombus in the left atrium, long axis (*top*) and apical four-chamber (*bottom*) views. (From DR Boughner, MD, University of Western Ontario, with permission.)

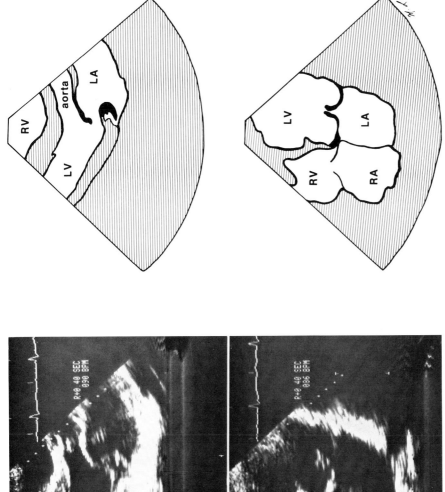

FIGURE 75. 2-D echocardiography findings in a patient with marked mitral valve prolapse, long axis (*top*) and apical four-chamber (*bottom*) views. (From DR Boughner, MD, University of Western Ontario, with permission.)

relationship between the severity of prolapse and the likelihood of cerebral events has emerged. The presence of MVP does not implicate, nor does the coexistence of an alternative explanation exonerate, MVP as a cause of stroke. Even with this proviso, MVP is probably the commonest cause of stroke in the young.

Bicuspid aortic valve may occasionally cause stroke. *Idiopathic hypertrophic subaortic stenosis* usually presents with cardiac complications or syncope but, in a series of 155 patients followed for an average of 5.5 years, 4 percent developed transient and 3 percent permanent strokes, usually from atrial fibrillation.[14] Despite technical and surgical advances in valve replacement and better anticoagulation, *valvular prostheses*, as a source of emboli, remain a risk for stroke.[4] Abnormal and artificial valves are vulnerable to *infection*, and cerebral embolism may follow an infection or tooth extraction.

Cardiomyopathies foster clots (Fig. 76) and, in developing countries, they commonly cause stroke in the young. Chagas' disease is uncommon in North America but indigenous to large areas of Latin America. Ten million inhabitants of a corridor of dry vegetation running from northeastern Brazil to northern Argentina are infected with the protozoan Trypanosoma cruzi.[15] In the acute phase, the parasite infects the blood and vital organs, especially the heart, producing fever and a systemic reaction. Most subjects survive but later fall victim to the slow destruction of their colon, heart, and autonomic ganglia. The apex of the myocardium often undergoes ischemic necrosis and interstitial fibrosis, sometimes becoming paper-thin (Fig. 77). Clots accumulate in this akinetic hollow and may be hurled as emboli by the irregular contractions of the denervated heart.

A monoclonal antibody has been developed that reacts with the parasite and with the neurons in the gastrointestinal tract and myocardial muscle.[16] Although no direct evidence has yet been produced for an antigen common to Trypanosoma cruzi and mammalian tissue, the prospect exists that some strokes may be prevented by suppressing immunologic mechanisms.

Large, apical *myocardial infarcts* favor thrombosis, embolizing to the cerebral arteries in 2 percent of cases. The peak incidence is about 2 weeks after the myocardial infarction.[4]

Atrial myxoma is a benign, rare heart tumor causing a mitral diastolic murmur and is associated with multiple emboli and raised plasma gammaglobulins.[17] Excision of the tumor removes this source of emboli.

Paradoxical embolism occurs when increased pressure in the right atrium allows thrombi from limb veins to cross the foramen ovale and embolize the systemic circulation.[18,19]

Migraine

Although migraine occurs in 15 to 19 percent of men and 25 to 29 percent of women[20] and is commonly associated with transient visual or sensory disturbances, permanent neurologic sequelae are rare. Evidence for cerebral infarction derives from clinical, pathologic, and, more recently, CT and angiographic studies.[21–27]

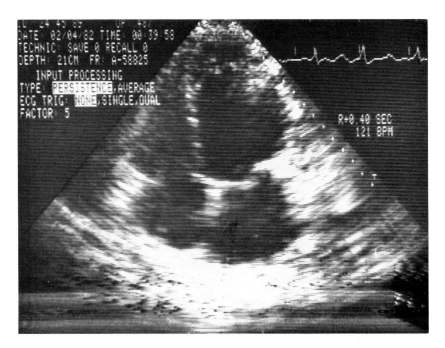

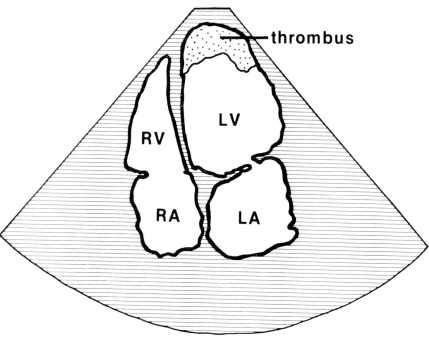

FIGURE 76. 2-D echocardiogram of a patient with cardiomyopathy and a left ventricular apical thrombus, apical four-chamber view. (From DR Boughner, MD, University of Western Ontario, with permission.)

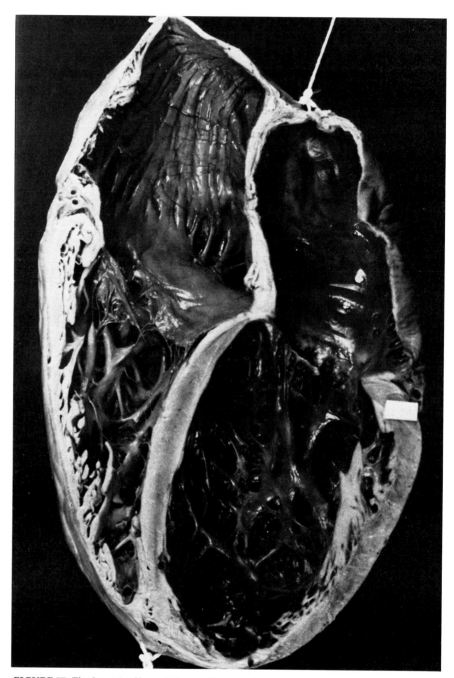

FIGURE 77. The heart in Chagas' disease. The apex is extremely thin and is the site for thrombus formation and cerebral and systemic embolization. (From Silver, MD, and Datta, BN: *Parasitic diseases of the heart.* In Silver, MD (ed): *Cardiovascular Pathology.* Churchill-Livingstone, New York, 1983, with permission.)

Abnormal CT scans were found in 80 percent of 46 cases of recurrent migraine in one study, with 17 percent showing cerebral atrophy and 13 percent infarction.[23] Similar data are reported elsewhere,[24,25] but patients with CT changes may not represent the average migraineur, since they have migraine severe or atypical enough to require hospitalization or further investigation.

Five of six migraine patients with cerebral infarction had arterial occlusions at angiography,[26] and the authors suggest that attributing cerebral infarction to migraine requires (1) an unequivocal history of migraine, (2) close timing of the neurologic deficit with the migraine attack, and (3) exclusion of other causes such as atheroma or embolization (echocardiography was negative in all their cases).

Disturbances of the cerebral circulation in migraine have been postulated for centuries.[28-30] Indirect evidence of cerebral blood flow (CBF) changes in migraine derives from bulging of a craniotomy defect during migraine,[31] the arrest of scotomata with vasodilators,[32] the analysis of visual symptoms,[33] angiography during a migraine attack,[34] and the measurement of cerebral spinal fluid pressure during migraine (although direct measurement of CBF during migraine was not performed until 1967).[35]

Vasospasm is the most usual explanation for cerebral infarction in migraine, but the evidence is thin. Dukes and Vieth[34] reported a case with cerebral "vasospasm" demonstrated by angiography, but the P_{CO_2} was not measured and the appearance might have been due to hyperventilation, common during migraine attacks.[36] However, CBF studies indicate decreased flow during the aura phase of classic migraine,[35,37] sometimes down to infarction levels.[36] CBF changes may be focal or diffuse[38,39] and occur in the symptomatic or opposite hemisphere, the decrease tending to be greater in the affected side.[40] The decrease in flow usually begins in the occipital area and moves forward at 3 mm/min, the same rate of the spreading depression of Leão across vascular territories.[41] Patients with common migraine do not show these changes, suggesting that it represents a disorder different from classic migraine.[42]

Platelet aggregation causing decreased cerebral perfusion is an alternative but unproven hypothesis.[43,44]

Atherosclerosis

Atherosclerotic stroke before the age of 45 is rare without associated risk factors, such as hypertension, diabetes, or hyperlipidemia.[45] Cigarette smoking, use of oral contraceptives, hypertension, and ECG abnormalities are special risk factors for stroke in young adults.[46]

Extensive atherosclerosis, unaccompanied by any recognizable risk factors, may also occur. Seneviratne and Ameratunga[47] reported 44 rural Ceylonese patients between the ages of 12 and 45 with ischemic stroke, including 19 men with internal carotid occlusions mostly due to atherosclerosis. They were not hypertensive, diabetic, or hypercholesterolemic but consumed a calorically marginal diet and possibly had carbohydrate-induced hyperlipidemia.

Arterial Dissection

Trauma to the main cervical arteries may cause dissection with luminal obstruction, aneurysm formation or hemorrhage,[48] or endothelial injury with thrombus formation and embolization (Fig. 78).

Rotation of the neck causes the axis to rotate around the atlas, stretching and compressing the vertebral arteries, and causing stroke

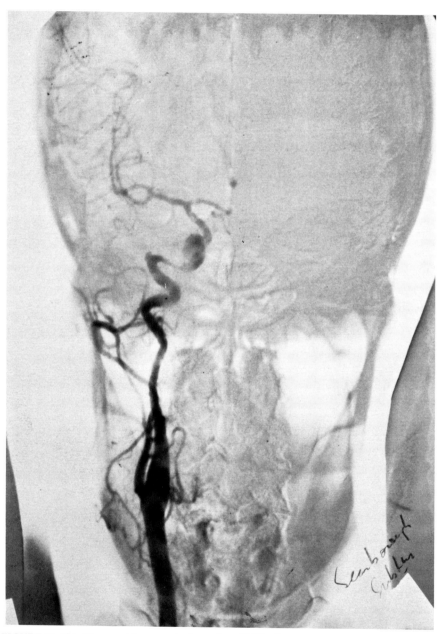

FIGURE 78. This 48-year-old woman had a series of "TIAs," consisting of blurring of the right visual field, and tingling and weakness of the right arm—each episode lasting several minutes. Carotid angiography showed extensive carotid dissection. Note the outpouching ("aneurysm"), which may be a source of emboli.

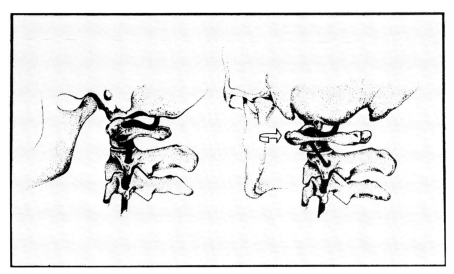

FIGURE 79. Vulnerability of the vertebral artery with rotation of the head. (From Barnett, HJM: *Progress towards stroke prevention: Robert Wartenberg lecture.* Neurology 30:1212, 1980, with permission.)

(Fig. 79), as in the sudden and vigorous, head-turning of chiropractic manipulation.[49-52] Its true incidence may be underestimated because of the lag of hours or days between endothelial damage, thrombus formation, and stroke. Occlusion of a single vertebral artery may be asymptomatic but may decrease the patient's future capacity to compensate for disease of the remaining vertebral artery.

Spontaneous arterial dissection can arise from fibrous dysplasia or atherosclerotic plaque,[53] causing headache, facial pain, parasympathetic palsy, and transient monocular blindness, followed by stroke. It may cause neck bruits.[54] Typical dissection patterns are shown in Figure 80.

Infections

The frequency of *neurosyphilis* is declining but the relative proportion of vascular neurosyphilis is rising in young people,[55] especially among homosexuals[56] and in patients with inadequately treated primary syphilis. There is increasing evidence that later stages of neurosyphilis should be treated with intravenous, and not intramuscular, antibiotics.[57] Meningovascular syphilis may cause diffuse cerebral angiopathy[58] or combined intracranial-extracranial arterial disease.[59]

In *falciparum malaria*, clumps of pigment and parasitized erythrocytes plug vessels, causing headache, confusion, somnolence, and seizures, and, occasionally, focal neurologic signs.[60]

Other infections such as tuberculosis may constrict cerebral arteries, but the cause of cerebral infarction due to infection remains uncertain[61] (Fig. 81).

Arteritis

Collagen vascular diseases such as lupus erythematosus, polyarteritis nodosa, and Wegener's granulomatosis all produce cerebral arteritis.

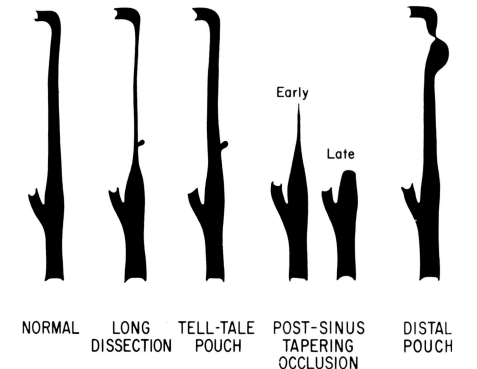

NORMAL   LONG   TELL-TALE   POST-SINUS   DISTAL
         DISSECTION   POUCH   TAPERING   POUCH
                                OCCLUSION

FIGURE 80. Angiographic profiles in carotid dissection (diagrammed). (From Fisher, Ojemann, and Robertson,[54] with permission.)

Patients with collagen vascular disease produce a lupus antibody that is an anticoagulant in vitro but that promotes coagulation and thrombosis in vivo.[62] Systemic lupus erythematosus causes small-vessel vasculitis, but occlusion of major cerebral vessels is rare.[63,64]

Isolated central nervous system angiitis can result in cerebral infarction associated with multiple narrowings of the cerebral arteries.[65]

Drug abuse of oral or intravenous amphetamines (commonly methamphetamines) can cause fibroid necrosis of the media and intima of medium-sized and small cerebral arteries.[66] These vessels may show "beading" and segmental changes in the lumen on angiography[67] in patients presenting with subarachnoid or intracranial hemorrhage[68] (Fig. 82).

Intravenous heroin can induce carotid siphon stenosis and "beading" of intracranial arteries.[69] Intravenous Talwin and Pyribenzamine ("T's," "blues") can cause deep cerebral infarcts or intracerebral hemorrhage.[70] Vascular damage may result from embolization of particulate matter injected intravenously, development of endocarditis and cerebral mycotic aneurysms, and induction of an autoimmune response.[66,70]

Fibromuscular dysplasia involves small to medium-sized branches of the renal, celiac, splenic, hepatic, cervical, and intracranial arteries. It is most often segmental and multifocal, but focal or tubular lesions also occur. It may involve the intima, usually the media, and occasionally the adventitia. Metabolic, ischemic, and immunologic causes have been pos-

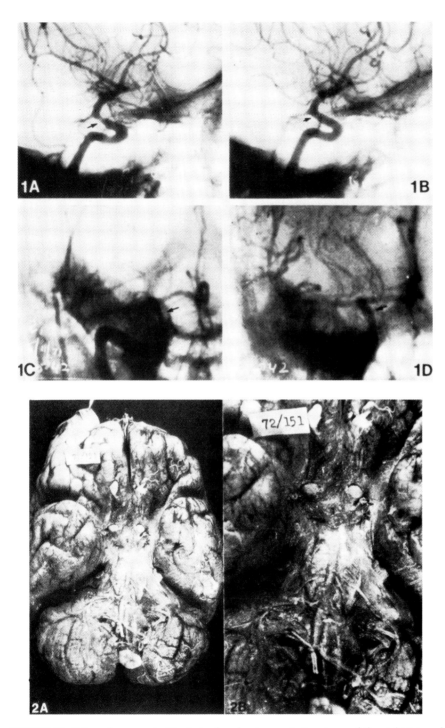

FIGURE 81. Tuberculous meningitis. Lateral and anteroposterior views of the right internal carotid artery, showing narrowing of the supraclinoid segment (*top*). Fifteen weeks later, the narrowing virtually disappeared (*bottom*), despite the fulminating and fatal course of the illness. (From Dalal, PM,[61] with permission.)

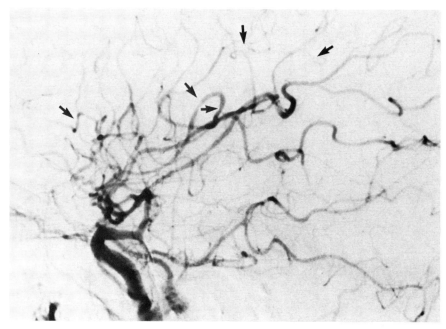

FIGURE 82. A 25-year-old man took four capsules of "street" amphetamine and experienced severe tremors, anxiety, palpitations, and sweating within half an hour. Fifteen minutes later he developed blinding headache, lethargy, neck stiffness, and a right homonymous hemianopia. CT shows a hematoma in the left frontal lobe and another in the left posterior temporal area associated with intraventricular and subarachnoid hemorrhage. Cerebral angiography the next day showed arterial "beading."

tulated.[71] It is often familial and is commoner in women but the cause is unknown. Cerebral angiography reveals it in the distal third of the extracranial internal carotid artery. It is asymptomatic and is found by chance in about 0.6 percent of angiograms.[72] It may cause dissecting aneurysms,[73] berry aneurysms, thrombus formation, and hemorrhagic and ischemic stroke.[71,74,75] Fibromuscular dysplasia producing a stenosing septum in the lumen may induce cerebral ischemic events.[74]

Moyamoya disease is a disease of unknown etiology that produces carotid occlusion with cerebral infarction in children but more commonly intracranial hemorrhages in adults.[76,77] It may represent the exaggerated vascular response of the young brain to major vessel occlusion from any cause.

The characteristic angiographic appearance of net-like vessels at the base of the brain produces a tangled mistiness of collaterals (moyamoya is Japanese for "a puff of smoke") (Fig. 83). The disease is not unique to Japanese patients.[77] Although in Japan the radiologic moyamoya appearance usually corresponds to a clinical entity, a similar appearance can be produced by other conditions.[78]

Takayasu disease is a progressive disease also of unknown etiology, affecting the aorta and major cervical arteries and leading to their stenosis and occlusion.[79] Mural thrombi may form on inflammatory lesions in the elastica of the aorta and carotid and subclavian arteries, causing embolism in the carotid, subclavian, or vertebrobasilar territories.

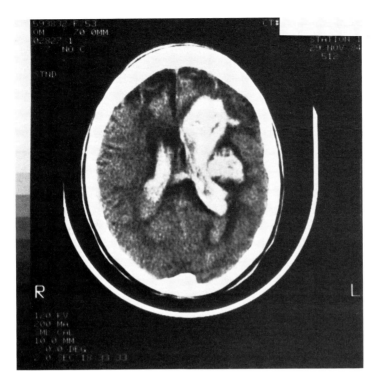

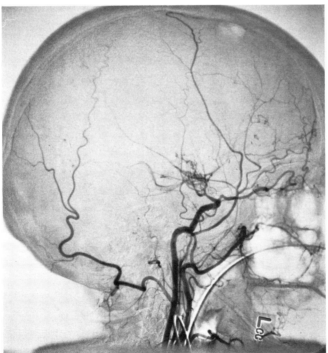

FIGURE 83. This Caucasian woman had a right hemiplegia at age 35, leaving her with a residual spastic hemiparesis. She was readmitted to the hospital 14 years later with a left cerebral hemorrhage (*top*). Subsequent cerebral angiography revealed bilateral moyamoya disease. (*bottom*).

Hematologic Disorders

In *sickle-cell disease,* neurologic complications are more common with the -SS form, but the -SC variant more commonly causes retinal complications. Complications usually occur during a crisis, when increased factor VIII activity and decreased fibrinolytic activity produce platelet-fibrin thrombi. Sickle-cell emboli, necrosis of vascular walls, and capillary and venous stasis cause hemorrhages and small arterial and venous occlusions. Occlusions of larger arteries with cerebral infarction are less common, occurring in about 4 percent of sickle-cell patients.[80,81]

Migraine and hemoglobinopathy together may predispose to stroke. In a Nigerian study, 60 percent of patients with complicated migraine had hemoglobin-AS compared with 20 percent of those with simple migraine.[81] Patients with hemoglobin-AS may develop cerebral infarcts, sometimes multiple, particularly when hypoxic.[82]

Pregnancy and Puerperium

Pregnancy does not protect against stroke; aneurysms and arteriovenous malformations sometimes bleed during pregnancy or rebleed during delivery. Eclampsia is fortunately waning, and only occasionally does it produce intracerebral hemorrhage. Venous thrombosis is declining, perhaps due to previous overdiagnosis.[83-85] A hypercoagulable state during the third trimester and puerperium may enhance the likelihood of arterial and venous stroke.

The incidence of cerebral arterial occlusion during pregnancy and puerperium is 1/20,000 live births, and mortality is three times that of nonpregnant women of the same age.[85]

Oral contraceptives alter platelet aggregation, enhance antithrombin III activity, decrease serum antithrombin levels, and elevate the levels of certain coagulation factors, especially factor VII.[86-89] These changes may be important in predisposing to stroke.

An apparent excess of neuro-ophthalmologic and neurologic complications noted in women on the "pill"[90] was confirmed epidemiologically.[91] The Collaborative Group for the Study of Stroke in Young Women[92] compared 598 nonpregnant women aged 15 to 44 years with stroke with a control group matched for age and race. Relative risks for thrombotic and hemorrhagic stroke were 2.0 and 1.8, respectively. Risks rose sharply with increasing blood pressure, heavy smoking (6.1 to 7.6), and migraine (from 2.0 to 5.9). The incidence of oral contraceptive use among stroke patients (47 percent) seems excessive, compared with 15 to 20 percent of the female population of childbearing age.[93] The Royal College of General Practitioners' Oral Contraception Study[94] prospectively compared 23,000 oral contraceptive users with an equal number of controls. The incidence of all cerebrovascular disease per 1000 woman-years, standardized for age, parity, social class, and smoking status, was 0.62 for pill users and 0.20 for controls. The risk for all types of vascular disease increased with smoking and with age over 35 years. Significantly, the combined incidence of cerebral thrombosis and cerebral embolism (the commonest type of stroke) was 0.19 in users of oral contraceptives and 0.01 in nonusers (giving a relative risk of 19 for users). Former oral contraceptive users had a combined incidence of cerebral thrombosis and embolism of 0.05, their stroke risk remaining elevated for at least 6 years.

While oral contraceptives increase the relative risk of stroke considerably, the absolute risk remains small and must be weighed against the potential consequences of not using them. Attributing stroke to oral contraceptive use is dependent upon first excluding all other likely causes, such as mitral valve prolapse.

Disseminated intravascular coagulopathy may result from head trauma, surgical operations, neurologic disturbances, eclampsia, diabetic ketoacidosis, and shock, which may damage tissue, including vascular endothelium, and discharge thromboplastin into the bloodstream. Phospholipids released by damaged red cells accelerate clotting, whereas fibrin and other degradation products and local consumption of clotting factors produce an anticoagulant tendency, resulting in ischemic or hemorrhagic strokes. In the young, hemorrhagic lesions predominate.[95]

Thrombotic thrombocytopenic purpura usually affects young patients, particularly women, who present with microangiopathic hemolytic anemia with prominent red cell fragmentation. Thrombocytopenia, fluctuating neurologic signs, and fever are also common.[96] Thrombotic thrombocytopenic purpura causes widespread noninflammatory thrombotic occlusions of arterioles and capillaries by fibrin and platelet aggregations. These occlusions can occur anywhere in the body, but especially in the brain and heart, resulting in multiple infarctions and, sometimes, petechial hemorrhages.[97] Treatment with plasmapheresis and antiplatelet agents remains unproven.[98]

Alcoholic Intoxication

Forty percent of adults with cerebral infarction were intoxicated with alcohol during the preceding 24 hours, a rate four to seven times greater in men and six to 15 times greater in women than in the Finnish population of the same age.[99] The Framingham data indicate a relationship between alcohol intake and stroke in men.[100] Alcoholism may increase the risk of stroke by raising blood pressure[101] and may precipitate cerebral infarction through dehydration, increased blood viscosity, and coagulability.[99] Unreported or forgotten trauma to cervical arteries remains a plausible but unproven mechanism. Ethanol produces graded contraction of rat cerebral arterioles and Altura postulates that alcohol-induced spasm of cerebral blood vessels contributes to alcohol-associated stroke.[102]

Venous Infarction

Cerebral venous infarction is rare compared with arterial stroke, but its true incidence may be underestimated since it is similar clinically to arterial infarction. Even when suspected, it may be missed unless the venous phase of cerebral angiography is studied.[103,104] Carcinoma, leukemia, polycythemia, sickle-cell crisis, trauma, dehydration, congestive heart failure,[105] sepsis, pregnancy and the puerperium, and the contraceptive pill[106] may precipitate cerebral venous thrombosis.[107,108]

Cerebral venous infarction, usually due to cortical vein thrombosis, is often hemorrhagic. Occlusion of the venous sinuses plugs the arachnoid villi, blocks reabsorption of cerebrospinal fluid, and increases intracranial pressure.

In cortical venous thrombosis, headache (from inflammation of pain-sensitive veins and dura) is usually the first symptom, followed by recurrent focal seizures and other signs such as aphasia and hemiparesis. Headache from increased intracranial pressure, with stupor and coma, indicate progressing cerebral edema and extension of the clot to adjacent dural sinuses. In sagittal sinus thrombosis, paraplegia occurs with seizures on alternating sides. Headache due to increased intracranial pressure and focal neurologic signs may also occur. The thrombus may extend into the superior cortical veins, producing additional focal symptoms and signs. Lateral sinus thrombosis produces increased intracranial pressure, and propagation of the thrombus to adjacent cortical veins causes seizures and contralateral weakness of the face and arm. This syndrome usually follows otitis or mastoiditis, which are less common since the advent of antibiotics.

Cavernous sinus thrombosis causes local signs of infection and exophthalmos, ophthalmoplegia, and hyperalgesia in the first division of the trigeminal nerve. Involvement of the cranial nerves coursing through the cavernous sinus (III, IV, V-1, and VI) is common and visual impairment may also occur. Cavernous sinus thrombosis usually follows infection of the face and paranasal sinuses. Its incidence has decreased with effective antibiotic treatment but opportunistic and fungal infections may supervene, especially in diabetic or immunosuppressed patients.[108]

Thrombosis of cerebellar veins produces hemorrhagic cerebellar infarction, which becomes an expanding mass in the posterior fossa, necessitating urgent surgical decompression.

CEREBRAL HEMORRHAGE

Arteriovenous Malformations

Arteriovenous malformations (AVMs) are abnormalities in embryonal development leading to a skein of tangled arteries and veins, usually without an intervening capillary bed. About 0.14 percent of the population harbor an AVM.[109] The peak incidence of ruptured AVMs is in patients of both sexes between the ages of 20 and 40 years.

Subarachnoid hemorrhage with intraparenchymal clot occurs more commonly than does subarachnoid hemorrhage alone.[110] Most AVMs occur in the distribution of the middle cerebral artery in a wedge that includes superficial abnormal vessels with the apex pointing centrally. The high blood flow through an AVM may siphon blood from distant areas of the brain, producing relative ischemia, a form of "intracranial steal."[111] About 10 percent of patients with AVMs will have an associated berry aneurysm.[109] Small capillary telangiectasias in the basal ganglia and brainstem usually remain asymptomatic, occasionally bursting into devastating hematomas.[112]

Arteriovenous malformations cause cerebral hemorrhages or seizures.[113] Only 1 percent of AVM patients presenting with seizures bled within 1 year, all surviving;[113] whereas 7 percent of patients presenting with hemorrhage bled again within 1 year, 0.9 percent dying.

Ruptured Berry Aneurysm

One quarter of North American patients with ruptured aneurysms die or become disabled through misdiagnosis or mismanagement each year.[114] The sudden severe headache of subarachnoid hemorrhage with neck stiffness is seldom misinterpreted, but the symptoms of the "warning leak" are often missed. According to Gillingham, 70 percent of patients admitted in stupor or coma from subarachnoid hemorrhage had at least one minor forewarning of the catastrophe. These patients present with occipital or neck pain radiating to the vertex or spine, occasionally with vomiting. Most patients have persisting headache or neck stiffness but can return to work in 48 hours.[115] When in doubt, lumbar puncture should be performed, if necessary in the emergency room.

Intracerebral Hemorrhage

In a young person, intraparenchymal hemorrhage from arteriovenous malformation, aneurysm, hypertension, coagulopathy, anticoagulants, and especially from drug abuse should be considered (see Fig. 82). Certain tumors may present with multiple intracranial hemorrhages, including malignant melanoma, hypernephroma, and choriocarcinoma.

HYPERTENSIVE ENCEPHALOPATHY

Sudden, severe hypertension as in pheochromocytoma may cause headache. In hypertensive encephalopathy there is visual blurring, nausea, and vomiting, owing to increased intracranial pressure. Convulsions and focal neurologic signs sometimes occur. Although its incidence is declining, this condition may arise at any age and it remains a problem in the second to fourth decades of life, especially in patients with acute nephritis or toxemia.[116]

CONCLUSION

Strokes in the young are due to different causes than in older age groups, since cerebral arteriosclerosis is unusual. The causes of ischemic stroke are cardiac embolism, migraine, trauma, arteritis, and coagulopathies. Atherosclerosis is only causal in young patients when there are unusually premature risk factors, such as hypertension, diabetes, and hyperlipidemia.

Young stroke patients have the greatest recovery potential and the greatest likelihood of finding a remediable lesion, which justifies extensive investigation. The less the expertise and confidence of the physician, the greater the need for complete investigation, including cerebral angiography.

Cerebral hemorrhage is more commonly due to an arteriovenous malformation or ruptured berry aneurysm than are the hypertensive and amyloid types of stroke seen in older patients. Special investigations such as CT scanning and angiography are essential in cerebral hemorrhage of the young, since surgery is more feasible in these cases.

REFERENCES

1. WALKER, AE, ROBINS, M, AND WEINFELD, FD: *Clinical findings.* In WEINFELD, FD (ED): *The National Survey of Stroke.* Stroke 12 (Suppl 1): I-15, 1981.

2. BHARUCHA, EP, AND UMERJI, RS: *Cerebrovascular disease in India.* Neurology (India) 10:137, 1962.

3. DALAL, PM: *Strokes in the young in west central India.* In GOLDSTEIN, M, ET AL (EDS): *Advances in Neurology,* Vol 25. Raven Press, New York, 1979, p 339.

4. BARNETT, HJM: *Heart in ischemic stroke—A changing emphasis.* Neurol Clin 1:291, 1983.

5. PORTAL, RW: *Mitral stenosis: The picture changes.* Br Med J 288:167, 1984.

6. STATISTICS CANADA: *Causes of death 1978.* Queen's Printer, Ottawa, 1980.

7. WOLF, PA, ET AL: *Duration of atrial fibrillation and imminence of stroke: The Framingham study.* Stroke 14:664, 1983.

8. BROWN, OR, KOLSTER, FE, AND DeMOTS, H: *Incidence of mitral valve prolapse in the asymptomatic normal* (abstr). Circulation (Suppl 2):77, 1975.

9. PROCACCI, PM, ET AL: *Clinical frequency and implications of mitral valve prolapse in the female population* (abstr). Circulation 51, 52 (Suppl 2):78, 1975.

10. BARNETT, HJM, ET AL: *Further evidence relating mitral-valve prolapse to cerebral ischemic events.* N Engl J Med 302:139, 1980.

11. BROWN, OR, ET AL: *Aortic root dilatation and mitral valve prolapse in Marfan's syndrome: An echocardiographic study.* Circulation 52:651, 1975.

12. LEBWOHL, MG, ET AL: *Pseudoxanthoma elasticum and mitral-valve prolapse.* N Engl J Med 307:228, 1982.

13. ROSENBERG, CA, ET AL: *Hypomastia and mitral-valve prolapse.* N Engl J Med 309:1230, 1983.

14. FURLAN, AJ, ET AL: *Cerebrovascular complications associated with idiopathic hypertrophic subaortic stenosis.* Stroke 15:282, 1984.

15. BUCHER, EH, AND SCHOFIELD, CJ: *Economic assault on Chagas disease.* New Scientist 101:321, 1981.

16. WOOD, JN, ET AL: *A monoclonal antibody defining antigenic determinants on subpopulations of mammalian neurones and Trypanosoma cruzi parasites.* Nature 296:34, 1982.

17. SANDOK, BA, VON ESTORFF, I, AND GIULIANI, ER: *Subsequent neurological events in patients with atrial myxoma.* Ann Neurol 8:305, 1980.

18. JONES HR JR, ET AL: *Cerebral emboli of paradoxical origin.* Ann Neurol 13:314, 1983.

19. LAUGHLIN, RA, AND MANDEL, SR: *Paradoxical embolism, case report and review of the literature.* Arch Surg 112:648, 1977.

20. WATERS, WE: *The Epidemiology of Migraine.* Böhringer Ingelheim, Bracknell, United Kingdom, 1974.

21. SYMONDS, C: *Migrainous variants.* Trans Med Soc Lond 67:237, 1952.

22. GUEST, IA, AND WOOLF, AL: *Fatal infarction of brain in migraine.* Br Med J 1:225, 1964.

23. CALA, LA, AND MASTAGLIA, FL: *Computerized axial tomography findings in a group of patients with migrainous headaches.* Proc Aust Assoc Neurol 13:35, 1976.

24. HUNGERFORD, GD, DU BOULAY, GH, AND ZILKHA, KJ: *Computerised axial tomography in patients with severe migraine: A preliminary report.* J Neurol Neurosurg Psychiatry 39:990, 1976.

25. MATHEW, NT, ET AL: *Abnormal CT-scans in migraine.* Headache 16:272, 1977.

26. RASCOL, A, ET AL: *Accidents ischemiques cérébraux au cours de crises migraineuses.* Rev Neurol 12:867, 1979.

27. CORBETT, JJ: *Neuro-ophthalmic complications of migraine and cluster headaches.* Neurol Clin 1:973, 1983.

28. WILLIS, T: *De Anima Brutorum.* Oxford, England, 1672.

29. LATHAM, PA: *Clinical lectures on nervous or sick headaches.* Br Med J 1:305, 336, 1872.

30. SCHILLER, F: *The migraine tradition.* Bull Hist Med 49:1, 1975.

31. GOLTMAN, AM: *The mechanics of migraine.* J Allergy Clin Immunol 7:351, 1935.

32. MARCUSSEN, RM, AND WOLFF, HG: *Studies on headache.* Arch Neurol Psychiatry 23:42, 1950.

33. HACHINSKI, VC, PORCHAWKA, J, AND STEELE, JC: *Visual symptoms in the migraine syndrome.* Neurology 23:570, 1973.

34. DUKES, HT, AND VIETH, RG: *Cerebral arteriography during migraine prodrome and headache.* Neurology 14:636, 1964.

35. O'BRIEN, MD: *Cerebral cortex perfusion rates in migraine.* Lancet 1:1036, 1967.

36. HACHINSKI, VC, ET AL: *Cerebral hemodynamics in migraine.* Can J Neurol Sci 4:245, 1977.

37. NORRIS, JW, HACHINSKI, VC, AND COOPER, PW: *Changes in cerebral blood flow during a migraine attack.* Br Med J 3:676, 1975.

38. SKINHØJ, E: *Hemodynamic studies within the brain during migraine.* Arch Neurol 29:207, 1973.

39. SIMARD, D, AND PAULSON, OB: *Cerebral vasomotor paralysis during migraine attack.* Arch Neurol 29:207, 1973.

40. SAKAI, F, AND MEYER, JS: *Regional cerebral hemodynamics during migraine and cluster headaches measured by the Xe-133 inhalation method.* Headache 18:122, 1978.

41. OLESEN, J, LARSEN, B, AND LAURITZEN, M: *Focal hyperemia followed by spreading oligemia and impaired activation of rCBF in classic migraine.* Ann Neurol 9:344, 1981.

42. LAURITZEN, M, AND OLESEN, J: *Regional cerebral blood flow during migraine attacks by xenon-133 inhalation and emission tomography.* Brain 107:447, 1984.

43. KALENDOVSKY, Z, AND AUSTIN, JH: *Changes in blood clotting systems during migraine attacks.* Headache 16:293, 1977.

44. COUCH, JR, AND HASSANEIN, RS: *Platelet aggregability in migraine.* Neurology 27:843, 1977.

45. LOUIS, S, AND MCDOWELL, F: *Stroke in young adults.* Ann Intern Med 66:932, 1967.

46. FOGELHOLM, R, AND AHO, K: *Ischemic cerebrovascular disease in young adults. i. Smoking habits, use of oral contraceptives, relative weight, blood pressure and electrocardiographic findings.* Acta Neurol Scand 49:415, 1973.

47. SENEVIRATNE, BIB, AND AMERATUNGA, B: *Strokes young adults.* Br Med J 3:791, 1972.

48. EASTON, JD, AND HART, RG: *Underestimated causes of stroke.* Ann Neurol 16:37, 1983.

49. PRATT-THOMAS, HR, AND BERGER, KE: *Cerebellar and spinal injuries after chiropractic manipulation.* JAMA 133:600, 1947.

50. EASTON, JD, AND SHERMAN, DG: *Cervical manipulation and stroke.* Stroke 8:594, 1977.

51. ROBERTSON, JT: *Neck manipulation as a cause of stroke.* Stroke 12:1, 1981.

52. SHERMAN, DG, HART, RG, AND EASTON, JD: *Abrupt change in head position and cerebral infarction.* Stroke 12:2, 1981.

53. BOGOUSSLAVSKY, J, REGLI, F, AND DESPLAND, PA: *Aneurysmes dissequants spontanés de l'artere carotide interne.* Rev Neurol 140:625, 1984.

54. FISHER, CM, OJEMANN, RG, AND ROBERTSON, GH: *Spontaneous dissection of cervico-cerebral arteries.* Can J Neurol Sci 5:9, 1978.

55. HEATHFIELD, KWG: *The decline of neurolues.* Practitioner 217:753, 1976.

56. CENTERS FOR DISEASE CONTROL: *Syphilis trends in the United States.* MMWR 1(30):441, 1981.

57. HOLMES, MD, BRANT-ZAWADSKI, MM, AND SIMON, RP: *Clinical features of meningovascular syphilis.* Neurology 34:553, 1984.

58. VATZ, KA, ET AL: *Neurosyphilis and diffuse cerebral angiopathy: A case report.* Neurology 24:472, 1974.

59. MERRITT, H, ADAMS, R, AND SOLOMON, H: *Neurosyphilis.* Oxford University Press, New York, 1946.

60. WYLER, DJ: *Malaria—Resurgence, resistance, and research.* N Engl J Med 308:875, 934, 1983.

61. DALAL, PM: *Observations on the involvement of cerebral vessels in tuberculous meningitis in adults.* In GOLDSTEIN, M, ET AL (EDS): *Advances in Neurology.* Vol 25. Raven Press, New York, 1979, p 149.

62. BOEY, ML, ET AL: *Thrombosis in systemic lupus erythematosus: striking association with the presence of circulating lupus anticoagulant.* Br Med J 287:1021, 1983.

63. TREVOR, RP, ET AL: *Angiographic demonstration of major cerebral vessel occlusion in systemic lupus erythematosus.* Neuroradiology 4:202, 1972.

64. ELLIS, SG, AND VERITY, MA: *Central nervous system involvement in systemic lupus erythematosus: A review of neuropathologic findings in 57 cases, 1955–1977.* Semin Arthritis Rheum 8:212, 1979.

65. CUPPS, TR, MOORE, PM, AND FAUCI, AS: *Isolated angiitis of the central nervous system.* Am J Med 74:97, 1983.

66. CITRON, BP, ET AL: *Necrotizing angiitis associated with drug abuse.* N Engl J Med 283:1003, 1970.

67. RUMBAUGH, CL, ET AL: *Cerebral angiographic changes in the drug abuse patient.* Radiology 101:335, 1971.

68. DELANEY, P, AND ESTES, M: *Intracranial hemorrhage with amphetamine abuse.* Neurology 30:1125, 1980.

69. BRUST, JCM, ET AL: *Aphasia in acute stroke.* Stroke 7:167, 1976.

70. CAPLAN, LR, HIER, DB, AND BANKS, G: *Stroke and drug abuse.* Stroke 82:869, 1982.

71. METTINGER, KL, AND ERICSON, K: *Fibromuscular dysplasia and the brain, observations on angiographic, clinical and genetic characteristics.* Stroke 13:46, 1982.

72. CORRIN, LS, SANDOK, BA, AND HOUSER, OW: *Cerebral ischemic events in patients with carotid artery fibromuscular dysplasia.* Arch Neurol 38:616, 1981.

73. POLLOCK, M, AND JACKSON, BM: *Fibromuscular dysplasia of the carotid arteries.* Neurology 21:1226, 1971.

74. SO, EL, ET AL: *Cephalic fibromuscular dysplasia in 32 patients, clinical findings and radiologic features.* Arch Neurol 38:619, 1981.

75. SANDOK, BA: *Fibromuscular dysplasia of the internal carotid artery.* Neurol Clin 1:17, 1983.

76. SUZUKI, J, AND TAKAKU, A: *Cerebrovascular 'Moyamoya' disease.* Arch Neurol 20:288, 1969.

77. SUZUKI, J, AND KODAMA, N: *Moyamoya disease—A review.* Stroke 14:104, 1983.

78. DEBRUN, G, ET AL: *Moyamoya, a nonspecific radiologic syndrome.* Neuroradiology 8:241, 1975.

79. DALAL, PM: *The aortic arch syndrome.* In SPILLANE, JD (ED): *Tropical Neurology.* Oxford University Press, London, 1973, p 92.

80. STOCKMAN, JA, ET AL: *Occlusion of large cerebral vessels in sickle-cell anemia.* N Engl J Med 287:846, 1972.

81. OSUNTOKUN, BO: *Undernutrition and infectious disorders as risk factors in stroke (with special reference to Africans).* In GOLDSTEIN, M, ET AL (EDS): *Advances in Neurology,* Vol 25. Raven Press, New York, 1979, p 161.

82. HANDLER, CE, AND PERKIN, GD: *Sickle cell trait and multiple cerebral infarctions.* J R Soc Med 75:550, 1982.

83. RASCOL, A, ET AL: *Accidents vasculaires cérébraux pendant la grossesse et le post-partum.* In BALLIÈRE, J-B (ED): *Maladies vasculaires cérébrales.* 2ième Conf de la Salpetrière, Paris, 1980.

84. AMIES, AG: *Cerebral vascular disease in pregnancy. I. Hemorrhage.* J Obstet Gynaecol 77:100, 1970.

85. CROSS, JN, CASTRO, PO, AND JENNETT, WB: *Cerebral strokes associated with pregnancy and the puerperium.* Br Med J 3:214, 1968.

86. POLLER, L, TABIOWO, A, AND THOMPSON, JM: *Effects of low-dose oral contraceptives on blood coagulation.* Br Med J 3:218, 1968.

87. LEFF, B, ET AL: *Effect of oral contraceptive use on platelet prothrombin converting (platelet factor 3) activity.* Thromb Res 15:631, 1979.

88. MEADE, TW, GREENBERG, G, AND THOMPSON, SG: *Progestogens and cardiovascular reactions associated with oral contraceptives and a comparison of the safety of 50- and 30-µg oestrogen preparations.* Br Med J 1:1157, 1980.

89. ZAHAVI, J, AND KAKKAR, VV: *β-thromboglobulin—A specific marker of in-vivo platelet release reaction.* Thromb Haemost 117:23, 1980.

90. WALSH, FB: *Oral contraceptives and neuro-ophthalmologic interest.* Arch Ophthalmol 74:628, 1965.

91. VESSEY, MP, AND DOLL, R: *Investigation of relation between use of oral contraceptives and thromboembolic diseases.* Br Med J 2:651, 1969.

92. COLLABORATIVE GROUP FOR THE STUDY OF STROKE IN YOUNG WOMEN: *Oral contraceptives and stroke in young women.* JAMA 231:718, 1975.

93. HART, RG, AND MILLER, VT: *Cerebral infarction in young adults: A practical approach.* Stroke 14:110, 1983.

94. ROYAL COLLEGE OF GENERAL PRACTITIONERS' ORAL CONTRACEPTION STUDY: *Incidence of arterial disease among oral contraceptive users.* J R Coll Gen Prac 33:75, 1983.

95. HAMILTON, PJ, STALKER, AL, AND DOUGLAS, AS: *Disseminated intravascular coagulation: A review.* J Clin Pathol 31:601, 1978.

96. SILVERSTEIN, A: *Thrombotic thrombocytopenic purpura, initial neurologic manifestations.* Arch Neurol 18:358, 1968.

97. MEACHAM, GC, ET AL: *Thrombocytic thrombocytopenic purpura, a disseminated disease of arterioles.* Blood 6:706, 1951.

98. MYERS, TJ, ET AL: *Thrombotic thrombocytopenic purpura: Combined treatment with plasmapheresis and antiplatelet agents.* Ann Intern Med 92:149, 1980.

99. HILLBOM, M, KASTE, M, AND RASI, V: *Can ethanol intoxication affect hemocoagulation with increased risk of infarction in young adults?* Neurology 33:381, 1983.

100. WOLF, PA, KANNEL, WB, AND VERTER, J: *Current status of risk factors for stroke.* Neurol Clin 1:317, 1983.

101. MITCHELL, PI, MORGAN, MJ, BOADLE, DJ, ET AL: *Role of alcohol in the aetiology of hypertension.* Med J Aust 2:198, 1980.

102. ALTURA, BM, ALTURA, BT, AND GEBREWOLD, A: *Alcohol-induced spasms of cerebral blood vessels: Relation to cerebrovascular accidents and sudden death.* Science 220:331, 1983.

103. KINGSLEY, DPE, ET AL: *Superior sagittal sinus thrombosis: An evaluation of the changes demonstrated on computed tomography.* J Neurol Neurosurg Psychiatry 41:1065, 1978.

104. AUERBACK, P: *Primary cerebral venous thrombosis in young adults: The diverse manifestations of an under-recognized disease.* Ann Neurol 3:81, 1978.

105. TOWBIN, A: *The syndrome of latent cerebral venous thrombosis: Its frequency and relation to age in congestive cardiac failure.* Stroke 4:419, 1973.

106. ATKINSON, EA, FAIRBURN, B, AND HEATHFIELD, KWG: *Intracranial venous thrombosis as complication of oral contraceptives.* Lancet 1:914, 1970.

107. KALBAG, RM, AND WOOLF, AL: *Cerebral Venous Thrombosis.* Oxford University Press, London, 1967.

108. HUMPHREY, PRD, CLARKE, CRA, AND GREENWOOD, RJ: *Cerebral venous thrombosis.* In HARRISON, MJG, AND DYKEN, ML: *Cerebral Vascular Disease.* Butterworths, London, 1983, p 309.

109. MITCHELSON, WS: *Natural history and pathophysiology of arteriovenous malformations.* Clin Neurosurg 26:307, 1979.

110. DRAKE, CG: *Cerebral arteriovenous malformations: Considerations for and experience with surgical treatment in 166 cases.* Clin Neurosurg 26:145, 1979.

111. HACHINSKI, VC, ET AL: *Symptomatic intracranial steal.* Arch Neurol 34:149, 1977.

112. AMINOFF, MJ: *Angiomas and fistulae involving the nervous system.* In ROSS RUSSELL, RW (ED): *Vascular Disease of the Central Nervous System.* Churchill-Livingstone, Edinburgh, 1983, p 296.

113. PERIET, G, AND NISHIOKI, H: *Arteriovenous malformations, an analysis of 545 cases of craniocerebral arteriovenous malformations and fistuli reported to the cooperative study.* J Neurosurg 25:467, 1966.

114. KASSELL, NF, AND DRAKE, CG: *Review of the management of saccular aneurysms.* Neurol Clin 1:73, 1983.

115. GILLINGHAM, FJ: *The management of ruptured intracranial aneurysms.* Scott Med J 12:377, 1967.

116. DINSDALE, HB: *Hypertensive encephalopathy.* Neurol Clin 1:3, 1983.

Chapter 10

CARDIAC DISEASE AND STROKE

The profession have long been aware of the concomitance of the diseases of the heart and diseases of the brain.
Samuel Solly, 1848

The heart and brain share close anatomic, epidemiologic, and pathologic relationships. Heart disease as a cause of stroke was recognized as long ago as the last century,[1] but discovery of the complex interrelationship of vascular disease of the heart and brain had to await development of diagnostic technology and epidemiologic strategies. Data from the Framingham Study[2-4] indicated the importance of hypertension, ischemic heart disease, and chronic atrial fibrillation as risk factors for ischemic stroke. The apparent low incidence of cardiac causes of stroke noted by clinicians did not concur with either the pathologic and angiographic data indicating the importance of extracranial arterial disease in stroke patients,[5,6] or with the high frequency of cardiac embolic sources found at autopsy.[7]

Demonstration by cardiac imaging techniques of the full spectrum of cardiac dysfunction in stroke was limited by the risks of angiocardiography and the technical difficulties of M-mode scanning. Two-dimensional echocardiography now often documents cardiac etiology for stroke when none was previously suspected.[8-10] Acute rheumatic heart disease has fortunately declined to a vanishing point[11] but, as the frequency of subsequent cardiac embolism decreases, that from prosthetic heart valves remains and mitral valve prolapse is increasingly recognized as a cause of cardioembolic stroke.[12]

Long-term ECG (Holter) monitoring in acute cerebrovascular lesions, especially subarachnoid hemorrhage, reveals a variety of cardiac arrhythmias, some fatal.[13,14] Their relationship to cardiac micronecrosis

CARDIAC DISEASE
AND STROKE

165

and the possible role of excessive plasma catecholamines secondary to autonomic disturbance remains speculative.[15]

THE INTERRELATIONSHIP OF VASCULAR DISEASE OF THE HEART AND BRAIN

Cardiovascular and cerebrovascular disease share more than etiology. Both represent disturbed arterial perfusion of critical organs which are exquisitely sensitive to hypoxia and ischemia. Experimental cerebral ischemia induced by systemic anoxia produces premature circulatory collapse from cardiac arrhythmias (Fig. 84). While brain perfusion is critically dependent upon cardiac function, the heart is highly sensitive to neural control, as sudden death from psychologic causes illustrates.[16–18]

Warnings of impending cardiac or cerebral necrosis (angina or TIAs) were initially attributed to vasospasm. However, cerebral vasospasm is an unusual cause of stroke, restricted to subarachnoid hemorrhage and

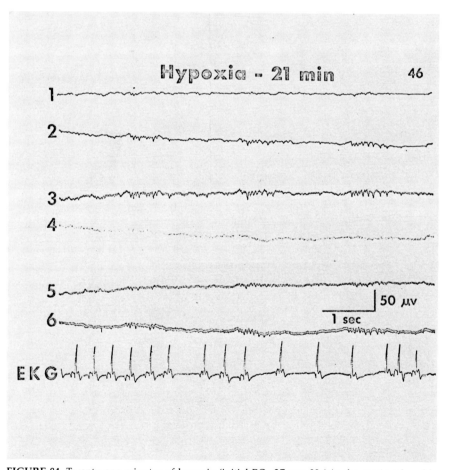

FIGURE 84. Twenty-one minutes of hypoxia (initial PO_2 27 mm Hg) in the cat (produced by inhaling 4 percent O_2 for 3 hours). EEG *(upper six tracings)* shows reduction in voltage. ECG shows variable tachycardias and heart block. Cardiac stimulants and pressor agents were necessary throughout the experiment to prevent fatal cardiovascular collapse. (From Norris, JW, and Pappius, HM: *Cerebral water and electrolytes—Effect of asphyxia, hypoxia and hypercapnia.* Arch Neurol 23:248, 1970, with permission.)

perhaps migraine, while coronary vasospasm (Prinzmetal's angina) occurring in an otherwise healthy vessel seldom progresses to frank myocardial infarction. More commonly, the lesion results from critical atherosclerotic stenosis of the conduit vessel, and arterial thrombus is infrequently found at autopsy. Arteriosclerosis develops later in life in the cerebral than in the coronary vessels, but its overall severity is similar in the individual.[19]

Epidemiologic Interrelationships

Vascular disease, the commonest disorder of both heart and brain, causes more than half of the deaths in the western world.[20] Although the incidence of ischemic heart disease did not initially share the dramatic decrease experienced by stroke, the incidence of both diseases has declined over 20 percent since 1968 (Fig. 85). Cardiovascular, cerebrovascular, and peripheral vascular disease often coexist,[21] sharing risk factors of degenerative arteriopathy. Hypertension is the most powerful determinant of morbidity and mortality while ischemic heart disease and diabetes are important secondary factors (Fig. 86).

Stroke and ischemic heart disease are risks for each other. The fivefold risk of stroke associated with coronary heart disease[2] was not due to mural thrombosis, since patients with strokes occurring within 6 months of myocardial infarction were excluded. Ischemic cardiac events are the commonest outcome in any form of cerebrovascular disease. Myocardial infarction is a commoner cause of death than stroke in patients with asymptomatic carotid bruits, previous stroke, transient ischemic attacks, and postcarotid endarterectomy.[22-25]

Left ventricular hypertrophy on ECG carries a ninefold risk of cerebral infarction, chest x-ray evidence of cardiac enlargement a threefold risk[2-4,26] (Fig. 87), and atrial fibrillation a fivefold risk—factors largely expressing coexistent hypertension. The risk profiles of cerebral and myocardial infarction differ. The male preponderance seen in ischemic heart disease is less prominent in stroke, especially in the early years.[23,27] The incidence of ischemic cerebral disease is maximal a decade later than ischemic heart disease.[20] Cigarette smoking and serum lipids are less certain risk factors of ischemic cerebral disease.[28]

In the Toronto Unit, the incidence of overall heart disease largely reflects the incidence of hypertension (Table 33). Hypertensive and ischemic heart disease together represented 87 percent of all cardiac disease encountered in ischemic and hemorrhagic stroke, while chronic rheumatic valvular heart disease accounted for only 1 percent.

CARDIAC CAUSES OF STROKE

Cerebral Embolism

Embolic stroke usually arises from thrombi on the left atrium, cardiac valves ("endocarditis"), or ventricular wall. Rarely, thrombi from plaques in the great vessels or from cardiac tumor are responsible. In some parts of the world, cardiomyopathies such as Chagas' disease are important causes.[29]

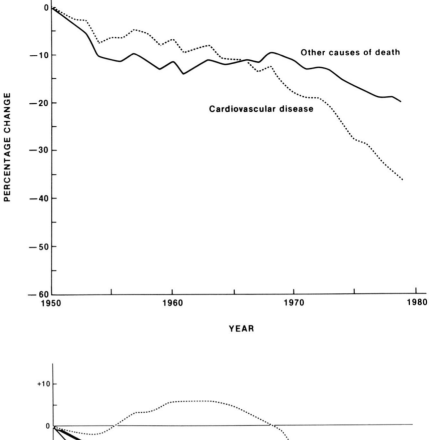

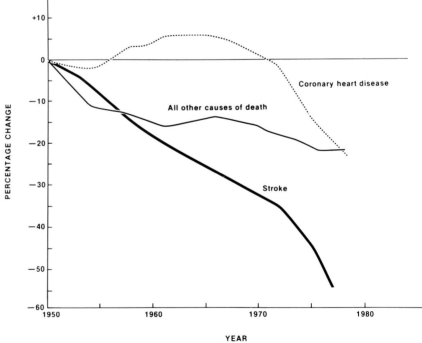

FIGURE 85. Declining incidence of cardiovascular *(top)* and cerebrovascular *(bottom)* disease, 1950 to 1980. (Adapted from Levy and Moskowitz,[20] with permission).

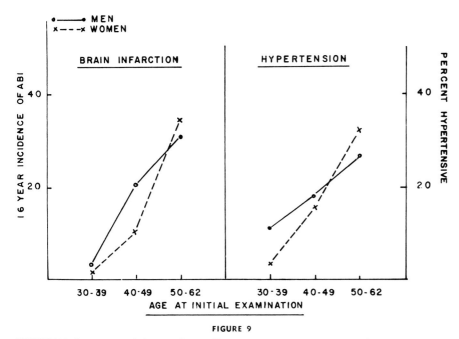

FIGURE 9

FIGURE 86. Age-sex trends in prevalence of hypertension versus incidence of atherothrombotic brain infarction. Men and women aged 30 to 62 at entry: Framingham Study. (From Levy and Moskowitz,[20] with permission.)

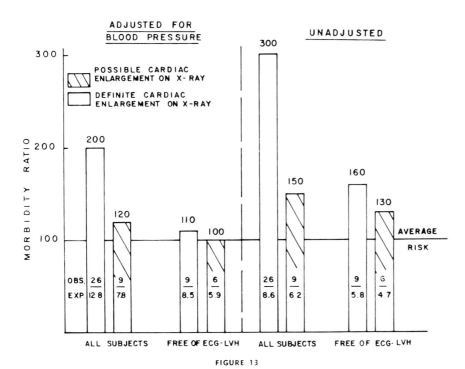

FIGURE 13

FIGURE 87. Risk of atherothrombotic brain infarction (16-year followup) according to prior cardiac enlargement on x-ray, ECG, and blood pressure. (From Levy and Moskowitz,[20] with permission.)

TABLE 33. Incidence of Heart Disease in 560 Consecutive Stroke Patients Admitted to the Toronto Acute Stroke Unit

	Hypertensive	Ischemic	Other*	Rheumatic	Total
Cerebral infarction	210	77	31	15	333/512
Cerebral hemorrhage	24	6	3	0	33/48

*Prolapsing mitral valve (7); prosthetic heart valves (3); cardiomyopathy (2); cor pulmonale, left atrial myxoma, and others (1 each).

Embolism from the heart has long been an underestimated cause of cerebral infarction, confirmed by the retrospective autopsy review of Blackwood and coworkers.[7] Half of 105 patients with cerebral infarction had associated cardiac disease, mostly due to endocarditis or rheumatic valvular disease. The high incidence of endocarditis and rheumatic valvular heart disease largely reflected childhood rheumatic fever of a bygone era. More recent data indicate that 20 to 30 percent of ischemic strokes are of cardiogenic origin, of which only a minority are due to rheumatic valvular heart disease (Table 34).[30-32]

The diagnostic difficulties posed by cerebral embolism result in a lower incidence (3 to 8 percent) of identified cardiac sources in clinical compared with pathologic studies.[23,33,34] No unequivocal criteria for differentiating "embolic" from "thrombotic" stroke have yet been defined.

TABLE 34. 136 Patients with Cerebral Infarcts due to Presumed Cardiac Embolism

Idiopathic atrial fibrillation	89 (65%)
Valvular disease	29 (21%)
Thyrotoxicosis and atrial fibrillation	3 (2%)
Myocardial infarction	9 (7%)
Other causes	6 (4%)

From Gautier,[30] with permission.

TABLE 35. Diagnosis of Cardiac Embolism

Essential criteria—Potential embolic source
  Atrial fibrillation (paroxysmal or chronic)
  Sick sinus syndrome
  Mitral stenosis (with or without atrial fibrillation)
  Prosthetic cardiac valve
  Endocarditis
  Myocardial infarction within 3 months of stroke
  Ventricular aneurysm
  Cardiomyopathy (with or without demonstrable clot)
  Mitral valve prolapse
  Annulus calcification
  Left atrial myxoma

Suggestive criteria
  Involvement of multiple vascular territories in the acute stage
  Seizure at onset
  Branch occlusion of cerebral arteries on arteriogram
  CT finding of multiple infarcts or hemorrhagic infarct
  Concurrent peripheral embolism

TABLE 36. Incidence of Cardiac Lesions in 222 Patients with Cerebral Infarction Admitted to the Toronto Acute Stroke Unit

Relationship	Number		Percent
None		175	79
Embolic source		44	20
Atrial fibrillation	26		
Mural embolism	4		
Prolapsed mitral valve syndrome	3		
Chronic rheumatic heart disease	3		
Subacute bacterial endocarditis	2		
Ventricular aneurysm	2		
Prosthetic heart valves	2		
Cardiomyopathy	1		
Atrial myxoma	1		
Presumed hemodynamic		3	1
Accidental surgical hypotension	2		
Paroxysmal ventricular tachycardia	1		

Even the role of carotid artery disease in generating artery-to-artery emboli is disputed, and the high incidence of embolic stroke in the Harvard Stroke Registry is largely due to defining "embolic stroke" by the presence of carotid artery disease (such as neck bruits).[35] It is essential that a source of emboli be present; in its absence there are a number of suggestive criteria (Table 35).

Twenty percent of patients in the Toronto Unit had an embolic source of acute cerebral infarction (Table 36). The diagnosis of cerebral embolism was made on demonstration of a potential embolic source such

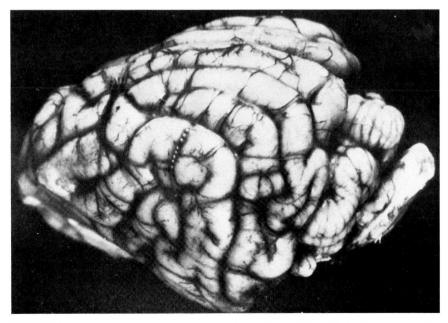

FIGURE 88. Streamlining in experimental cerebral embolism. Eight of 11 steel bearings injected into the common carotid artery of the dog aligned in a single cortical artery. (From Whisnant,[36] with permission.)

as atrial fibrillation or mural thrombosis. Further systemic emboli or random cerebral ischemic episodes confirm this diagnosis but may still underestimate the true incidence, since multiple emboli may all converge in the same vessel (Fig. 88).[36]

Systemic embolism from atrial fibrillation with rheumatic heart disease is well recognized, but chronic atrial fibrillation without valvular heart disease is less commonly suspected.[34] In the Framingham Study,[4] the fivefold risk of ischemic stroke in patients with atrial fibrillation alone increased to 17-fold in the presence of rheumatic heart disease, and, as the duration of atrial fibrillation increased, so did the frequency of stroke. In a clinicopathologic review of 333 cases, Hinton and associates found a high incidence of systemic emboli from atrial fibrillation of any origin, particularly when due to mitral valve or ischemic heart disease.[37]

Cardiac Arrhythmias

Cardiac arrhythmias occur in 42 to 61 percent of patients with acute ischemic or hemorrhagic stroke who are monitored by long-term ECG.[38-42] Over half the cardiac arrhythmias recorded in the Toronto Unit were ectopic beats,[40] a benign disorder usually reflecting the patient's age. Eighteen percent had atrial fibrillation, and 4 percent had other serious arrhythmias of embolic potential, such as sinoatrial disorder (Table 37).[43]

Cardiac arrhythmias may be a cause or effect of ischemic stroke. They are equally frequent in hemorrhagic stroke, and even more frequent in subarachnoid hemorrhage,[44] so denying a causal effect. In the Toronto Unit, cardiac arrhythmias were equally profuse in stroke patients with and without cardiac disease,[42] suggesting an effect independent of coexistent cardiovascular disease.

Episodic cardiac arrhythmias may be an underestimated cause of ischemic stroke; and sick sinus syndrome, atrial fibrillation, and certain tachycardias may predispose to left atrial thrombus with subsequent embolism.[41] Certainly, a large minority of ischemic strokes have no apparent cause, even after extensive investigation.

TABLE 37. Incidence of Cardiac Arrhythmias
(Predominant Arrhythmia for Each Patient) in Patients
Admitted to the Toronto Unit

	Arrhythmias				
Cerebral Lesion	Ectopics	AFib	Misc	No Arrhythmias	Total
Cerebral infarction	73	42	10	117 (48%)	242
Cerebral hemorrhage	7	6	1	16 (53%)	30
Controls	12	8	0	70 (78%)	90

Ectopics = Both supraventricular and ventricular ectopic beats
AFib = Atrial fibrillation
Misc = Other arrhythmias, including sick sinus syndrome and supraventricular and ventricular tachycardias
Controls = Nonstroke patients admitted to the Unit

Mural Thrombosis

Systemic embolism is evident in only 1 to 2 percent of all patients with myocardial infarction,[45] although pathologic studies indicate that 21 to 67 percent have mural thrombosis,[46] suggesting higher mortality in patients with larger myocardial infarcts.

Mural thrombi were detected by angiocardiography in 10 percent of 228 cases of transmural myocardial infarction[46] and were more frequent in patients with anterior wall infarctions, cardiomegaly, and disturbed left ventricular function with apical stasis. They were not associated with hypertension or congestive cardiac failure. In 70 consecutive cases of transmural myocardial infarction, 17 percent had ventricular clot on two-dimensional echocardiography. Severe dyskinesia of the apical wall was found associated with and prior to the development of these mural thrombi (Fig. 89).[8] Anterior wall infarctions more commonly produce mural thrombosis than do those in other areas of the left ventricle, and they are often larger. High creatine-kinase levels in myocardial infarction patients who suffered stroke also suggest that stroke risk relates directly to infarction size.[45]

There is no consensus on management. Routine two-dimensional echocardiography of patients with cerebral ischemic episodes has an unrewarding yield.[47] Prophylactic anticoagulation in acute myocardial infarction should be reserved for high-risk patients with severe apical

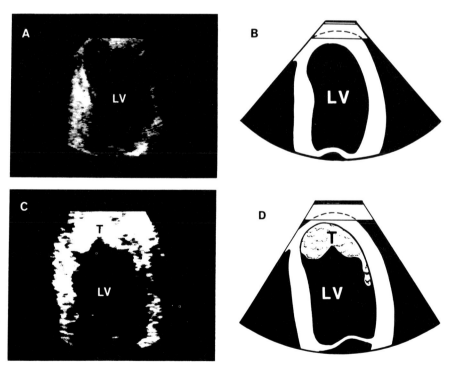

FIGURE 89. Echocardiographic images of apical views in a patient 7 days (*A* and *B*) and 11 days (*C* and *D*) following myocardial infarction, showing the formation of thrombus (T) in the left ventricle (LV). (From Asinger, et al,[8] with permission.)

hypokinesia, identified by two-dimensional echocardiography, preferably prior to the development of thrombi.[8] Low-risk patients with inferior or anterior infarction and normal or hypokinetic segments do not warrant anticoagulants.

Although the incidence of stroke in patients with myocardial infarction is low, myocardial infarction in acute stroke patients may be as frequent as 13 to 14 percent.[48] "Acute myocardial ischemia" was reported in 13 percent of acute stroke patients admitted to a geriatric unit, but clinical evidence was absent in 71 percent of patients, the diagnosis resting solely on ECG and cardiac enzyme changes.[49] Diffuse cardiac damage unrelated to myocardial ischemia may occur secondary to stroke; these cardiologic findings might be an effect and not the cause of the stroke.

Ventricular Aneurysm

Ventricular aneurysm most commonly results from myocardial infarction but occasionally complicates obstructive cardiomyopathy. Clinical evidence of systemic embolism is found in about 5 percent of patients with ventricular aneurysm, but, at autopsy, mural thrombi are found in about

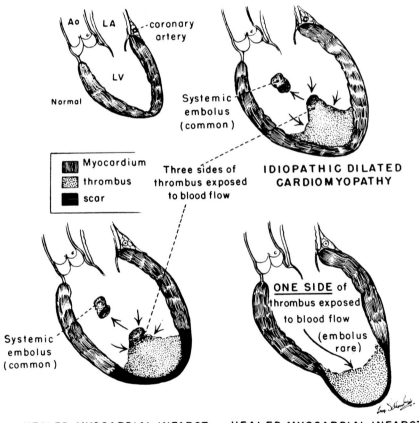

FIGURE 90. Liability of mural thrombi to embolize, depending upon the underlying cardiac pathology. (From Cabin and Roberts,[50] with permission.)

half.[50] The relatively low rate of systemic embolism is probably due to the frequent accommodation of the thrombus within the aneurysmal cavity, which presents a smooth flat surface to ventricular blood flow, minimizing fragmentation of the clot (Fig. 90).

Angiocardiography is unjustifiably dangerous in these patients and only ultrasound techniques such as 2-D echo can effectively evaluate the incidence of intracardiac clot. Increasing detection of intraventricular thrombus by this technique has resulted in successful surgical aneurysmectomy,[51] encouraging 2-D echo screening of these patients, superseding long-term anticoagulant therapy.[52]

Mitral Valve Prolapse and Cerebral Ischemia

Mitral valve prolapse (MVP) is a myxomatous degeneration of the valve leaflet that leads to redundancy and prolapse of the valve during systole and occurs in 5 to 10 percent of the population,[53] predominantly in women (Fig. 91). In the study of Barnett and coworkers,[54] the frequency of MVP in patients over age 45 was similar to that in controls (5.7 percent versus 7.1 percent), but below this age it was significantly higher (40 percent versus 6.8 percent), suggesting that its effect is diluted by large numbers of older patients in whom extracranial arterial disease predominates as a cause of stroke.

Symptomatic MVP is distinctly unusual. Only 26 (2 percent) of 40 focal cerebral ischemic events could be attributed solely to this mechanism in 1138 MVP patients diagnosed by echocardiography at the Mayo Clinic.[55] The true frequency of thromboembolic events in the population with MVP is much lower, probably only 1 per 6000 per year.[53]

MVP is not always benign but may cause progressive mitral regurgitation, sudden death from ventricular arrhythmias, and systemic embolism from bacterial endocarditis[12,55] or left atrial thrombus.[56] Decreased platelet survival is a sensitive indicator of thrombosis in many clinical states. It is shortened in 46 percent of patients with otherwise asymptomatic MVP, suggesting a direct effect of the valvular lesion. Shortened platelet survival in all patients with MVP and stroke suggests a thromboembolic relationship.[57]

No management for asymptomatic MVP has yet been decided, beyond amelioration of putative risk factors.[12] In MVP with embolic complications, antithrombotic therapy is a rational but untested approach. Long-term anticoagulant treatment is unjustified, since most patients are young, but short-term anticoagulants or platelet antiaggregants have been recommended.[12,55] Prophylactic antibiotic therapy is indicated in surgical procedures such as tooth extractions, just as in any other cardiac valvular lesion.

Mitral Annulus Calcification

Massive calcium deposits in the mitral annulus produce platelet or possibly calcific emboli, an alleged source of cerebral emboli.[58] Seen most commonly in patients over 60 years, it produces a harsh systolic murmur conducted to the neck and axilla, similar to that of calcific aortic sclerosis.

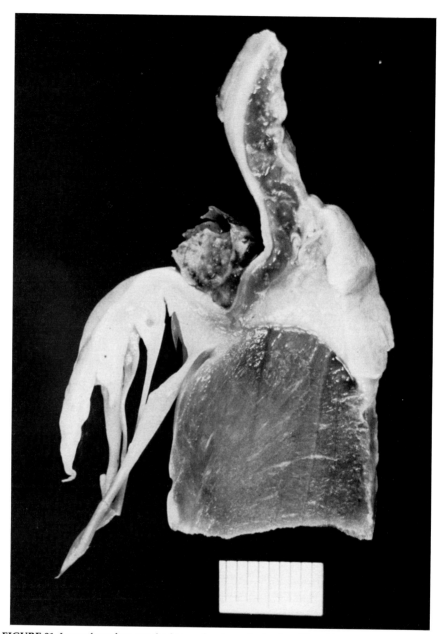

FIGURE 91. Large thrombus attached to prolapsing mitral valve. (From Barnett, HJM: *Embolism in mitral valve prolapse.* Ann Rev Med 33:497, 1982, with permission.)

It is best diagnosed by echocardiography though it may be discovered on oblique views of the chest x-ray.

Infective Endocarditis

Subacute bacterial endocarditis (SBE) has changed considerably since Osler described his famous triad of fever, heart murmur, and hemiplegia. Antibiotics have all but eliminated acute rheumatic fever and patients with chronic rheumatic valvular diseases are aging (Fig. 92), so the effect

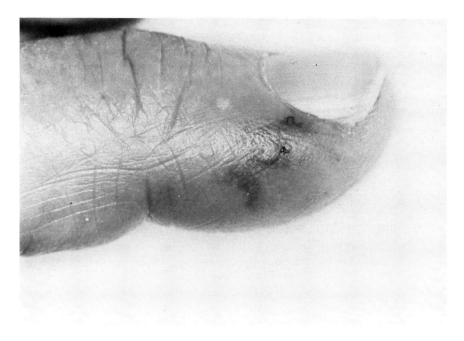

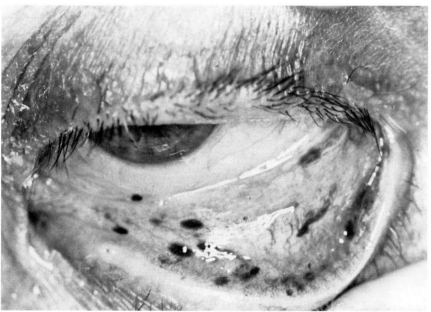

FIGURE 92. A previously healthy 75-year-old woman had an influenzal illness 1 week prior to admission. On the day of admission, she developed a fever of 103°F and sudden right hemiplegia. There were no signs of bacterial endocarditis except for an apical systolic murmur, but after taking blood cultures, intravenous ampicillin therapy was started. Several hours later, she developed multiple petechiae in skin *(top)* and mucosa *(bottom)* and multiple basal and apical cardiac murmurs. She lapsed into coma, dying on the 13th day. Blood cultures grew profuse S. aureus resistant to ampicillin.

CARDIAC DISEASE AND STROKE

177

of SBE is not so devastating and noninfective endocarditis is now commoner.[59,60]

Bacterial endocarditis is an unusual cause of stroke, though stroke is probably its commonest neurologic complication. Only 1.6 percent of patients with cerebral infarcts in our series had associated subacute bacterial endocarditis (see Table 36). Neurologic complications occur in 30 to 50 percent of patients with infective endocarditis, of which 14 to 39 percent represent focal cerebral ischemia.[59,61,62] The mortality rate in these patients is much higher than in the nonneurologic group (50 percent in those with cerebral infarction and 90 percent in those with hemorrhage).[62] In the Massachusetts General Hospital series, 84 (39 percent) of 218 patients had neurologic complications, of whom 37 were embolic strokes, 30 being fatal. Seizures occurred in 24 patients, presumably secondary to embolism, though in three patients no cerebral lesion was found at autopsy.[59]

Systemic emboli arise more commonly from mitral valve lesions than from other valvular lesions, possibly because sluggish flow in the left atrium favors larger friable vegetations, which do not occur in the left ventricle due to high pressure flow. Mortality is higher in acute compared with subacute bacterial endocarditis since the rate of embolism is much higher (30 percent versus 7 percent).[63] Also, the organisms are more virulent; S. aureus and E. coli are implicated in acute endocarditis, whereas streptococci account for most subacute infections.

Hemorrhagic stroke due to mycotic aneurysm is rare (4.6 percent in Pruitt's series), since endocarditic vegetations embolizing into an arterial bifurcation usually produce infarction. If the arterial wall is weakened by bacterial invasion but arterial patency is maintained, an aneurysm may arise, later causing subarachnoid or intracerebral hemorrhage. Ischemic stroke may occasionally be due to "proliferative endarteritis" around a septic embolus. Serial blood cultures most reliably establish the diagnosis. Echocardiography can identify vegetations as small as 2 mm and may establish the diagnosis in patients with consistently negative blood cultures.[64] Emergency broad-spectrum antibiotic therapy should be delayed until samples for blood (and sometimes CSF) culture have been obtained. Culture findings will determine the definitive antibiotic. Though anticoagulation may prove disastrous due to fatal hemorrhagic complications, it may be justified in the presence of effective antibiotic therapy.[65] Valve replacement in infective endocarditis is indicated in severe congestive heart failure (48 percent), uncontrolled sepsis (28 percent), and persistent embolization (24 percent).[66]

Nonbacterial Thrombotic Endocarditis (NBTE)

Originally described as "marantic" or "terminal" endocarditis, NBTE was believed a rare agonal complication, usually silent but occasionally causing systemic embolism. It is uncommon (0.7 to 2 percent)[67,68] but should always be suspected when ischemic stroke occurs in patients with malignancy.[69] The true clinical incidence (as opposed to autopsy findings) has only emerged with progress in echocardiography.[70] The diagnostic value of early detection of the syndrome is debatable, since NBTE is com-

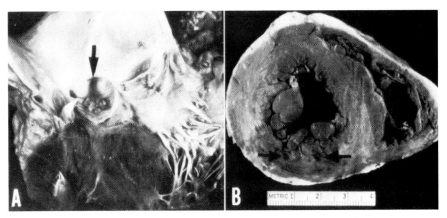

FIGURE 93. Cardiac vegetations in "marantic endocarditis." (From Olney,[67] with permission.)

monly an agonal event in patients with widespread cancer. However, patients must be managed individually since the syndrome may occur with small or nonmetastasizing resectable tumors. The heart valves are normal, and immune complexes elicited by the malignancy produce systemic coagulopathies such as hyperfibrinogenemia, hypofibrinogenemia, thrombocytopenia, and decreased levels of factors V, VIII, and XIII.[71,72]

Nonbacterial thrombotic endocarditis is probably a manifestation of disseminated intravascular coagulation[73,74] and small-vessel thrombotic occlusion may occur side by side with embolic events. Sometimes only a consumption coagulopathy is found[75] with low platelet count and fibrinogen level. It is most commonly associated with mucin-secreting adenocarcinoma,[76] especially pancreatic and pulmonary, and may coexist with the syndrome of "thrombophlebitis migrans" (Trousseau's syndrome), so that arterial and venous occlusions may be concurrent. However, various nonneoplastic disorders predominate in some series.[68,77] The mitral valve is most commonly affected, although, despite multiple and massive systemic embolism, the valve may be devoid of thrombi at autopsy. Cardiac murmurs are unusual and the lesions may escape 2-D–echo detection since the vegetations are small and friable, unlike those in bacterial endocarditis (Fig. 93). Cerebral embolism is commonly accompanied by systemic embolism.[75]

The clinical onset may be "stuttering" due to frequent small emboli preceding the major cerebral event, which often declares itself by a seizure. Microinfarcts scattered throughout the brain in addition to the main cerebral embolus may blur the clinical neurologic picture, superimposing an acute confusional state.

Anticoagulation remains the treatment of choice, although antiplatelet agents may prove of the same value as in patients with cardiac prosthetic valves, in whom a similar dyscrasia may occur.

Paradoxical Embolism

Emboli, usually from venous thrombosis of the legs, may cross an intracardiac defect and enter the systemic circulation, especially with an increase in right atrial pressure, as may follow pulmonary embolism.

Diagnosis rests upon the presence of venous thrombosis or pulmonary embolism, arterial embolism without a cardiac embolic source, and a right-to-left cardiac shunt (commonly via an atrial or ventricular septal defect, a patent foramen ovale or ductus arteriosus).[78] Usually discovered at postmortem, diagnosis during life may lead to prophylactic cardiac surgery.[79]

Cardiomyopathies

Dilated, hypertrophic, and restrictive cardiomyopathies pose a worldwide problem. Dilated cardiomyopathy occurs in all continents but prevails in Asia. Its annual incidence is about 10 per 100,000,[80] with a mortality of 70 percent over 10 years.[81] The dilated heart muscle is pale, flabby, and hypertrophied, and thrombi clump on the thickened endothelium in over half of cases.[29] Among cardiomyopathies, the dilated varieties are the most prone to systemic emboli and stroke.

"Hemodynamic" Stroke

Enthusiasm for the concept of focal cerebral ischemia due to cardiac or systemic hypotension ("hemodynamic crises")[82] waned with the discovery of cerebral autoregulation. Tilt-table experiments with TIA patients produced symptoms of global cerebral ischemia instead of reproducing their attacks.[83] Only 1 percent of patients with a pacemaker who had bradycardia had focal neurologic signs attributable to the arrhythmia; the rest experienced syncope.[84] Only 5.2 percent of 135 survivors of cardiac arrest had new infarcts at autopsy, and the severity of the infarct did not relate to the degree of cerebral arteriosclerosis.[85]

Hemodynamic causes probably account for 1 to 5 percent of carotid ischemic stroke (see Table 36),[86] and a larger proportion of vertebrobasilar ischemia. Perfusion imaging of the vertebral arteries during head turning at autopsy indicates that total occlusion of a vertebral artery may occur in a spondylotic cervical spine.[87,88] Barnett[86] believes that the "special case" of vertebrobasilar ischemia has been exaggerated and may arise from the difficulty in distinguishing vertebrobasilar TIAs from syncopal symptoms. Most would agree that the great majority of focal cerebral ischemic symptoms, whatever the territory, are thromboembolic.

EFFECTS OF STROKE ON THE HEART

Experimentally, intracranial hemorrhage, raised intracranial pressure,[89] or direct stimulation of certain areas of the central or peripheral nervous system[44] produce a variety of cardiac changes, including arrhythmias and focal myocardial damage.[90] Neurosurgical manipulation of the circle of Willis also produces acute ECG changes and cardiac arrhythmias.[91]

ECG changes in stroke were first reported in patients with subarachnoid hemorrhage in whom tall or inverted T waves and prolonged Q-T intervals suggested subendocardial ischemia.[92,93] Systematic examination of patients with cerebral infarction showed that over two thirds had ischemic ECG changes, originally attributed to coincidental arteriosclerosis (Fig. 94).[38]

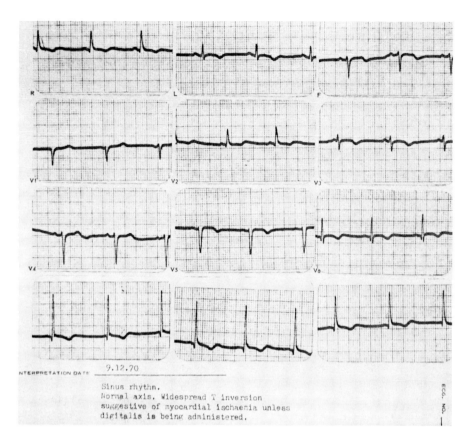

9.12.70

INTERPRETATION DATE

Sinus rhythm.
Normal axis. Widespread T inversion
suggestive of myocardial ischaemia unless
digitalis is being administered.

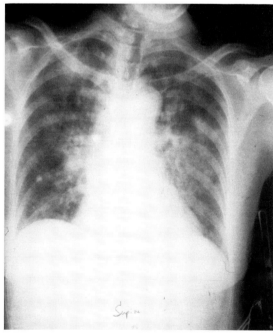

Sup.ne

FIGURE 94. A 50-year-old woman collapsed unconscious and arrived in the emergency room several hours later. She was later found to have a subarachnoid hemorrhage, confirmed by lumbar puncture. ECG *(top)* showed classic signs of bradycardia, prolonged Q-T interval, and inverted T waves. Chest x-ray *(bottom)* showed severe neurogenic pulmonary edema.

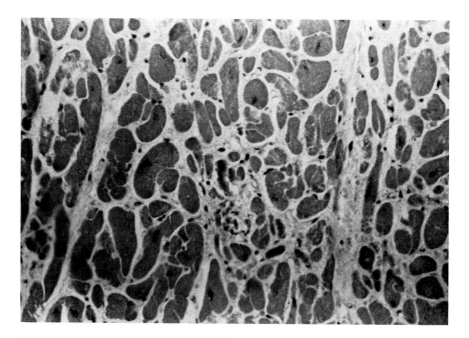

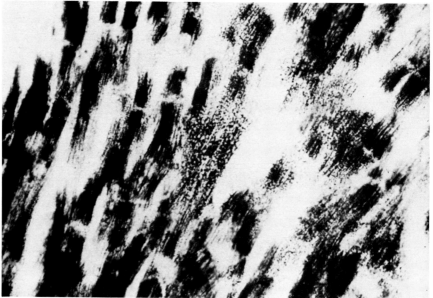

FIGURE 95. *Top,* Hematoxylin-and-eosin section of heart showing an area of focal myocardial necrosis. Patient died on day 4 after brainstem infarction.

  Bottom, Succinic dehydrogenase section showing coarse irregular granularity of myofibrils. Patient died of coning secondary to a glioma. (From A Kolin, MD, University of Toronto, with permission.)

  Arrhythmias are seen significantly more commonly in stroke patients, compared with those without stroke, matched for age and heart disease.[42,94] Prolonged ECG ("Holter") monitoring reveals a great variety of arrhythmias,[38,39] some coincidental, some causal, and some consequential to the stroke (Table 37). The commonest arrhythmias, ectopic beats, are probably an index of coincidental arterial disease. A small number of arrhythmias, including paroxysmal atrial fibrillation and sinoatrial disorders, are potential causes of systemic embolism. Some arrhythmias are consequential, similar to those produced experimentally. They are at least as frequent in hemorrhagic as ischemic stroke (Table 37) and are sometimes associated with transtentorial herniation.[94] Cardiac arrhythmias such as ventricular fibrillation may cause sudden death in patients with subarachnoid hemorrhage.[14]

Subendocardial hemorrhages noted by Koskelo and associates[95] in three subarachnoid hemorrhage patients with "ischemic" ECG changes were attributed to a sudden rise in left ventricular cardiac pressure secondary to increased intracranial pressure. This produced subendocardial ischemia with subsequent hemorrhage. They noted the similarity to the cardiac findings both experimentally and clinically in other lesions with raised intracranial pressure. Reichenbach and Benditt[96] suggested that the diffuse micronecrotic mottling throughout the myocardium (myofibrillar degeneration) seen in subarachnoid hemorrhage patients could account for these ECG changes. Focal myocytolysis has been observed in both ischemic and hemorrhagic stroke[97,98] (Fig. 95).

Other cerebral lesions characterized by raised intracranial pressure also produce these myocardial lesions,[99] but they are not seen in patients dying suddenly from a violent death nor are they present more than 2 weeks after the acute intracranial event.[100] They appear within 12 hours of the ictus and then resolve over the ensuing days or weeks. This correlates with changes in serum cardiac enzymes (including cardiospecific CPK-MB). Unlike the acute rise and fall of serum CPK-MB levels within 36 hours seen in patients with acute myocardial infarction, the enzyme

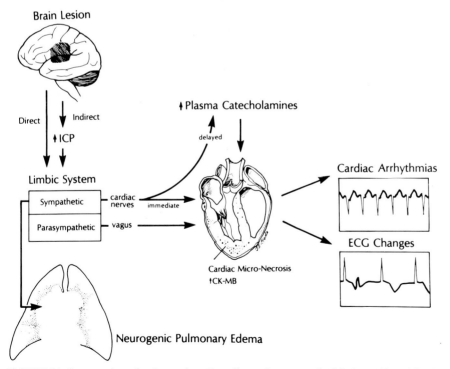

FIGURE 96. Suggested mechanisms of cardiac effects of acute cerebral lesions. (From Norris, JW: *The effects of cerebrovascular lesions upon the heart.* Neurol Clin 1:87, 1983, with permission.)

levels in stroke rose gradually over the first few days, reaching their peak by about 7 days and returning to normal by the second week.[98]

Infusion of noradrenaline or its congeners into experimental animals or focal stimulation of certain parts of the limbic system in animals produces similar cardiac pathology.[90] Tomomatsu[101] found raised urinary catecholamine levels in 19 patients with a variety of hemorrhagic and ischemic strokes, a finding later confirmed with more precise plasma assays in ischemic and hemorrhagic stroke.[102] These changes were especially striking in subarachnoid hemorrhage.[103,104]

The cycle of events is becoming clearer (Fig. 96). In any acute intracranial event with raised intracranial pressure, the autonomic nervous system produces catecholamines acutely in the heart via the cardiac nerves, or subacutely as an index of generalized sympathetic hyperactivity, increasing plasma catecholamines. The ischemia produced by excessive catecholamine activity damages the myofibrillary mitochondria and may progress to diffuse cardiac micronecrosis or possibly to myocardial infarction.

Some of the resulting cardiac arrhythmias may be life threatening in acute stroke patients as well as in those with other forms of acute cerebral lesions, including head injury. Estanol and coworkers[14] suggested that sudden death in subarachnoid hemorrhage is often from this cause. The acute rise in plasma catecholamines could also explain death in epileptic seizures.[105] Beta-receptor blockade may protect against these serious neurogenic cardiac effects[106] but this promising approach has not been fully explored yet.

CONCLUSION

Cardiac abnormalities in stroke may be causal, coincidental, or consequential. Epidemiologic studies demonstrate that cardiac disease and stroke represent risks for each other.

The changing incidence of vascular diseases demands re-evaluation of the relationship of stroke to disordered cardiac function. Chronic rheumatic valvular and hypertensive heart disease have declined sharply in the last two decades and the incidence of all types of vascular disease continues to fall. Mitral valve prolapse is increasingly recognized as a significant cause of cerebral embolism, especially in the young.

The interdependence of heart and brain in pathophysiology, epidemiology, and management is an area of increasing interest and importance, inviting close cooperation between neurologic and cardiologic research.

REFERENCES

1. REDDY J: *On paralysis with aphasia.* Can Med J 8:407, 1871–1872.
2. KANNEL, WB, *Current status of the epidemiology of brain infarction associated with occlusive arterial disease.* Stroke 2:295, 1971.
3. KANNEL, WB, WOLF, PA, AND VERTER, J: *Manifestations of coronary disease predisposing to stroke.* JAMA 250:2942, 1983.

4. WOLF, PA, ET AL: *Epidemiologic assessment of chronic atrial fibrillation and risk of stroke: The Framingham Study.* Neurology 28:973, 1978.

5. FISHER, CM: *Occlusion of the internal carotid artery.* Arch Neurol 65:346, 1951.

6. LASCELLES, RG, AND BURROWS, EH: *Occlusion of the middle cerebral artery.* Brain 88:85, 1965.

7. BLACKWOOD, W, ET AL: *Atheromatous disease of the carotid arterial system and embolism from the heart in cerebral infarction: A morbid anatomical study.* Brain 92:897, 1969.

8. ASINGER, RW, ET AL: *Incidence of left-ventricular thrombosis after acute transmural myocardial infarction.* N Engl J Med 305:297, 1981.

9. MELTZER, R, AND ROELANDT, J: *2-D echo for left ventricular thrombi.* Chest 80:118, 1981.

10. MINTZ, GS, AND KOTLER, MN: *Clinical value and limitations of echocardiography—Its use in the study of patients with infectious endocarditis.* Arch Intern Med 140:1022, 1980.

11. PORTAL, RW: *Mitral stenosis: The picture changes.* Br Med J 288:167, 1984.

12. BARNETT, HJM: *Heart in ischemic stroke—A changing emphasis.* Neurol Clin 1:291, 1983.

13. BYER, E, ASHMAN, R, AND TOTH, LA: *Electrocardiograms with large upright T waves and long Q-T intervals.* Am Heart J 33:796, 1947.

14. ESTANOL, BV, AND MARIN, OSM: *Cardiac arrhythmias and sudden death in subarachnoid hemorrhage.* Stroke 6:382, 1975.

15. NORRIS, JW: *The effects of cerebrovascular lesions upon the heart.* Neurol Clin 1:87, 1983.

16. ENGEL, GL: *Sudden and rapid death during psychological stress. Folklore or folk wisdom?* Ann Intern Med 74:771, 1971.

17. SKINNER, JE: *Heart attack trigger.* Psychol Today (July) 124, 1980.

18. SCHWARTZ, PJ, AND LOWELL STONE, H: *The role of the autonomic system in sudden coronary death.* Ann NY Acad Sci 1982.

19. SOLBERG, LA, ET AL: *Distribution of cerebral atherosclerosis by geographic location, race, and sex.* Lab Invest 18:604, 1968.

20. LEVY, RI, AND MOSKOWITZ, J: *Cardiovascular research: Decades of progress, a decade of promise.* Science 217:121, 1982.

21. KANNEL, WB, ET AL: *Vascular disease of the brain—Epidemiologic aspects: The Framingham study.* Am J Publ Health 55:1355, 1965.

22. NORRIS, JW, AND D'ALTON, JG: *Outcome of patients with asymptomatic carotid bruits.* In REIVICH, M, AND HURTIG, HI (EDS): *Cerebrovascular Diseases.* Raven Press, New York, 1983, p 63.

23. WHISNANT, JP, ET AL: *Natural history of stroke in Rochester, Minnesota, 1945 through 1954.* Stroke 2:11, 1971.

24. GOLDNER, JC, WHISNANT, JP, AND TAYLOR, WF: *Long-term prognosis of transient cerebral ischemic attacks.* Stroke 2:160, 1971.

25. ENNIX, CL, ET AL: *Improved results of carotid endarterectomy in patients with symptomatic coronary disease: An analysis of 1546 consecutive carotid operations.* Stroke 10:122, 1979.

26. WOLF, PA, ET AL: *Duration of atrial fibrillation and imminence of stroke: The Framingham study.* Stroke 14:664, 1983.

27. CHAMBERS, BR, ET AL: *Prognostic profiles in acute stroke.* Can J Neurol Sci 11:335, 1983.

28. SCHOENBERG, BS: *Risk factors for cerebrovascular disease.* In ROSE, FC (ED): *Clinical Neuroepidemiology.* Pitman, Tunbridge Wells, United Kingdom, 1980, p 151.

29. WHO: *Cardiomyopathies.* WHO Tech Rep Ser 697, 1984.

30. GAUTIER, JC: *Arterial pathology in cerebral ischemia and infarction.* In GREENHALGH, RM, AND ROSE, FC (EDS): *Progress in Stroke Research.* Pitman, Tunbridge Wells, United Kingdom, 1979, p 28.

31. CASTAIGNE, P, ET AL: *Internal carotid artery occlusion. A study of 61 instances in 50 patients with post-mortem data.* Brain 93:231, 1970.

32. LHERMITTE, F, ET AL: *Ischemic accidents in the middle cerebral artery territory.* Arch Neurol 19:248, 1968.

33. MATSUMOTO, N, ET AL: *Natural history of stroke in Rochester, Minnesota, 1955 through 1969: An extension of a previous study, 1945 through 1954.* Stroke 4:20, 1973.

34. EASTON, JD, AND SHERMAN, DG: *Management of cerebral embolism of cardiac origin.* Stroke 11:433, 1980.

35. MOHR, JP, ET AL: *The Harvard Cooperative Stroke Registry: A prospective registry.* Neurology 28:754, 1978.

36. WHISNANT, JP: *Multiple particles injected may all go to the same cerebral artery branch.* Stroke 13:720, 1982.

37. HINTON, RC, ET AL: *Influence of etiology of atrial fibrillation on incidence of systemic embolism.* Am J Cardiol 40:509, 1977.

38. REINSTEIN, L, ET AL: *Cardiac monitoring in the acute stroke patient.* Arch Phys Med 53:311, 1972.

39. LAVY, S, ET AL: *The effect of acute stroke on cardiac functions as observed in an intensive stroke care unit.* Stroke 5:775, 1974.

40. NORRIS, JW, FROGGATT, GM, AND HACHINSKI, VC: *Cardiac arrhythmias in acute stroke.* Stroke 9:392, 1978.

41. ABDON, NJ, ET AL: *Is occult atrial disorder a frequent cause of non-hemorrhagic stroke? Long-term ECG in 86 patients.* Stroke 13:832, 1982.

42. MYERS, MG, ET AL: *Cardiac sequelae of acute stroke.* Stroke 13:838, 1982.

43. FAIRFAX, AJ, LAMBERT, CD, AND LEATHAM, A: *Systemic embolism in chronic sino-atrial disorder.* N Engl J Med 295:190, 1976.

44. WEIDLER, DJ: *Myocardial damage and cardiac arrhythmias after intracranial hemorrhage, a critical review.* Stroke 5:759, 1974.

45. THOMPSON, PL, AND ROBINSON, JS: *Stroke after acute myocardial infarction: Relation to infarct size.* Br Med J 2:457, 1978.

46. HAMBY, RI, ET AL: *Coronary artery disease and left ventricular mural thrombi: Clinical, hemodynamic and angiocardiographic aspects.* Chest 66:488, 1974.

47. LOVETT, JL, ET AL: *Two-dimensional echocardiography in patients with focal cerebral ischemia.* Ann Intern Med 95:1, 1981.

48. ROGERS, FB: *Unsuspected cardiac infarction with cerebrovascular accidents.* J Am Geriatr Soc 3:714, 1955.

49. CHIN, PL, KAMINSKI, J, AND ROUT, M: *Myocardial infarction coincident with cerebrovascular accidents in the elderly.* Age Ageing 6:4, 1977.

50. CABIN, HS, AND ROBERTS, WC: *Left ventricular aneurysm, intra-aneurysmal thrombus and systemic embolus in coronary heart disease.* Chest 77:586, 1980.

51. LEWIN, RF, ET AL: *Two-dimensional real-time echocardiographic detection of a left ventricular aneurysm associated with mobile pedunculated thrombi.* Chest 77:704, 1980.

52. SIMPSON, MT, ET AL: *Prevalence of mural thrombi and systemic embolization with left ventricular aneurysm. Effect on anticoagulation therapy.* Chest 77:463, 1980.

53. HART, RG, AND EASTON, JD: *Mitral valve prolapse and cerebral infarction.* Stroke 13:429, 1982.

54. BARNETT, HJM, ET AL: *Further evidence relating mitral-valve prolapse to cerebral ischemic events.* N Engl J Med 302:139, 1980.

55. SANDOK, BA, AND GIULIANI, ER: *Cerebral ischemic events in patients with mitral valve prolapse.* Stroke 13:448, 1982.

56. KNOPMAN, DS, ET AL: *Indications for echocardiography in patients with ischemic stroke.* Neurology 32:1005, 1982.

57. STEELE, P, ET AL: *Platelet survival time and thromboembolism in patients with mitral valve prolapse.* Circulation 60:43, 1979.

58. DE BONO, DP, AND WARLOW, CP: *Mitral-annulus calcification and cerebral or retinal ischaemia.* Lancet 2:383, 1979.

59. PRUITT, AA, ET AL: *Neurologic complications of bacterial endocarditis.* Medicine 57:329, 1978.

60. WEINSTEIN, L, LERNER, P, AND CHEW, W: *Clinical and bacteriological studies on the effect of 'massive' doses of penicillin G on infection caused by gram negative bacilli.* N Engl J Med 271:5251, 1964.

61. HARRISON, MJG, AND HAMPTON, JR: *Neurological presentation of bacterial endocarditis.* Br Med J 2:148, 1967.

62. JONES, HR, SIEKERT, RG, AND GERACI, JE: *Neurological manifestations of bacterial endocarditis.* Ann Intern Med 71:21, 1969.

63. MORGAN, WL, AND BLAND, EF: *Bacterial endocarditis in the antibiotic era.* Circulation 19:753, 1959.

64. RUBENSON, DS, ET AL: *The use of echocardiography in diagnosing culture-negative endocarditis.* Circulation 64:641, 1981.

65. FREEDMAN, LR: *Infective Endocarditis and Other Intravascular Infections.* Medical Book Co, New York, 1982, pp 13, 108, 180.

66. BOYD, AD, ET AL: *Infective endocarditis—An analysis of 54 surgically treated patients.* J Thorac Cardiovasc Surg 73:23, 1977.

67. OLNEY, BA, ET AL: *The consequences of the inconsequential: Marantic (nonbacterial thrombotic) endocarditis.* Am Heart J 98:513, 1979.

68. BILLER, J, ET AL: *Nonbacterial thrombotic endocarditis. A neurologic perspective of clinicopathologic correlations of 99 patients.* Arch Neurol 39:95, 1982.

69. CASE RECORDS OF THE MASSACHUSETTS GENERAL HOSPITAL: *Case 27-1980.* N Engl J Med 303:92, 1980.

70. SIEGEL, RJ, ET AL: *Marantic endocarditis. Diagnosis by 2-D echocardiography.* Chest 80:118, 1981.

71. LEHTO, VP, STENMAN, S, AND SOMER, T: *Immunohistological studies on valvular vegetations in nonbacterial thrombotic endocarditis (NBTE).* Acta Pathol Microbiol Immunol Scand (Sect A) 90:207, 1982.

72. EDITORIAL *Non-bacterial thrombotic endocarditis.* Br Med J 1:197, 1978.

73. REAGAN, TJ, AND OKAZAKI, H: *The thrombotic syndrome associated with carcinoma. A clinical and neuropathologic study.* Arch Neurol 31:390, 1974.

74. KIM, HS, SUZUKI, M, AND LIE, JT: *Nonbacterial thrombotic endocarditis (NBTE) and disseminated intravascular coagulation (DIC).* Arch Pathol Lab Med 101:65, 1977.

75. KOOIKER, JC, MACLEAN, JM, AND SUMI, SM: *Cerebral embolism, marantic endocarditis, and cancer.* Arch Neurol 33:260, 1976.

76. MIN, K-W, GYORKEY, F, AND SATO, C: *Mucin-producing adenocarcinomas and nonbacterial thrombotic endocarditis.* Cancer 45:2374, 1980.

77. MACDONALD, RA, AND ROBBINS, SL: *The significance of nonbacterial thrombotic endocarditis: An autopsy and clinical study of 78 cases.* Ann Intern Med 46:255, 1957.

78. MEISTER, SG, ET AL: *Paradoxical embolism—Diagnosis during life.* Am J Med 53:292, 1972.

79. JONES, HR, ET AL: *Cerebral emboli of paradoxical origin.* Ann Neurol 13:314, 1983.

80. TORP, A: *Incidence of congestive cardiomyopathy.* In GOODWIN, JF, ET AL (EDS): *Congestive Cardiomyopathy.* AB Hässle, Mölndal, Sweden, 1981, p 18.

81. KUHN, H, ET AL: *Prognosis and possible presymptomatic manifestations of congestive cardiomyopathy (COCM).* Postgrad Med J 54:451, 1978.

82. MEYER, JS, AND DENNY-BROWN, D: *The cerebral collateral circulation. 1. Factors influencing collateral blood flow.* Neurology 7:447, 1957.

83. KENDELL, RE, AND MARSHALL, J: *Role of hypotension in the genesis of transient focal cerebral ischaemic attacks.* Br Med J 5353:344, 1963.

84. REED, RL, SIEKERT, RG, AND MERIDETH, J: *Rarity of transient focal cerebral ischemia in cardiac dysrhythmia.* JAMA 223:893, 1973.

85. TORVIK, A, AND SKULLERUD, K: *How often are brain infarcts caused by hypotensive episodes?* Stroke 7:255, 1976.

86. BARNETT, HJM: *Progress towards stroke prevention: Robert Wartenberg lecture.* Neurology 30:1212, 1980.

87. TISSINGTON TATLOW, WF, AND BAMMER, HG: *Syndrome of vertebral artery compression.* Neurology 7:331, 1957.

88. TOOLE, JF, AND TUCKER, SH: *Influence of head position upon cerebral circulation. Studies in blood flow in cadavers.* Arch Neurol 2:616, 1960.

89. GRAF, CJ, AND ROSSI, NP: *Catecholamine response to intracranial hypertension.* J Neurosurg 49:862, 1978.

90. GREENHOOT, JH, AND REICHENBACH, DD: *Cardiac injury and subarachnoid hemorrhage. A clinical, pathological, and physiological correlation.* J Neurosurg 30:521, 1969.

91. POOL, JL: *Vasocardiac effects of the circle of Willis.* Arch Neurol 78:355, 1957.

92. BURCH, GE, MEYERS, R, AND ABILDSKOV, JA: *A new electrocardiographic pattern observed in cerebrovascular accidents.* Circulation 9:719, 1954.

93. BYER, E, ASHMAN, R, AND TOTH, LA: *Electrocardiograms with large, upright T waves and long Q-T intervals.* Am Heart J 33:796, 1947.

94. NORRIS, JW, HACHINSKI, VC, AND MYERS, MG: *Cardiac lesions following acute stroke.* In MEYER, JS, LECHNER, H, AND REIVICH, R (EDS): *Cerebral Vascular Disease 2.* Excerpta Medica, Amsterdam, 1978, p 292.

95. KOSKELO, P, PUNSAR, S, AND SIPILA, W: *Subendocardial haemorrhage and ECG changes in intracerebral bleeding.* Br Med J 1:1479, 1964.

96. REICHENBACH, DD, AND BENDITT, EP: *Catecholamines and cardiomyopathy.* Hum Pathol 1:125, 1970.

97. DIMANT, J, AND GROB, D: *Electrocardiographic changes and myocardial damage in patients with acute cerebrovascular accidents.* Stroke 8:448, 1977.

98. NORRIS, JW, ET AL: *Serum cardiac enzymes in stroke.* Stroke 10:548, 1979.

99. CONNOR, RCR: *Focal myocytolysis and fuchsinophilic degeneration of the myocardium of patients dying with various brain lesions.* Ann NY Acad Sci 156:261, 1970.

100. KOLIN, A, AND NORRIS, JW: *Myocardial damage from acute cerebral lesions.* Stroke 15:990, 1984.

101. TOMOMATSU, T, ET AL: *ECG observations and urinary excretion of catecholamines in cerebrovascular accident.* Jpn Circ J 28:884, 1964.

102. MYERS, MG, ET AL: *Plasma norepinephrine in stroke.* Stroke 12:200, 1981.

103. PEERLESS, SJ, AND GRIFFITHS, JC: *Plasma catecholamines following subarachnoid hemorrhage.* Ann R Coll Physicians Surg (Can) 5:48, 1972.

104. BENEDICT, CR, AND LOACH, AB: *Clinical significance of plasma adrenaline and noradrenaline concentrations in patients with subarachnoid hemorrhage.* J Neurol Neurosurg Psychiatry 41:113, 1978.

105. SIMON, RP, AMINOFF, MJ, AND BENOWITZ, NL: *Changes in plasma catecholamines after tonic-clonic seizures.* Neurology 34:255, 1984.

106. NEIL-DWYER, G, ET AL: *Effect of propanolol and phentolamine on myocardial necrosis after subarachnoid haemorrhage.* Br Med J 2:990, 1978.

Chapter 11

INVESTIGATION

We must look for help to what we know by investigation.
Celsus

Intelligent use of laboratory investigations is almost as valuable as clinical acumen, particularly as the two are closely related. The hospital chart sometimes documents the quandary of the perplexed physician: the history and examination are detailed in a few lines, followed by pages of often conflicting and irrelevant laboratory reports. The platitude that laboratory investigations cannot substitute for a good clinical examination bears repeating, since the error is committed daily throughout the world. The "standard" automated battery of tests often available in large centers may also mislead, since it removes deduction from patient evaluation, producing inexplicable results.

Every investigation has costs, advantages, and limitations. "Noninvasive" investigations do not exist, since they are all intrusions into someone's time, comfort, safety, or pocketbook. Their benefits should exceed their costs. Screening procedures for common or important conditions should have a high "sensitivity" (the ability to detect disease when it is present) and those valuable in one part of the world may not be justifiable elsewhere as sensitivity depends upon the prevalence of the disease. What is routine in a university hospital may be undreamt of in the rural clinic.

Basic investigations (such as erythrocyte sedimentation rate and urinalysis) should generally be performed on all stroke patients. They are nonspecific but monitor systemic factors such as hydration and the state of the systemic circulation.

Special investigations such as lumbar puncture, CT, and angiography give information about cerebral function and the cerebrovascular system. They should be performed only on selected patients in whom therapeutic benefit is likely.

Research investigations such as PET scanning have not yet achieved useful clinical application and are not available for routine management of stroke. Their use may have future impact.

BASIC INVESTIGATIONS

Certain investigations are justified in most patients (Table 38).

Hematology

Abnormally high *hemoglobin* levels double the risk of stroke, and hypertension increases this risk,[1] whereas low hemoglobin levels protect against stroke.[2] Polycythemia reflecting adaptation to high altitudes carries no risk for stroke.[3] A high *hematocrit* level is said to increase the chance of a more severe stroke,[4] although during the acute phase the hematocrit may be physiologically elevated due to dehydration and hemoconcentration.

Leukocytosis indicates possible infection such as subacute bacterial endocarditis, since cerebral infarction or hemorrhage does not raise the white cell count. Low leukocyte levels may signal bone marrow depression, and abnormally high white cell counts suggest leukemia.

Blood film examination identifies the abnormal erythrocytes of sickle-cell disease, and the parasitized red blood cells of falciparum malaria. Atypical lymphocytes and monocytes characterize infectious mononucleosis, a rare cause of stroke in the young. Neutrophilia may indicate a bacterial infection, whereas lymphocytosis suggests viral disease. When platelets fall below 40,000 per cubic mm, spontaneous bleeding is common.

The *erythrocyte sedimentation rate* is a sensitive, nonspecific test, unaffected by uncomplicated stroke. An elevated sedimentation rate suggests a systemic cause for the stroke such as temporal arteritis, collagen disease, or bacterial endocarditis.

TABLE 38. Basic Investigation of Stroke Patients

Hematology
  Hemoglobin (or hematocrit)
  White cell count
  Blood film
  Erythrocyte sedimentation rate
Biochemistry
  Serum electrolytes
  Blood urea nitrogen
  Serum creatine kinase (preferably the CK-MB isoenzyme)
  Fasting and/or 2-hr p.c. blood sugar
Urinalysis
Electrocardiogram
Radiology
  Chest x-ray
  CT of brain (alternatively skull x-ray or radioisotope brain scan)

Biochemistry

Serum electrolytes are often abnormal. The commonest cause for low serum potassium is diuretic therapy, since cardiac failure is common in stroke patients. Inappropriate ADH syndrome (serum osmolality inappropriately low compared with the urine) is unusual in stroke. *Blood urea nitrogen* determinations screen for renal disease and hydration. *Serum cardiac enzyme* levels are often elevated in the first few days in stroke patients (Table 39), the increased levels most commonly reflecting muscle trauma,[5] but elevated *creatine kinase* levels indicate myocardial damage when the cardiac isoenzyme fraction (CPK-MB) is raised.[5]

Hyperglycemia detected on admission and due to diabetes must be distinguished from reactive hyperglycemia, which occurs acutely in nondiabetic patients[6] but normalizes within 2 to 3 weeks. In nonketotic hyperosmolar states, hyperglycemia may spare unconsciousness but produce focal neurologic signs easily mistaken for an acute cerebrovascular event. *Hypoglycemia* can produce a focal neurologic picture (including hemiparesis) that is indistinguishable from stroke;[7] 50 ml of 50 percent glucose should be given these patients after blood samples are taken.

Elevated *blood lipid* levels are a risk for stroke only in patients under 55 years.[8] Serologic *screening for syphilis* is of doubtful value. None of 1729 patients admitted to the Toronto Unit had positive serology, although VDRL estimation was routine. *Urinalysis* detects urinary infection, diabetes, renal failure, and dehydration.

Electrocardiography (ECG)

Stroke patients often have abnormal ECGs due to the following:

1. Coincidental heart disease, usually hypertensive or ischemic
2. Heart disease causing stroke, including arrhythmias such as atrial fibrillation and sick sinus syndrome, and myocardial infarction with mural thrombosis and cerebral embolism

TABLE 39. Serum Cardiac Enzyme Levels in 214 Stroke Patients Admitted to the Toronto Unit

Lesion	CK	LDH	SGOT
Cerebral infarct (n = 137)	7.2 ± 0.7*	206 ± 5.1	17.0 ± 0.5
Brainstem infarct (n = 25)	7.4 ± 1.3*	176 ± 8.7	17.1 ± 1.4
Cerebral hemorrhage (n = 23)	11.0 ± 2.2†	245 ± 17.8	20.7 ± 1.6‡
TIA (n = 39)	4.9 ± 0.7	192 ± 8.3	18.2 ± 1.2
Controls (n = 64)	4.7 ± 0.6	188 ± 7.2	15.7 ± 7.3

CK = Creatine kinase, LDH = Lactic dehydrogenase, SGOT = Serum glutamic-oxaloacetic transaminase.

* Difference from controls: $p = 0.05$
† Difference from controls: $p > 0.001$
‡ Difference from controls: $p > 0.005$

From Norris, et al,[5] with permission.

3. The stroke causing the ECG abnormalities, most often T-wave inversion, S-T depression and elevation, and Q-T interval prolongations[9]

Detection of abnormalities may justify serial ECGs, in conjunction with serial cardiac enzymes, to exclude acute myocardial infarction.

LONG-TERM ECG MONITORING. Monitoring the ECG of the acute stroke patient may detect paroxysmal arrhythmias, which are unsuspected causes of both TIA and cerebral infarction. In the Toronto Unit, 22 percent of 272 patients with cerebral infarction had serious cardiac arrhythmias, including atrial fibrillation, sick sinus syndrome, and ventricular tachycardia.[10] Practical considerations modify the ideal of long-term ECG monitoring of all stroke patients.

Radiology

A *chest x-ray* may show cardiac enlargement, indicating hypertension or cardiac valvular disease, or heart failure or aspiration pneumonia. Most tumors metastasizing to the brain also lodge in the lungs and are visible on chest x-ray.

A *skull x-ray* can help when a CT scan is unavailable. The pineal gland calcifies in most adults, marking midline structures. A pineal shift in the first hours after a stroke suggests hemorrhage and, in the first few days, cerebral infarction due to cerebral edema becoming maximal at 2 to 4 days.[11,12] A skull x-ray may show abnormal calcification in arteriovenous malformation, brain tumor, and cysticercosis.

SPECIAL INVESTIGATIONS

Lumbar puncture is useful when CT scanning is not available. It may confirm intracranial bleeding if the CT is negative or unavailable although the CSF may be clear in intracerebral hemorrhage (Fig. 97) which has not leaked to the spinal subarachnoid space.

Lumbar puncture is contraindicated in stroke patients with drowsiness, coma, papilledema, or other signs of raised intracranial pressure, since it may precipitate transtentorial herniation ("coning"). One third of cerebral infarction patients have a mild elevation of CSF protein.[13] In 80 percent of intracerebral hemorrhage cases and in hemorrhagic infarction, the CSF may be bloodstained and xanthochromic. Xanthochromia appears within 6 hours and is best demonstrated by comparing the CSF supernatant with water. Leukocyte pleocytosis is seen in one third of cerebral infarction cases, two thirds of cerebral hemorrhage cases,[14] and commonly in stroke from septic emboli and marantic endocarditis.

Electroencephalography is not much help in the diagnosis of stroke, especially when CT scanning is available. Epileptogenic foci are seldom seen in patients having seizures with their acute stroke, although they may appear later. Slow waves may mirror a focal lesion but not its cause. The EEG aids in localizing and determining the nature of the lesion.[15]

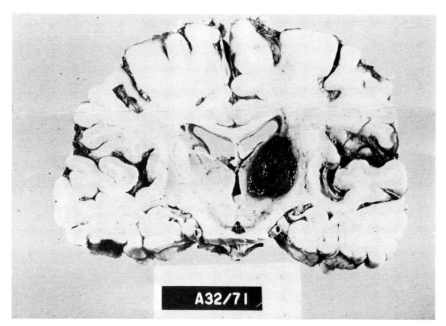

FIGURE 97. Coronal section of the brain showing a large thalamic hemorrhage. The CSF was clear.

Capsular and brainstem infarcts do not change the EEG except in the "locked-in" syndrome, when there may be a continuously awake EEG pattern,[7] or alpha coma and an unreactive EEG.

Computerized Tomography

The investigation and understanding of stroke comprise two eras: before and after CT scanning. These two eras coexist uneasily throughout the world.

CT scanning is a superior diagnostic tool to cerebral angiography in cerebral hemorrhage, since it is positive in virtually all cases.[16,17] A positive CT scan in cerebral infarction reveals the exact location and size of the lesion and the degree of cerebral edema and midline shift. It supersedes the most astute clinician armed with all the diagnostic aids of the pre-CT era.

Cerebral infarcts appear in a vascular territory (Fig. 98, *top*) as low-density areas with initially well-defined boundaries that sharpen in 2 weeks. CT scan is positive in only 5 percent of cases in the first 4 hours, 50 percent by the first day, and 95 percent by the eighth day.[17,18] Necrosis and cavitation (usually after 4 weeks) produce well-defined low-density areas in a recognizable vascular territory, often with retraction of tissue and dilation of part of the ventricular system (Fig. 98, *bottom*). Occasionally, an intracranial artery freshly occluded by a thrombus appears as an abnormally dense structure in the unenhanced CT (Fig. 99).

Enhancement of the lesion with intravenously injected contrast medium occurs usually between the first and fourth weeks,[19,20] but some-

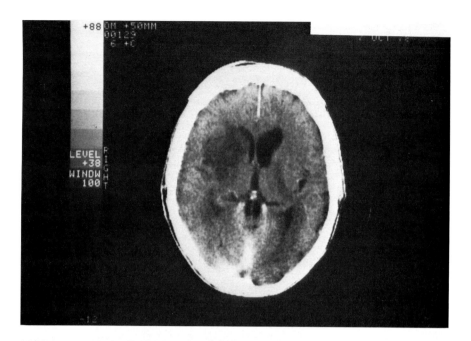

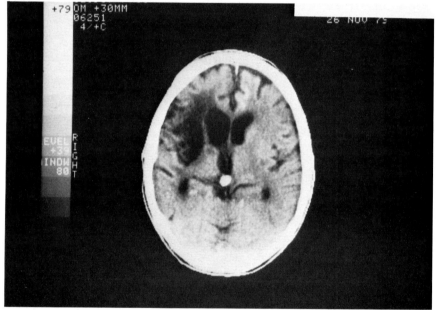

FIGURE 98. *Top,* Infarction in the middle cerebral artery territory. *Bottom,* Postinfarction gliosis of the right cerebral hemisphere, producing retraction of cerebral tissue and enlargement of the lateral ventricle.

times as early as the first day or as late as several months (Fig. 100).[19] It correlates well with a positive isotope brain scan. Contrast enhancement distinguishes cerebral infarcts from primary and secondary tumors and white-matter edema.[21]

Neuropathologic examinations suggest that cerebral infarcts less than 5 mm are difficult to detect on CT,[22] although detection may improve with the greater resolution of newer CT scanners.

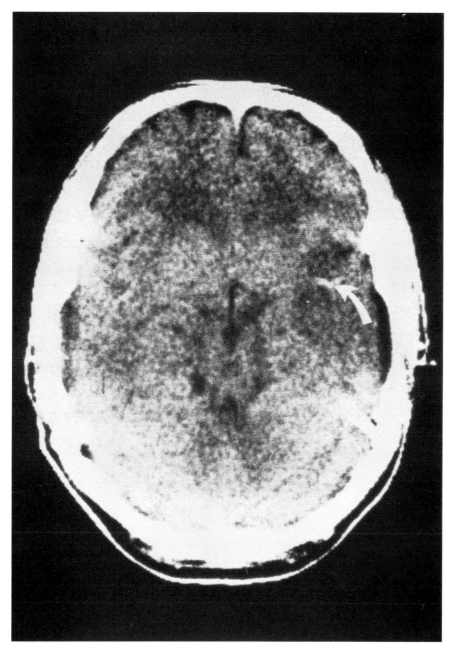

FIGURE 99. Unenhanced CT scan of a 41-year-old man who, on cerebral angiography, had occlusion of the left internal carotid artery in the neck. Note the high-density area corresponding to the trifurcation of the left middle cerebral artery *(arrow)* and the surrounding hypodense area in its vascular territory. (From Gacs, G, et al: Stroke 14:756, 1983, with permission.)

CT is negative in about 80 percent of *TIAs*[23] but may show focal translucency.[18] All patients with presumed TIA should have CT to exclude other structural lesions such as cerebral hemorrhage, tumor, or subdural hematoma.

The diagnosis of *intracranial hemorrhage* represents the single most important use of CT in stroke (Fig. 101), in which the increased density

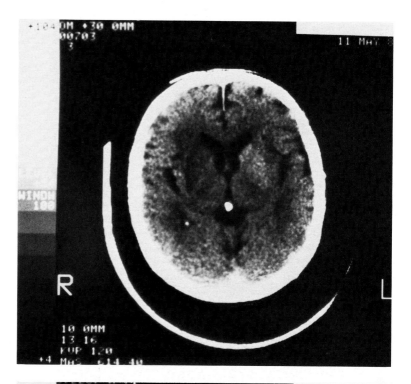

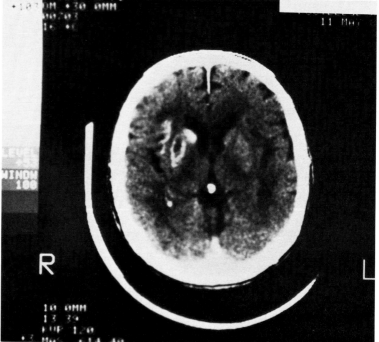

FIGURE 100. Inconspicuous infarction of the right basal ganglia *(top)* shows enhancement after contrast *(bottom)* 5 days after the stroke.

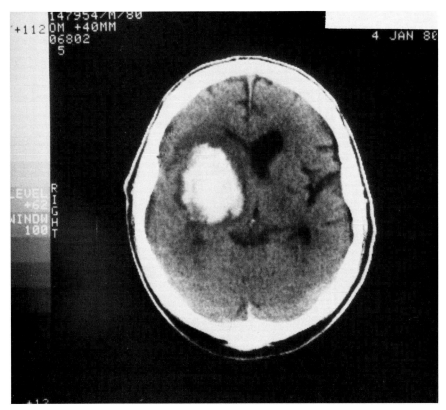

FIGURE 101. Hypertensive hemorrhage with a halo of edema in the right basal ganglia.

is related to globin, calcium content, and hematocrit. Gradual attenuation of density occurs at the periphery as the hematoma resolves, and clot retraction produces decreased density owing to serum extrusion. Cerebral edema, usually appearing by the fourth day, may persist for weeks. Enhancement is probably due to blood-brain barrier permeability and not to luxury perfusion.

The location of the hemorrhage suggests its etiology. Frontal hemorrhages often arise from aneurysms; trigone and parieto-occipital hematomas, as a complication of anticoagulant therapy; and basal ganglia and posterior fossa hemorrhages in hypertension.[24] Intraventricular rupture is not as ominous as once thought, provided CSF circulation remains normal. A CT scan with contrast may show an arteriovenous malformation or a tumor obscured by hematoma. The clinical presentation of small paraputaminal and thalamic hemorrhages can mimic middle cerebral artery territory infarcts. Most lobar hematomas have a good prognosis and do not require surgery unless they result from an arteriovenous malformation or an aneurysm.

Complications of CT scanning include anaphylactic and allergic reactions from contrast medium. Good hydration minimizes the chance of contrast-induced renal failure. Serial studies create a radiation hazard, especially in patients undergoing other radiologic investigations such as angiography.[16]

INVESTIGATION

197

The various *limitations* of CT scanning are listed below.

1. Clinical decisions are often made during the first 48 hours, when the CT is often still negative.
2. Different lesions share the same CT appearance. For example, a residual cerebral hematoma is indistinguishable from an old infarct.
3. CT scan detects changes in brain density and not in brain function, and so has no diagnostic value in conditions with no structural equivalent.
4. The extent of the CT lesion may correlate poorly with clinical signs, and the scan may show a deep infarct when cerebral blood flow measurements demonstrate additional areas of ischemia.
5. Partial volume effect, by averaging out adjacent high- and low-density areas, may obscure hemorrhagic infarcts. This effect and artifact from adjacent bone befog the base of the brain and the brainstem, making it difficult to detect blood in the basal cisterns.
6. Hematomas are difficult to visualize in anemic patients (hemoglobin less than 7 g/100 ml), or if hematomas are isodense and bilateral.

Magnetic Resonance (MR)

Using a principle known for decades, cerebral images are produced by bouncing radio waves from protons, the emitted energy depending on its environment. Horizontal, sagittal, and coronal views can be constructed from three-dimensional data (Fig. 102).

MR is particularly promising in stroke diagnosis,[25] since resolution of gray and white is superior to that of CT scanning and since cerebral infarction is evident much earlier, usually within 2 to 6 hours (Fig. 103).[26,27] It does not visualize bone, and areas normally obscured by bone on CT scan are easily imaged by MR.

Although MR lacks the radiation hazards of x-ray methods, there are dangers. The movement of clips and metal prostheses in the body produced by the powerful magnetic fields may prove fatal, and people wearing metallic objects may be dragged into the machinery. Also, good patient cooperation is essential to avoid movement artifact.

Cerebral Angiography

Visualization of the aortic arch and of the cervical and cerebral vessels is fundamental to the understanding of cerebrovascular disease. Direct puncture and retrograde injection of arteries have been largely replaced by femoral catheterization under local anesthesia with selective injection of the four major arteries leading to the brain.

All views should be in two planes to avoid missing lesions visible in only one plane (Fig. 104). Films of the head as well as of the neck

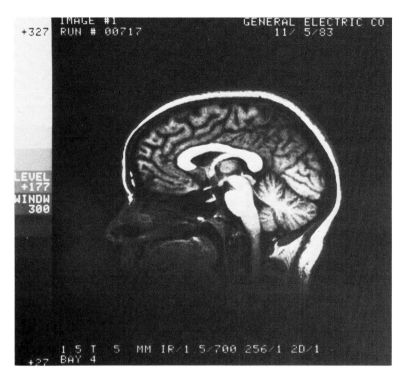

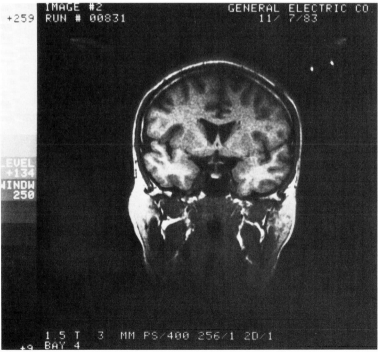

FIGURE 102. Magnetic resonance images of a normal subject; sagittal *(top)*, and coronal *(bottom)* sections. (From General Electric, with permission.)

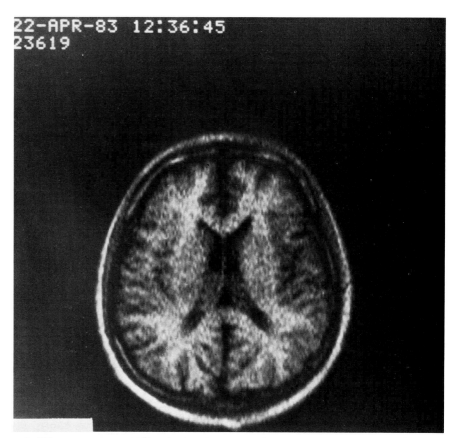

FIGURE 103. Magnetic resonance image of infarction in the left middle cerebral artery territory. (From Technicare, with permission.)

should be taken to demonstrate intracranial (Fig. 105) and tandem lesions. Sufficient films should be obtained of all phases (arterial, capillary, and venous) so that the early filling of veins suggestive of cerebral infarction or the lack of filling of cerebral sinus or vein occlusion are not missed.

Cerebral angiography may reveal ulceration (Fig. 106), thromboembolism (Fig. 107), stenosis, occlusion (Fig. 108), tortuosity, ectasia, anomalies, dissection (Fig 109; see also Fig. 82), fibrous dysplasia, webs, multiple occlusions, and profuse collaterals (see Fig. 83).

In *cerebral infarction* there may be an avascular area with vessel displacement due to edema, late filling of arteries or emptying of veins, absence of normal capillary blush, or early filling veins. The sooner after stroke an angiogram is performed, the more likely it is to show an occlusion.[28] Isolated occlusion of the middle cerebral artery in the presence of a normal internal carotid artery suggests cardiac embolism (Fig. 110).

In *cerebral hemorrhage* the cardinal sign is vessel displacement. In the anteroposterior view, lateral displacement of the lenticulostriate arteries suggests a deeply located hemorrhage, while medial displacements of the lenticulostriate arteries characterizes a superficial hematoma in the area of the external capsule. Rarely, contrast material is visualized leaking from a ruptured vessel. The angiogram may also show an aneu-

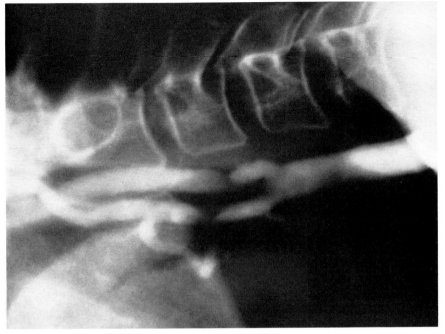

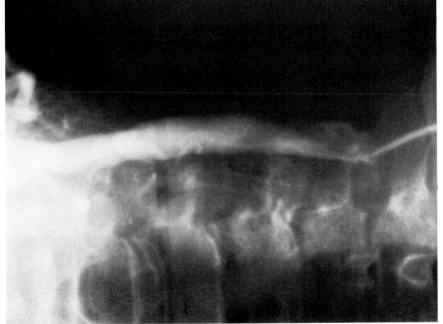

FIGURE 104. Normal-appearing anteroposterior view (*left*) with critical stenoses in the lateral view (*right*) of the carotid arteries.

INVESTIGATION

201

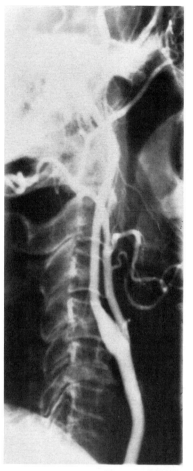

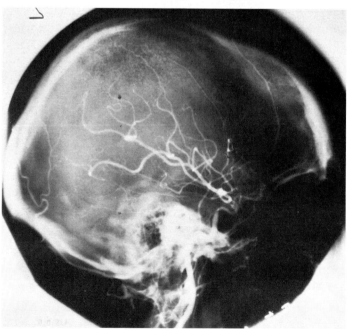

FIGURE 105. Carotid siphon stenosis and normal carotid bifurcation in a patient with TIAs.

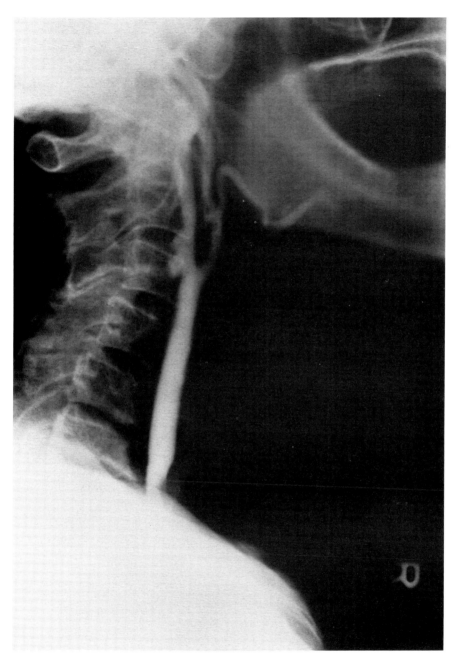

FIGURE 106. Deep ulcer craters in the internal carotid artery missed by carotid Doppler since no stenosis is present.

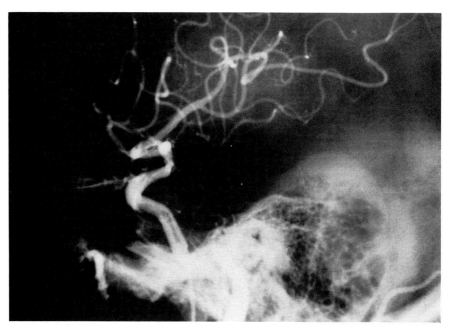

FIGURE 107. Embolism to the carotid siphon from an internal carotid artery bifurcation thrombus.

rysm, arteriovenous malformation (Fig. 111), or tumor responsible for the hemorrhage.

Cerebellar hemorrhage produces forward displacement of branches of the vertebrobasilar system and often hydrocephalus, shown as ventricular enlargement on the venous phase of carotid angiography.

Lesions in the Carotid System

Stenosis, ulceration, and occlusion are common, especially at the carotid bifurcation, the carotid siphon being the second most common site for atherosclerosis. Patients with arterial stenosis greater than 50 percent or with ulceration carry a higher risk of symptoms.[29]

Most cerebral angiograms are performed to identify a surgically correctable lesion, and surgical planning depends on assessing the global circulation of the brain. Visualization of collaterals and cross-filling of one side of the brain to the other become important (Fig. 112).

Lesions in the Vertebrobasilar System

Compared with the carotid system, stenoses and ulcerations are less commonly seen in the vertebral arteries. Occlusions are relatively more common, especially in the basilar artery and the posterior cerebral arteries (Fig. 113). The basilar bifurcation needs to be visualized, because it is often the recipient of emboli.

The chief indication for *cerebral angiography* is the search for a surgically treatable lesion. In ischemic cerebrovascular disease this consists mainly in identifying a stenosis or ulceration that is relevant to the

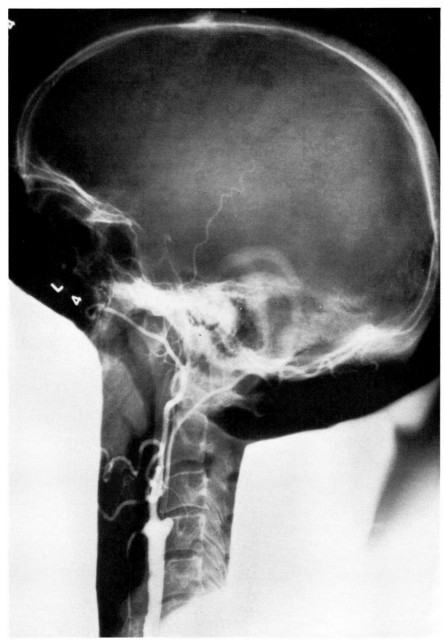

FIGURE 108. Internal carotid artery occlusion. Only the external carotid artery and its branches can be seen distal to the bifurcation.

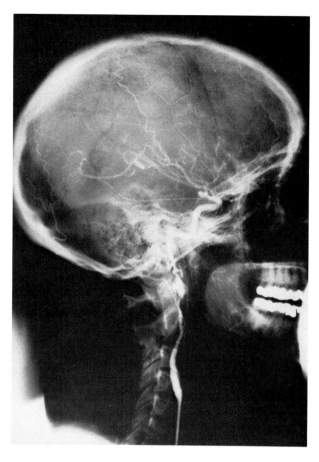

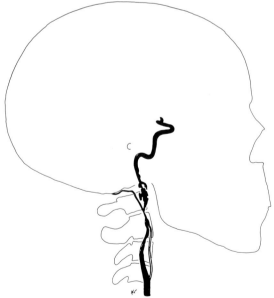

FIGURE 109. This 35-year-old legal secretary had sudden sharp pain in the right side of the neck, followed a few minutes later by dysphasia and right hemiparesis.

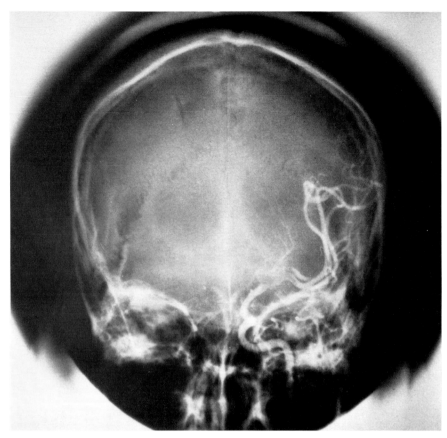

FIGURE 110. Middle cerebral artery occlusion in a patient with a normal carotid bifurcation, suggesting a cardiac source of emboli.

patient's symptoms. Vertebrobasilar ischemic disease seldom justifies cerebral angiography, since surgical management is of dubious value. In hemorrhagic stroke, aneurysms and arteriovenous malformations comprise the main treatable lesions. At times, cerebral angiography proves diagnostic for medically treatable conditions such as multiple small-vessel occlusions suggesting cardiac embolization, mycotic aneurysms implying infected emboli, and irregular constrictions denoting arteritis. Diagnostic angiography is particularly rewarding in the young, in whom the range of etiologic possibilities for stroke is broader than in elderly individuals.

The *complication* rate of carotid angiography varies according to the expertise of the arteriographer, the state of the patient, the extent of atherosclerosis in the vessels, and the nature and duration of the procedure. Serious complications (death or stroke) occur in 1 to 2 percent of cases and "minor" complications in 5 to 6 percent.[30-33]

Complications of direct puncture include dislodging a thrombus or atheromatous debris, subintimal injection of contrast causing critical stenosis, and local hematomas that compress the trachea. With the retrograde technique, occlusion of the brachial artery occurs in about 7 per-

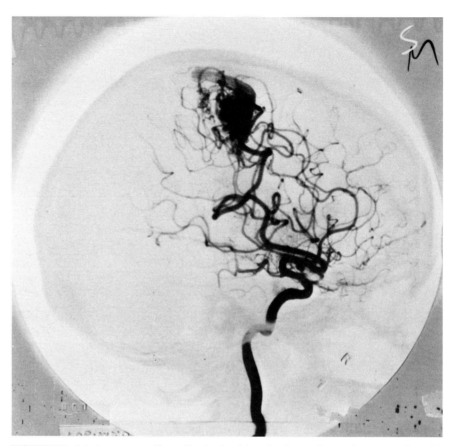

FIGURE 111. Arteriovenous malformation in the right rolandic area in a patient presenting with focal motor seizures of the leg.

cent of cases.[32] Complications relate to the number of injections, the volume of contrast used and the presence of brainstem abnormalities. Local hematomas often occur with the transfemoral route, and there is risk of dislodging atheromatous material from the aorta. Patients with atherosclerosis are probably more susceptible to complications.[32]

In a prospective study, 8.5 percent of 1517 patients undergoing cerebral angiograms had complications within 24 hours, with neurologic complications in 2.6 percent (0.33 percent of them permanent). Age, raised serum creatinine levels, and the use of multiple arterial catheters were associated with serious neurologic complications.[34] In our center, in 600 consecutive angiograms (including direct puncture of the cervical artery as well as the transfemoral route), there were one death and five strokes[33] (Table 40).

Digital Subtraction Arteriography

Although intravenous arteriography was first attempted in 1939,[35] only in the late 1970s did computer technology, imaging systems, and electronic enhancement allow interpretable pictures.[36-38] Digital arteriograms

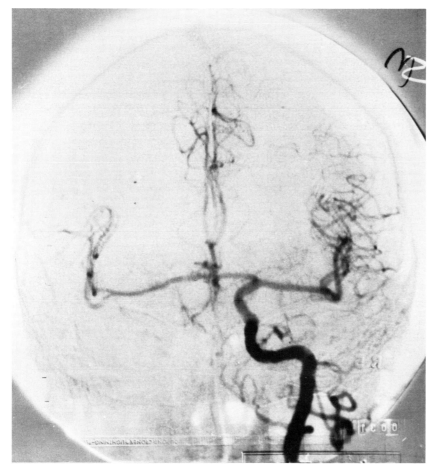

FIGURE 112. Cross-filling of the right hemisphere in a patient with right internal carotid artery occlusion.

can be performed intravenously (IV-DSA) (Fig. 114) or intra-arterially (IA-DSA).

INTRAVENOUS DIGITAL SUBTRACTION ARTERIOGRAPHY (IV-DSA). This technique requires less contrast, radiation, materials, and personnel than does conventional angiography, and by avoiding arterial puncture it becomes an out-patient procedure. About 40 to 60 ml contrast material is injected through a catheter into an antecubital vein or the superior vena cava over 30 to 45 minutes (Fig. 115).

Simultaneous display of vessels in the head and neck produces overlapping images, sometimes obscuring arterial lesions. The patient must remain still for up to 8 seconds to prevent movement artifact and, when contrast medium arrives at the lungs, it produces discomfort, coughing, and swallowing, especially in confused or uncooperative patients.

Even the best IV-DSA has poorer resolution than conventional angiography, and complications, although fewer, remain a small but con-

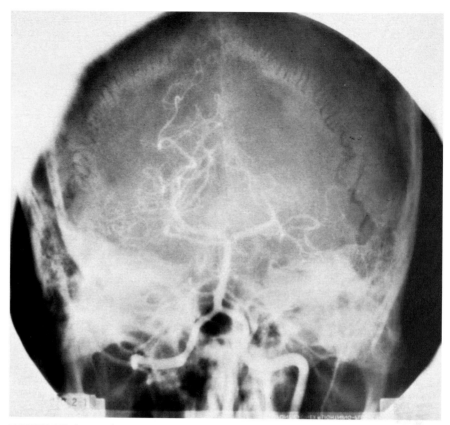

FIGURE 113. Asymptomatic occlusion of the posterior cerebral artery

stant menace. One in 70,000 patients will have a fatal reaction due to anaphylaxis or renal failure.[39]

Value of IV-DSA in Acute Cerebrovascular Disease. The carotid bifurcation images well in over 90 percent of patients, and arterial ulceration is usually clearly depicted, including that of the carotid artery[40] (Fig. 116).

TABLE 40. Reported Rates of Neurologic Complications of Cerebral Angiography

Investigator	Type of Angiography*	Incidence of Complications (%)		Indications
		Transient	Permanent	
Feild et al, 1962[93]	PC	1.4	0.68	All relevant diseases
Blain and Resch, 1966[94]	VT	22.0	0	Vascular occlusive disease
Faught et al, 1979[32]	FC	12.2	5.2	Stroke and TIA
Reisner et al, 1980[95]	VT	1.2	0.67	Vascular disease
Eisenberg et al, 1980[96]	FC	1.3	0	Hemispheric TIA or amaurosis fugax
Norris and D'Alton, 1983[33]	VT	1.3	0.5	Cerebrovascular disease
Earnest et al, 1983[34]	VT	2.3	0.33	Unspecified

*PC = Percutaneous carotid; FC = Femoral catheter; VT = Various techniques.

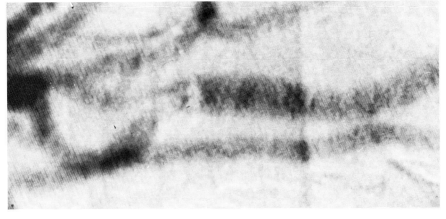

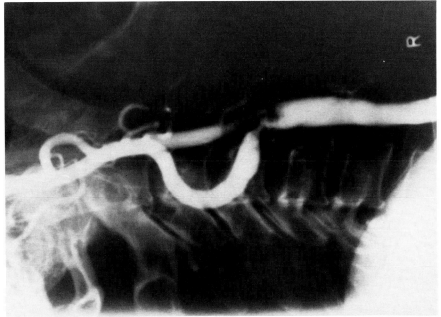

FIGURE 114. Comparison of severe carotid bifurcation stenosis visualized by conventional (*left*) and digital intravenous angiography (*right*).

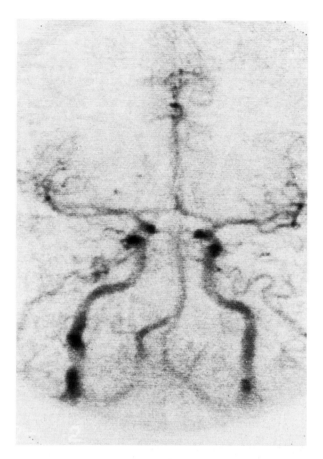

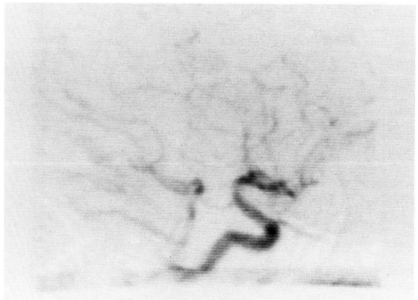

FIGURE 115. The intracranial circulation by digital intravenous angiography, anteroposterior *(top)* and lateral *(bottom)* views.

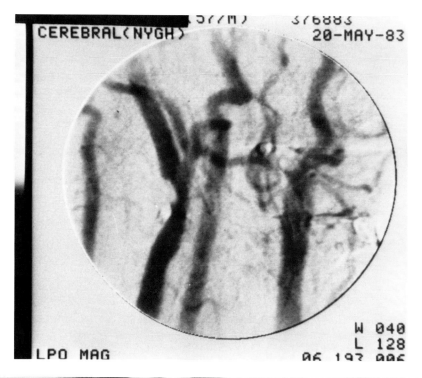

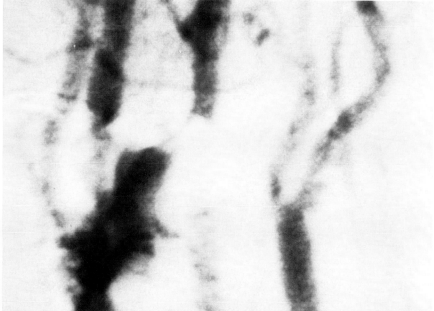

FIGURE 116. *Top,* Right internal carotid artery stenosis visualized by intravenous digital subtraction angiography.
    Bottom, Ulcerated plaque of the internal carotid artery.

Proximal vertebral artery occlusive disease generally lies outside the normal viewing field, though aortic arch views can demonstrate aortic or subclavian stenosis.[40] Occlusion of major intracranial arteries is usually identifiable, although the procedure is technically unsatisfactory in 11 percent of cases.[40]

The technique is valuable for pre- and postoperative evaluation of carotid endarterectomy and for assessing the results of extracranial/intracranial bypass surgery. Since all vessels fill simultaneously with contrast, real-time images are obtained and vertebral steal is easily seen. Using the pattern of cortical artery filling as an index of cerebral blood flow, this technique also compares favorably with xenon-133 inhalation.[40]

DSA was 95 percent sensitive, 99 percent specific, and 97 percent accurate, compared with conventional angiography, in visualizing the carotid bifurcation in 100 patients; but it missed four of eight cases of carotid ulceration.[41] IV-DSA produces false-positive results, which impairs surgical planning, and may result in surgery performed on normal carotid arteries. If conventional angiography is planned anyway, then IV-DSA is redundant.

When carotid Doppler, IV-DSA, and conventional angiography were compared, IV-DSA was found the most accurate in detecting minor stenoses and ulceration, and in differentiating occlusion from high-grade stenosis.[42]

INTRA-ARTERIAL DIGITAL SUBTRACTION ANGIOGRAPHY (IA-DSA). IA-DSA has replaced the intravenous method in some centers, and the better resolution of the intra-arterial technique may make it the new standard of arterial imaging. Greater simplicity and fewer complications make it an out-patient procedure, and only 5 to 10 ml of contrast medium is injected into the aorta. It also obviates the catheterization of the four major cervical vessels, decreasing embolic risks.

Radioisotope Scanning

When the blood-brain barrier is impaired by cerebrovascular or other lesions, the iodine- or technetium-labeled albumin injected intravenously leaks into the brain, producing an area of increased density.

Radioisotope scanning ("nuclear brain scan") has largely been replaced by CT in stroke diagnosis. It is less sensitive and less specific than CT and gives no information on midline shift, hydrocephalus, or ventricular blood. It does not readily differentiate infarcts from hemorrhage, nor from other structural lesions such as cerebral tumor.

Cerebral infarction appears as an area of increased density within a vascular distribution (Fig. 117). The isotope brain scan is positive in 25 percent of patients during the first week and in 75 percent by the third week.[43] The abnormal area resolves in the ensuing weeks, the opposite of cerebral tumor, which becomes increasingly positive and does not conform to a vascular territory. Delayed arrival of isotope in a hemisphere suggests carotid stenosis or occlusion or intracranial obstruction but is not a reliable index of cerebral perfusion. Increased perfusion in the

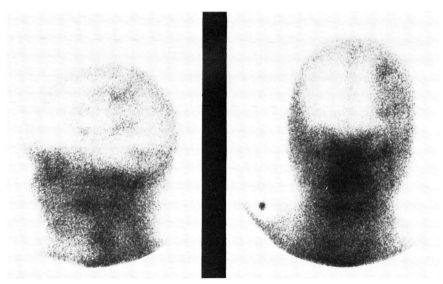

FIGURE 117. Isotope brain scan of an infarction in the left middle cerebral artery territory.

infarcted hemisphere ("hot stroke") may occur with cerebral embolism.[44] Patients with cerebral infarction and abnormal brain scans, especially if persistent, have a worse prognosis than those with normal scans.[45]

Cerebral hemorrhage may be manifested as a "ring" lesion, often sparing the cortex, and appearing more like a tumor or abscess than like a cerebral infarct. Acute *subdural hematoma* may not show on brain scan, but the chronic hematoma almost always produces a positive scan. *Tumors* most often appear subcortically, are not confined to a vascular territory, and have less well-defined margins than do infarcts. Sometimes they have a "donut-like" appearance, though this is more characteristic of abscesses.

Isotope brain scanning has few *complications* but many *limitations.* Brain scanning may miss lesions in the posterior fossa, lesions in the base of the brain, or bilateral subdural hematomas. Its spatial resolution is about 2 cm, well below that of CT. Lesions may not appear for days, or ever. When ⁹⁹Tc-pertechnetate and CT scans were compared in stroke patients, both located superficial lesions equally well 3 weeks after stroke, but ⁹⁹Tc scanning missed 18 of 32 deep infarcts identified by CT.[46]

Carotid Doppler Ultrasonography

A moving column of blood cells changes the frequency of reflected sound and the frequency difference between the transmitted and reflected sound waves represents the "Doppler shift" (Fig. 118). Arterial stenosis increases blood velocity, increasing the Doppler shift from the normal range of 2 to 4 kHz (Fig. 119) to levels reaching 20 kHz in severe stenoses. This technique is most accurate with high-grade stenoses but is insensitive to luminal narrowing less than 35 percent[47,48] (see Table 41).

For optimal accuracy, this method should be combined with *periorbital directional Doppler.* Normally, the direction of orbital blood flow is

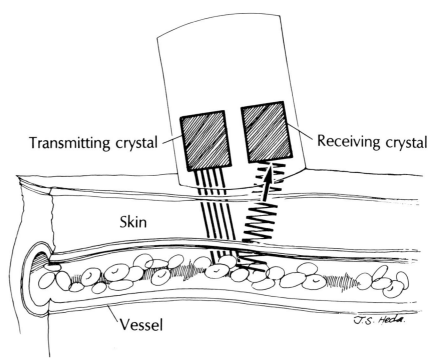

FIGURE 118. The Doppler principle. The difference between the transmitted and reflected ultrasound frequency is the "Doppler shift." The faster the blood flow (arterial stenosis) the greater the difference, and the higher the "shift" frequency. (From D'Alton and Norris,[48] with permission.)

Transmitting crystal

Receiving crystal

Skin

Vessel

J.S. Heda.

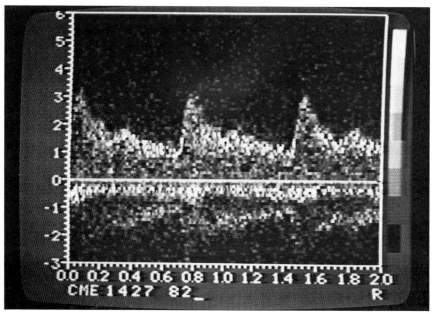

FIGURE 119. Normal Doppler sonogram. (From D'Alton and Norris,[48] with permission.)

TABLE 41. Results of Carotid Doppler Examination and Angiography in 123 Patients (246 Carotid Arteries)

Stenosis (%) Detected by Doppler Examination	No. of Arteries					
	Stenosis (%) Detected by Angiography					
	100	75–99	50–74	35–49	0–34	Total
100	14	2	0	0	0	16
75–99	8	53	5	3	4	73
50–74	1	5	6	1	3	16
35–49	0	0	4	6	3	13
0–34	1	1	8	7	111	128
Total	24	61	23	17	121	246

From D'Alton, and Norris,[48] with permission.

toward the eye from the brain (Fig. 120). If the internal carotid artery is occluded, the flow reversal is easily detected by the Doppler probe. The display of the common carotid artery and its branches, used for monitoring sites of high frequency, is not anatomically exact or equivalent to an arteriogram. It acts only as a guide to localizing Doppler shifts in the

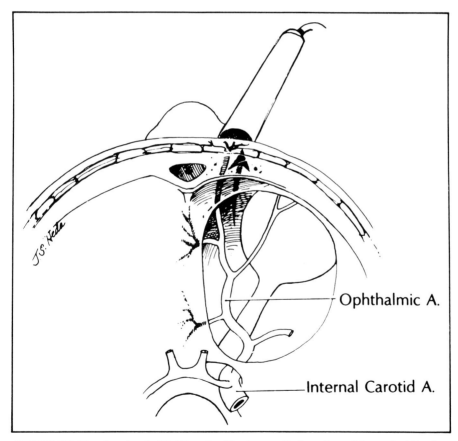

Ophthalmic A.

Internal Carotid A.

FIGURE 120. Directional periorbital Doppler. Blood normally flows toward the probe (direction of *arrow*), but in internal carotid artery occlusion the flow is reversed as external carotid collaterals attempt to perfuse the brain. (From D'Alton and Norris,[48] with permission.)

arterial system. The degree of arterial narrowing is determined by the peak Doppler frequency shift, turbulence, and the direction of blood flow in periorbital vessels. Precision is enhanced by spectral analysis and by color-coded display of Doppler signals.

VALUE OF CAROTID DOPPLER. In patients with TIAs, finding carotid artery stenosis, especially if "critical" (greater than 75 percent), should urge carotid angiography; and a normal Doppler or angiogram should prompt echocardiography.

Finding carotid stenosis in a patient with stroke will not affect the patient's management unless recovery is sufficient to consider carotid endarterectomy.

Carotid Doppler cannot detect intracranial or nonstenosing ulcerated arterial lesions, nor should it be a substitute for angiography (see Fig. 108). Doppler visualizes the vertebrobasilar system poorly and is of limited value there, except in subclavian steal.

In patients with *asymptomatic neck bruits,* when harmless lesions such as external carotid or other arterial stenosis cause the bruit, the patient can be reassured. Whether those patients with internal carotid artery lesions should be investigated further is controversial.[48-53]

Arterial patency after carotid endarterectomy or extracranial/intracranial bypass surgery can be assessed repeatedly and safely, without angiography.

B-Mode (Real-Time) Scanning

Imaging the pulsating artery identifies the carotid branches and often detects ulceration, plaques, and low-grade stenoses, but detection of high-grade stenosis is technically more difficult with this method than with carotid Doppler.

Difficulty in imaging increases with the depth of the structure. B-mode scanning can image neither the petrous portion of the internal carotid artery nor high carotid bifurcations. Lesions with the same acoustic impedance as blood are invisible ("sonolucent") to real-time imaging, and averaging of signals from a plaque with those of overlying normal tissues impairs definition of the lumen.[43] A tight stenosis is difficult to distinguish from occlusion, since the signal is so weak in both cases.

Duplex scanning, a Doppler probe combined with B-mode scanning,[54] is promising with nonstenotic lesions. Problems include a technical failure rate of about 20 percent, failure to distinguish total from subtotal occlusion, and an underestimation of significant stenotic lesions.[55,56]

Echocardiography

Echocardiography is indicated when the history or examination suggest a cardiogenic embolic source, especially a valvular lesion or a myocardial infarct. While routine echocardiography seldom yields new information in the absence of a positive history or physical examination, it is sometimes the only way of making a diagnosis, particularly in the young.[57] It has no known harmful effects and demonstrates lesions of the cardiac valves, the presence of akinetic segments, and thrombi on the valves or the heart chambers (see Fig. 74) as small as 0.5 cm.[58]

The right heart may be inaccessible to ultrasound examination in obese or thin patients, and in those with obstructive lung disease or enlarged cardiac chambers. If the cardiac septum or other area is visualized in only one plane, akinetic segments may be missed. Small vegetations and thrombi are sometimes beyond the resolution of the technique, and failure to demonstrate thrombi in the heart chambers may merely indicate their departure to the brain.

RESEARCH INVESTIGATIONS

Special Hematology

Hemoglobin electrophoresis is indicated if a hemoglobinopathy is suspected. Patients with sickle-cell anemia and Hb-SS die early and are prone to stroke, but those with sickle-cell trait (Hb-AS) have a better prognosis and fewer strokes.[59]

Platelet function and *coagulation* often change after TIA and cerebral infarction,[60] although it remains uncertain whether this reflects cause or effect. Although their clinical usefulness remains unproven, determination of beta-thromboglobulin[61] and platelet factor IV[62] may prove helpful in determining stroke risk or occurrence. The need for bleeding and clotting times, and prothrombin and cryoglobulin levels is dictated by the clinical situation.

Special CSF Determinations

The concentration of compounds in the lumbar cerebrospinal fluid (CSF) varies inversely with CSF turnover. Bedridden patients have slow CSF circulation and decreased clearance of substances that may reflect immobility rather than brain activity or injury. CSF–homovanillic acid provides an uncontaminated index of brain dopamine activity since it is not synthesized in the spinal cord. The CSF-HVA was decreased in brainstem infarct patients and widely scattered in hemisphere infarct cases, suggesting alteration of dopamine metabolism in acute stroke.[63] Other catecholamines, serotonin, aldolase, lactic dehydrogenase, enolase, cAMP, and adenylate kinase do not warrant routine lumbar puncture.[64–68] Spectrophotometry of the CSF can be helpful in detecting bleeding into the CSF.[69]

Polysomnography

Many systems, from brainstem to cortex, participate in the elaboration of sleep. Stroke disrupts this highly organized process in proportion to its extent.[70]

Evoked Responses

Visual, auditory, and somatosensory stimuli produce characteristic brainwaves that can be recorded noninvasively and can give information oth-

INVESTIGATION

219

erwise difficult to obtain, such as auditory evoked response in brainstem lesions. Evoked responses have become a growth industry out of proportion to their clinical usefulness and should only be performed when information relevant to the management of the patient may be obtained.[71]

Brain Electric Activity Mapping (BEAM)

This method combines information from EEG and evoked responses into color-coded tomographic maps.[72] Abnormalities have been demonstrated when the CT scan was normal, but this technique has not yet been evaluated in stroke.

Neuro-Otologic Evaluation.

Electronystagmography and other neuro-otologic evaluations can be helpful in specific cases of brainstem infarction or when an objective record of transient ocular abnormalities is required, such as in transient global amnesia.[73]

Dynamic CT Scanning

Measurement by CT of the distribution and density in the brain of intravenous contrast material provides an index of the cerebral circulation but not of cerebral perfusion. The vascular volume of the brain is variable—about 5 percent—and the cerebral blood volume can double without affecting the flow. CT scan will measure transit times but, because of relatively slow circulation in the brain (3 to 8 seconds), the in- and outflow phases of the contrast medium bolus overlap.[74] Numerous brain "slices" must be taken to obtain reasonable estimates of the transit time, thus increasing radiation hazards. Under ideal conditions, CT techniques produce cerebral blood flow values obtained by other methods but, with impairment of the blood-brain barrier, the assumptions used for the calculations become invalid and quantitation impossible.[75] Consequently, dynamic CT scanning is least reliable in the pathologic conditions of greatest clinical interest.

Cerebral blood flow can be measured through xenon inhalation and dynamic CT scanning.[76,77] Unfortunately, the need for analgesic and near-anesthetic doses of xenon (30 to 70 percent) make it difficult to study the cerebral circulation under physiologic conditions.

Estimation of Cerebral Blood Flow

The gamma-emitter xenon-133 is introduced into the cerebral circulation by intracarotid or intravenous injection, or by inhalation. Although the direct carotid route is technically the best, the others are preferred as less invasive. The speed of cerebral washout of the isotope is proportional to the cerebral blood flow. Regional flow in each hemisphere is measured using a probe bank of up to 240 probes.[78]

This technique, introduced using krypton-85, gave a new, dynamic dimension to cerebral function.[79] Regional cerebral blood flow (rCBF) reflects metabolism and function, mapping cortical activities such as speech, listening, and calculation.[78]

Failure of resolution of subcortical structures and the need for carotid puncture seriously limit this method. Although it can be performed during clinically indicated carotid angiography, it increases the danger of cerebral embolism.

It was valuable in studying the pathogenesis of stroke,[80] migraine,[81-83] and multi-infarct dementia,[84-86] and it helped delineate the thresholds of cardiac ischemia for carotid clamping or ligature.[87] It is now largely superseded by more dynamic tomographic imaging such as position emission tomography and single-photon emission tomography.

Single-Photon Emission Tomography

Combining the xenon-133 cerebral blood flow technique with tomography measures subcortical as well as cortical blood flow,[88] but it is limited by poor resolution and high radioisotope doses. The technique is being developed with various isotopes but seems unlikely to add to the knowledge obtained by conventional CBF methods and PET scanning.

Positron Emission Tomography (PET)

High-resolution tomographic imaging of cerebral function can be obtained using positron-emitting isotopes and positron-sensitive detectors, which rotate in a gantry around the head[89] (Fig. 121). The resolution of PET scanning is about 1 cm and is unlikely to become less than 5 mm, the average distance traveled by a positron before it collides with an electron and annihilates.

This is an expensive and cumbersome technique, as the short half-life of the isotopes requires a nearby cyclotron and a large team of experts. Its expense and complexity will limit its clinical use, but it remains a technique of enormous potential in elucidating the pathophysiology of stroke.

Oxygen-15 allows measurement of oxygen metabolism, 2-deoxy-glucose reflects glucose metabolism, and labeled carbon dioxide provides an index of cerebral blood flow.[90,91] The simultaneous measurement of cerebral blood flow and metabolism has proven valuable in investigating the pathogenesis of stroke[90] and dementia.[92]

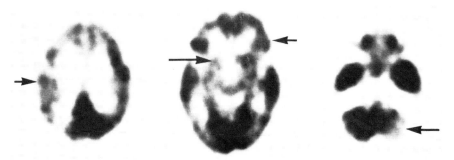

FIGURE 121. PET scans of a patient with only evidence of cerebral atrophy on CT scan, who had multiple areas of focal decrease in glucose metabolism *(arrows)*, suggesting multi-infarct dementia. (From Kuhl, DE: *The effects of aging and stroke on patterns of local cerebral glucose utilization.* In Reivich, M, and Hurtig, HI (eds): *Cerebrovascular Diseases.* Raven Press, New York, 1983, p 25, with permission.)

CONCLUSION

Clinical judgment should guide investigation. Every diagnostic test should offer potential benefit greater than its actual cost, risk, or inconvenience. These considerations may indicate a different strategy for each individual. Increasing the number of laboratory tests in patients with difficult diagnoses will confuse more than clarify, unless they are performed logically.

The physician should decide beforehand what action will follow a positive test, and treatable causes should be sought. Unusual problems merit full investigation, especially in young patients in whom an extraordinary etiology is more probable.

Clinical reassessment is often more enlightening than further tests. Careful and repeated clinical evaluation should always precede investigations of a diagnostic puzzle or unexplained clinical deterioration.

REFERENCES

1. KANNEL, WB, ET AL: *Hemoglobin and the risk of cerebral infarction: The Framingham study.* Stroke 3:409, 1972.
2. ELWOOD, PC, ET AL: *Mortality and anemia in women.* Lancet 1:891, 1974.
3. BANCALARI, E, ET AL: *Hospital incidence of cerebrovascular diseases in high altitude.* In MEYER, JS, ET AL (EDS): *Cerebral Vascular Disease 4.* Excerpta Medica, Amsterdam, 1983, p 22.
4. HARRISON, MJG, ET AL: *Effect of haematocrit on carotid stenosis and cerebral infarction.* Lancet 2:114, 1981.
5. NORRIS, JW, ET AL: *Serum cardiac enzymes in stroke.* Stroke 10:548, 1979.
6. MELAMED, E: *Reactive hyperglycemia in patients with acute stroke.* J Neurol Sci 29:267, 1976.
7. PLUM, F, AND POSNER, JB: *The Diagnosis of Stupor and Coma,* ed 3. FA Davis, Philadelphia, 1980.
8. GORDON, T, ET AL: *High density lipoprotein as a protective factor against coronary heart disease: The Framingham study.* Am J Med 62:707, 1977.
9. WEIDLER, DJ, *Myocardial damage and cardiac arrhythmias after intracranial hemorrhage. A critical review.* Stroke 5:759, 1974.
10. NORRIS, JW: *Effect of cerebrovascular lesions on the heart.* Neurol Clin 1:87, 1983.
11. SHAW, CM, ET AL: *Swelling of the brain following ischemic infarction with arterial occlusion.* Arch Neurol 1:161, 1959.
12. NG, LKY, AND NIMMANNITYA, J: *Massive cerebral infarction with severe brain swelling.* Stroke 1:158, 1970.
13. MERRITT, HH: *A Textbook of Neurology,* ed 6. Lea & Febiger, Philadelphia, 1979, p 173.
14. SÖRNÄS, R, OSTLUND, H, AND MÜLLER, R: *Cerebrospinal fluid cytology after stroke.* Arch Neurol 26:489, 1972.
15. PRIMAVERA, A, ET AL: *Letter to the Editor. The EEG in lacunar strokes.* Stroke 15:579, 1984.
16. KINKEL, W: *Computerized tomography in clinical neurology.* In BAKER, AB (ED): *Clinical Neurology,* Vol 4. Harper and Row, Philadelphia, 1983.
17. ABRAMS, HL, AND MCNEIL, BJ: *Medical implications of computed tomography ("CAT scanning").* N Engl J Med 298:255, 1978.
18. AULICH, A, FENSKE, A, AND WENDE, S: *Computerized axial tomography for diagnosis and follow-up studies of acute cerebral infarcts and hemorrhagic infarctions.* In MEYER, JS, LECHNER, H, AND REIVICH, M: *Cerebral Vascular Disease.* Excerpta Medica, Amsterdam, 1977, p 184.
19. NORTON, GA, KISHORE, PRS, AND LIN, J: *CT contrast enhancement in cerebral infarction.* AJR 131:881, 1978.
20. WEISBERG, LA: *Computerized tomographic enhancement patterns in cerebral infarction.* Arch Neurol 37:21, 1980.
21. KINKEL, W: *Clinical neurology.* In BAKER, AB (ED): *Computerized Tomography in Clinical Neurology,* Vol 1. Harper & Row, Philadelphia, 1983.

22. TOHGI, H, ET AL: *A comparison between the computed tomogram and the neuropathological findings in cerebrovascular disease.* J Neurol 224:211, 1981.

23. LADURNER, G, ET AL: *A correlation of clinical findings and CT in ischaemic cerebrovascular disease.* Eur Neurol 18:281, 1979.

24. ROPPER, AH, AND DAVIS, KR: *Lobar cerebral hemorrhages: Acute clinical syndromes in 26 cases.* Ann Neurol 8:141, 1980.

25. BUONANNO, FS, ET AL: *Proton NMR imaging in experimental ischemic infarction.* Stroke 14:178, 1983.

26. DOYLE, RH, ET AL: *Imaging of the brain by nuclear magnetic resonance.* Lancet 2:53, 1981.

27. SPETZLER, RF, ET AL: *NMR imaging: Preliminary laboratory and clinical evaluation of focal cerebral ischemia.* J Cereb Blood Flow Metab (Suppl)3:87, 1983.

28. BLADIN, PF: *A radiologic and pathologic study of embolism of the internal carotid-middle cerebral arterial axis.* Radiology 32:615, 1964.

29. GROTTA, JC, ET AL: *The significance of carotid stenosis or ulceration.* Neurology 34:437, 1984.

30. HASS, WK, ET AL: *Joint study of extracranial arterial occlusion: ii. Arteriography, techniques, sites, and complications.* JAMA 203:961, 1968.

31. MANI, RL, ET AL: *Complications of catheter cerebral arteriography: Analysis of 5000 procedures.* AJR 131:861, 1978.

32. FAUGHT, E, TRADER, SD, AND HANNA, GR: *Cerebral complications of angiography for transient ischemia and stroke: Prediction of risk.* Neurology 29:4, 1979.

33. NORRIS, JW, AND D'ALTON, JG: *Outcome of patients with asymptomtic carotid bruits.* In REIVICH, M, AND HURTIG, HI (EDS): *Cerebrovascular Diseases.* Raven Press, New York, 1983, p 63.

34. EARNEST, F, IV, ET AL: *Complications of cerebral angiography: Prospective assessment of risk.* AJNR 4:1191, 1983.

35. ROBB, GP, AND STEINBERG, I: *Visualization of the chambers of the heart, the pulmonary circulation, and the great blood vessels in man.* AJR 41:1, 1939.

36. BRANT-ZAWADZKI, M, ET AL: *Digital subtraction cerebral angiography by intraarterial injection: Comparison with conventional angiography.* AJNR 3:593, 1982.

37. CHILCOTE, WA, ET AL: *Digital subtraction angiography of the carotid arteries: A comparative study in 100 patients.* Radiology 139:287, 1981.

38. CRUMMY, AB, ET AL: *Computerized fluoroscopy: Digital subtraction for intravenous angiocardiography and arteriography.* AJR 135:1131, 1980.

39. FURLAN, AJ, ET AL: *Digital subtraction angiography in the evaluation of cerebrovascular disease.* Neurol Clin 1:55, 1983.

40. LITTLE, JR, ET AL: *Intravenous digital subtraction. Angiography in brain ischemia.* JAMA 247:3213, 1982.

41. FURLAN, AJ, ET AL: *Digital subtraction angiography in the evaluation of cerebrovascular disease.* Neurol Clin 1:55, 1983.

42. TURNIPSEED, WD, ET AL: *A comparison of standard cerebral arteriography with noninvasive Doppler imaging and intravenous angiography.* Arch Surg 117:419, 1982.

43. CHIU, LC, ET AL: *Computed tomography and brain scintigraphy in ischemic stroke.* AJR 127:481, 1976.

44. YARNELL, P, BURDICK, D, AND SANDERS, B: *The "hot stroke."* Arch Neurol 30:65, 1974.

45. NARVA, EV: *Radionuclide brain scanning and rapid sequential scintiphotography in patients with cerebral infarction.* Dissertation, University of Turku, Finland, 1980.

46. OLSEN, TS, ET AL: *Brain scintigraphy with Tc^{99}-pertechnetate in the evaluation of patients with cerebrovascular lesions.* Acta Neurol Scand 67:229, 1983.

47. BARNES, RW, ET AL: *Doppler cerebrovascular examination: Improved results with refinements in technique.* Stroke 8:468, 1977.

48. D'ALTON, JG, AND NORRIS, JW: *Carotid Doppler evaluation in cerebrovascular disease.* Can Med Assoc J 129:1184, 1983.

49. YATSU, FM, AND HART, FG: *Asymptomatic carotid bruit and stenosis: A reappraisal.* Stroke 14:301, 1983.

50. QUINONES-BALDRICH, WJ, AND MOORE, WS: *Letter: Asymptomatic carotid stenosis: Rationale for management.* Arch Neurol (in press).

51. YATSU, F, AND FIELDS, WS: *Asymptomatic carotid stenosis: Rationale for management.* Arch Neurol (in press).

52. HACHINSKI, VC: *Editorial comment: Asymptomatic carotid stenosis: Rationale for management.* Arch Neurol (in press).

53. CHAMBERS, BR, AND NORRIS, JW: *Asymptomatic carotid stenosis: Rationale for management.* Arch Neurol (in press).

54. ACKERMAN, RH: *A perspective on noninvasive diagnosis of carotid disease.* Neurology 29:615, 1979.

55. HENNERICI, M, AND FREUND, H-J: *Efficacy of CW-Doppler and duplex system examinations for the evaluation of extracranial carotid disease.* J Clin Ultrasound 12:155, 1984.

56. FISHER, CM, KARP, H, AND ADAMS, RD: *Cerebrovascular diseases.* In HARRISON, TR, ET AL: *Principles of Internal Medicine,* ed 3. McGraw-Hill, New York, 1958.

57. BARNETT, HJM: *Heart in ischemic stroke—A changing emphasis.* Neurol Clin 1:291, 1983.

58. LOVETT, JL, ET AL: *Two-dimensional echocardiography in patients with focal cerebral ischemia.* Ann Intern Med 95:1, 1981.

59. PORTNOY, BA, AND HERION, JC: *Neurological manifestations in sickle-cell disease.* Ann Intern Med 76:643, 1972.

60. DOUGHERTY, JH, LEVY, AND WEKSLER, BB: *Platelet activation in acute cerebral ischaemia.* Lancet 1:821, 1977.

61. ZAHAVI, J, AND KAKKAR, VV: *B-thromboglobulin—a specific marker of in-vivo platelet release reaction.* Thromb Haemost 44:23, 1980.

62. GAWEL, MJ: *Activation of coagulation and fibrinolytic systems after stroke.* In PLUM, F, AND PULSINELLI, W (EDS) *Cerebrovascular Diseases.* Raven Press, New York, p 225.

63. HACHINSKI, VC, ET AL: *Cerebrospinal fluid homovanillic acid in cerebral infarction.* J Neurol Transmission (Suppl 14):45, 1978.

64. MEYER, JS, ET AL: *Disordered neurotransmitter function demonstrated by measurement of norepinephrine and 5-hydrotryptamine in CSF of patients with recent cerebral infarction.* Brain 97:655, 1974.

65. WOLINTZ, AH: *Serum and cerebrospinal fluid enzymes in cerebrovascular disease.* Arch Neurol 20:54, 1969.

66. DONNAN, GA, ET AL: *CSF enzymes in lacunar and cortical stroke.* Stroke 14:266, 1983.

67. HEIKKINEN, ER, ET AL: *Cerebrospinal fluid concentration of cyclic AMP in cerebrovascular diseases.* Eur Neurol 14:129, 1976.

68. TERENT, A, AND RONQUIST, G: *Cerebrospinal fluid markers of disturbed brain cell metabolism in patients with stroke and global cerebral ischemia.* Acta Neurol Scand 62:327, 1980.

69. SÖDERSTRÖM, CE: *Diagnostic significance of CSF spectrophotometry and computer tomography in cerebrovascular disease.* Stroke 8:606, 1977.

70. HACHINSKI, VC, MAMELAK, M, AND NORRIS, JW: *Prognostic value of sleep morphology in cerebral infarction.* In MEYER, JS, LECHNER, H, AND REIVICH, M (EDS): *Cerebral Vascular Diseases 2.* Excerpta Medica, Amsterdam, 1979, p 287.

71. EISEN, A, AND CRACCO, RQ: *Overuse of evoked potentials: Caution.* Neurology 33:618, 1983.

72. DUFFY, FH, BURCHFIELD, JL, AND LOMBROSO, CT: *Brain electrical activity mapping (BEAM): A method for extending the clinical utility of EEG and evoked potential data.* Ann Neurol 5:309, 1979.

73. LONGRIDGE, NS: *Brain stem dysfunction in transient global amnesia.* Stroke 10:473, 1979.

74. TRAUPE, H, ET AL: *Hyperperfusion and enhancement in dynamic computed tomography of ischemic stroke patients.* J Comput Assist Tomogr 3:627, 1979.

75. PHELPS, ME, AND KUHL, DE: *Pitfalls in the measurement of cerebral blood volume with computed tomography.* Radiology 121:375, 1976.

76. DRAYER, BP, ET AL: *Xenon enhanced CT for analysis of cerebral integrity, perfusion, and blood flow.* Stroke 9:123, 1978.

77. GUR, D: *In-vivo mapping of local cerebral blood flow by xenon-enhanced computerized tomography.* Science 215:1267, 1982.

78. LASSEN, NA, INGVAR, DH, AND SKINHØJ, E: *Brain function and blood flow.* Sci Am 239:62, 1978.

79. INGVAR, DH: *Functional landscapes of the dominant hemisphere.* Brain Res 107:181, 1976.

80. FIESCHI, C, AND LENZI, GL: *Cerebral blood flow and metabolism in stroke patients.* In ROSS RUSSELL, RW (ED): *Vascular Disease of the Central Nervous System,* ed 2. Churchill-Livingstone, Edinburgh, p 101.

81. O'BRIEN, MD: *Cerebral blood changes in migraine.* Headache 10:139, 1971.

82. SKINHØJ, E: *Hemodynamic studies within the brain during migraine.* Arch Neurol 29:95, 1973.

83. OLESEN, J, LARSEN, B, AND LAURITZEN, M: *Focal hyperemia followed by spreading oligemia and impaired activation of rCBF in classic migraine.* Ann Neurol 9:344, 1981.

84. O'Brien, MD, and Mallett, BL: *Cerebral cortex perfusion rates in dementia.* J Neurol Neurosurg Psychiatry 33:497, 1970.

85. Simard, D, et al: *Regional cerebral blood flow and its regulation in dementia.* Brain 94:273, 1971.

86. Hachinski, VC, et al: *Cerebral blood flow in dementia.* Arch Neurol 32:632, 1975.

87. Jennett, WB, Harper, AM, and Gillespie, FC: *Measurement of regional cerebral blood flow during carotid ligation.* Lancet 2:1162, 1966.

88. Stokely, EM, et al: *A single photon dynamic computer assisted tomograph (DCAT) for imaging brain function in multiple cross sections.* J Comput Assist Tomogr 4:230, 1980.

89. Walker, MD (ed): *Research issues in positron emission tomography.* Ann Neurol (Suppl)15:S1, 1984.

90. Wise, RJS, et al: *Serial observations on the pathophysiology of acute stroke.* Brain 106:197, 1983.

91. Sokoloff, L: *Circulation and energy metabolism of the brain.* In Siegel, GJ, et al (eds): *Basic Neurochemistry*, ed 3. Little, Brown, Boston, 1981, p 471.

92. Frackowiak, RSJ, and Wise, RJS: *Positron tomography in ischemic cerebrovascular disease.* Neurol Clin 1:183, 1983.

93. Feild, JR, Robertson, JT, and DeSaussure, RL, JR: *Complications of cerebral angiography in 2000 consecutive cases.* J Neurosurg 19:775, 1962.

94. Blain, JG, and Resch, JA: *Complications of angiography in the stroke patient.* Geriatrics 21:149, 1966.

95. Reisner, H, Samec, P, and Zeiler, K: *On the complication rate of cerebral angiography.* Neurosurg Rev 3:23, 1980.

96. Eisenberg, RL, Bank, WO, and Hedgcock, MW: *Neurologic complications of angiography for cerebrovascular disease.* Neurology 30:895, 1980.

Chapter 12

MANAGEMENT

The tendency to improvement, by cerebral compensation,
and by spontaneous disappearance of indirect symptoms,is very marked and
makes it difficult to estimate
the actual influence of treatment that is employed;
at the same time it renders these cases
as a tempting field for the assumptions of the quasi-therapist.
William Gowers

The naive view that stroke is a product of irreversibly dead brain has generated a nihilistic attitude to treatment. Considerable potential for recovery lies in the area surrounding the acute lesion, where cell damage is reversible. The volume and degree of cellular necrosis within this invisible halo may explain the unpredictable and variable recovery of stroke patients with apparently similar lesions.

The brain has a limited repertoire of responses to injury, irrespective of the underlying cause. The term "stroke" encompasses a variety of totally different pathologies, and the principles of management depend upon knowing the precise underlying cause (for example, the hemiplegia of subarachnoid hemorrhage is managed differently from that of cerebral embolism). Trials conducted without CT or MR confirmation of the underlying pathology are unreliable since evaluating therapy in such a heterogeneous group of "stroke" patients runs the risk of dismissing as ineffective a treatment that might be beneficial to a diagnostic subgroup.

A profusion of unproven therapies persists in spite of the conflicting conclusions of early drug studies. It is popular to decry these pioneering trials, but methodology is a developing science and even now is beyond the province of most clinicians. Unfortunately, the legacy of these years has established fashions in therapy, raising unjustified objections to critical reappraisals of accepted remedies. For instance, the use of aspirin in patients with TIA is now so widespread that it is almost impossible to redesign a trial involving this drug. Anticoagulant and steroid therapies are so established in medical practice that a significant number of physicians would refuse to cooperate in such trials.

Our understanding of stroke is changing. The simple view that thrombosis in a cerebral artery causes stroke has given way to a more dynamic concept. Progress in research has revealed a complex interrelationship of cellular, biochemical, and hemodynamic changes. Combined with modern methodologic and biostatistical techniques, the prospect is good for finding specific treatments for stroke.

GENERAL MEASURES

Optimal Nursing Position

The suggestion that patients with acute cerebral infarction should be nursed supine for the first week[1] was supported by the explanation that cerebral autoregulation is lost in the ischemic brain, making cerebral perfusion passively dependent on systemic blood pressure.[2] Transient but dramatic worsening of the neurologic deficit from "positional cerebral ischemia" occurred in acute stroke patients when they sat up, rapidly reversing when they lay down again.[2] All had occlusive vascular disease on angiography. However, such cases are exceptional and no data exist to support the idea of an optimal position for all patients. Since the first week is critical in the active rehabilitation of the acute stroke patient[3] and is the time when the patient is most susceptible to pneumonia and deep venous thrombosis, we favor nursing the patient in the upright position, and early mobilization.

Ensure Oxygenation

Maintaining an airway is the primary step in unconscious patients and in alert patients with respiratory problems. The airway must be suctioned when necessary and the adequacy of ventilation monitored clinically and by blood gas analysis when required. Endotracheal intubation or assisted respiration is rarely indicated. Nurses, often alarmed by abnormal respiratory patterns such as Cheyne-Stokes respiration, commonly apply an oxygen mask. This may be therapeutic for the nursing staff and the patient's relatives but is of little value to the patient. No evidence supports routine oxygenation or tracheostomy in stroke.

Maintain Circulation

Hypotension is rarely a problem in uncomplicated strokes. It is preferable to err on the side of hypertension in ischemic stroke since regional perfusion is passively dependent on systemic blood pressure.[4] In hemorrhagic stroke, more stringent control of blood pressure is necessary, on the assumption that rebleeding can be precipitated by unexpected increases in blood pressure.

Exclude Hypoglycemia

Administration of 50 ml of 50 percent glucose in the emergency department is more often recommended than performed in patients with stupor, coma, or focal neurologic deficits. Hemiplegia from hypoglycemia is indistinguishable from that of vascular origin, and focal signs are the result of selective cerebral vulnerability due to a variable vascular supply. Hypoglycemic "stroke" is usually accompanied by stupor or coma and reverses within minutes with intravenous glucose. In view of the possible adverse affects of glucose[5] on the ischemic brain, such treatment is potentially dangerous but, in emergencies, reversing the deficit is clearly the lesser of the two evils.

Stop Seizures

Seizures at onset occur in only 4 percent of ischemic or hemorrhagic strokes and are commonest in embolic stroke.[6] Status epilepticus is rare in stroke. Early control of seizures is essential, since hypoxia secondary to convulsions increases cerebral damage. In rare cases, seizures result from the syndrome of inappropriate ADH secondary to the stroke.[7]

A 5- to 10-mg intravenous bolus of diazepam is probably the single most effective treatment, while monitoring breathing carefully to avoid respiratory depression, which sometimes occurs at relatively low doses of this drug. A bolus of 300 mg intravenous phenytoin given over 5 minutes is effective for subacute control of seizures. Since seizures are infrequent and seizure-prone stroke patients cannot be identified, prophylactic anticonvulsants are not indicated.

Treat Infection

Elevated ESR, white cell count or temperature usually indicate intercurrent infection from pneumonia or urinary tract infection. Patients lying comatose for hours or days before hospital admission often arrive with aspiration pneumonia and developing pressure areas. Fever without an obvious source of infection should prompt a search for subacute bacterial endocarditis, temporal arteritis, brain abscess, or encephalitis.

Restore Water and Electrolyte Balance

Dehydration, often present on arrival at hospital, is commonly aggravated by delays during admission. This should be corrected immediately by intravenous infusion of glucose-saline, since increased blood viscosity may increase regional ischemia.[8]

The syndrome of inappropriate ADH in stroke does not occur for several days[7] so low sodium levels at admission usually result from over-enthusiastic intravenous infusions. Low potassium levels, usually secondary to prior diuretic administration, are corrected by potassium supplements.

Sedation

Sedation is rarely indicated in acute stroke patients and iatrogenic drowsiness or stupor may mask neurologic deterioration from other causes. Confusion or agitation rarely result from stroke and indicate some other cause, such as electrolyte imbalance or postictal states. Barbiturates should especially be avoided since their effects are prolonged, unpredictable, and dangerous.

Prevent Pulmonary Embolism

During the first 10 days, about 50 percent of stroke patients will develop deep venous thrombosis (DVT) in the paralyzed leg and about 7 percent in the unaffected leg.[9,10] Obesity, concurrent heart failure, and smoking were not risk factors and the only significant predisposing factor was varicose veins. Pulmonary embolism, demonstrated by autopsy or clinical and chest x-ray evidence, occurred in 15 percent of stroke patients.[10]

Routine anticoagulation of stroke patients to prevent DVT has not gained universal acceptance, though a strong case can be made for minidose heparin therapy (5000 Units twice daily subcutaneously). McCarthy and coworkers,[11] using minidose heparin and ^{131}I leg scanning, found a significantly reduced incidence of DVT, but the subsequent incidence of pulmonary embolism was not assessed.

TREATMENT OF ISCHEMIC STROKE

No specific drug treatment for cerebral infarction is of proven value and many time-hallowed methods are useless or harmful and should be abandoned. Besides the few established and the many useless therapies, there are numerous promising treatments awaiting critical evaluation.

Effective Therapy

Osmotherapy

The effectiveness of hyperosmolar agents such as hypertonic glucose, glycerol, urea, and mannitol in rapidly reducing raised intracranial pressure has been well established since the historic reports of Weed and McKibben in 1919.[12] These drugs produce an osmotic gradient between blood and brain, reducing brain volume and increasing cerebral blood flow.[13] Since the action depends upon the blood-brain barrier acting as a semipermeable membrane, normal brain shrinks to accommodate osmotically inert infarcted brain. Unfortunately, after some hours the plasma solutes equilibrate with brain, and the osmotic effect is lost. Later, the damaged brain takes in solute with water, and "rebound" occurs as the damaged area expands.

These agents are most effective in patients in whom stupor or coma is due to cerebral distortion or compression by infarcted brain. The therapeutic effect is short-lived. With repeated administration, serious electrolyte disturbances occur and hypervolemia may tip the balance in patients with renal or cardiac failure. It is best reserved for cases in which further diagnostic procedures are necessary as a preliminary to decompressive surgery.

Mannitol is commonly used, usually 200 ml of 25 percent solution intravenously. Glycerol may be equally effective and can be given orally, the recommended dose being 1.5 g/kg/24 hr orally or 1.2 g/kg/24 hr intravenously.[14,15] Diuretic therapy reduces experimental cerebral edema produced by cryogenic lesions,[16] but we are not aware of any controlled studies on cerebrovascular lesions.

Anticoagulant Therapy

Anticoagulants have no role in the treatment of completed cerebral infarction except in patients with cerebral embolism and perhaps stroke-in-evolution.

In *cerebral embolism*, the decision to anticoagulate depends on the balance of the risk of cerebral or systemic hemorrhagic complications against the risk of further embolism. No prospective or controlled studies are available to tip this balance but decisions must nevertheless be made. Headache, abrupt loss of consciousness, a stuttering onset, and seizures are hallmarks of embolic stroke[17] but the definitive diagnosis requires proof of a source of cardiac (Table 42) or other emboli. The angiographic appearance of a "tail" of retrograde clot behind the arterial obstruction is also helpful (see Fig. 63).

According to data derived before CT scanning was available, about 50 to 70 percent of patients die or suffer a major stroke with their first cerebral embolus.[18,19] The chance of recurrent embolism is 13 to 15 percent within the first week[20,21] and 30 to 40 percent within the first month in chronic rheumatic heart disease,[17,22] and the risk from acute myocardial infarction with mural thrombosis is similar.[23] Anticoagulant therapy reduces these risks by 25 to 50 percent,[17] and, in a large cooperative randomized open trial of anticoagulant prophylaxis in acute myocardial infarction,[24] embolic complications were significantly reduced, stroke

TABLE 42. Major Cardiac Embolic Sources

Rheumatic heart disease, with or without atrial fibrillation
Acute myocardial infarction with mural thrombus
Cardiomyopathies
Prosthetic cardiac valves
Mitral valve prolapse
Cardiac arrhythmias such as sino-atrial disease
    or paroxysmal chronic atrial fibrillation from any cause
Endocarditis (bacterial and aseptic)
Left ventricular aneurysm
Atrial myxoma

incidence decreasing to 0.8 percent compared with 3.8 percent in the untreated group. No intracranial bleeding occurred in either group.

Differing definitions of *stroke-in-evolution* make previous studies difficult to evaluate. "Progression" is defined sometimes as "over minutes,"[25] sometimes as 2 hours,[26] but more commonly as 6 hours,[27] and resolution of the definition is overdue.[28] Anticoagulant therapy enjoyed considerable popularity in the 1960s on the assumption that progressing stroke was synonymous with progressing carotid or vertebrobasilar thrombosis.[29] Disenchantment with this treatment supervened as it became clearer that the effects of progressive "thrombosis" were indistinguishable from those of progressive cerebral edema. Properly conducted trials are urgently needed, since most studies were carried out before CT scanning and adequate statistical methods were available.

As in any deteriorating stroke, other causes for progression should be sought, such as drug effects, hyponatremia from SIADH, or hypoglycemia. After excluding alternative pathologies by CT scan, isotope brain scan, or lumbar puncture, heparin is infused intravenously. If a known source of emboli is present (such as mural thrombosis) and the progression is stepwise, suggesting repeated cerebral emboli, then heparin treatment is urgently indicated, after CT scan or lumbar puncture has excluded intracranial hemorrhage.

Fibrin activation is increased in stroke-in-evolution, while platelet factors are unchanged. Plasma beta-thromboglobulin, a marker of platelet activity, is normal in patients with completed "partial" strokes and in strokes progressing within 7 days of onset.[30] Serum FgE (a fibrin-fibrinogen degradation product) is elevated in all three groups, particularly in patients with progressing stroke.

The *risks of anticoagulant therapy* in stroke have been overemphasized. In experimental ischemic stroke, anticoagulants produce more hemorrhagic infarcts than in controls,[31-33] but there is little clinical confirmation, and intracranial hemorrhage is not a serious risk.[18,20,25,34]

The cerebrospinal fluid in anticoagulated patients may be hemorrhagic within 48 hours of the stroke, but, since the risk of recurrent embolism is high in the first days of stroke, anticoagulant treatment should start as soon as the diagnosis is firmly established.

An intravenous bolus of 5000 IU heparin should precede 1000 IU hourly by continuous infusion, adjusting the dose to maintain the partial thromboplastin time about twice the normal value. Anticoagulant therapy should continue for at least 1 year in mural embolism and for life in mitral stenosis with atrial fibrillation.

Experimental Therapy

Barbiturate Therapy

Barbiturate anesthesia, by decreasing cerebral metabolism and rapidly lowering intracranial pressure,[35] has potential for reducing ischemic brain damage, but its early promise has not been fulfilled. Its protective effect against cerebral anoxia has been known since the 1960s,[36] massive doses also protecting against experimental focal and global cerebral isch-

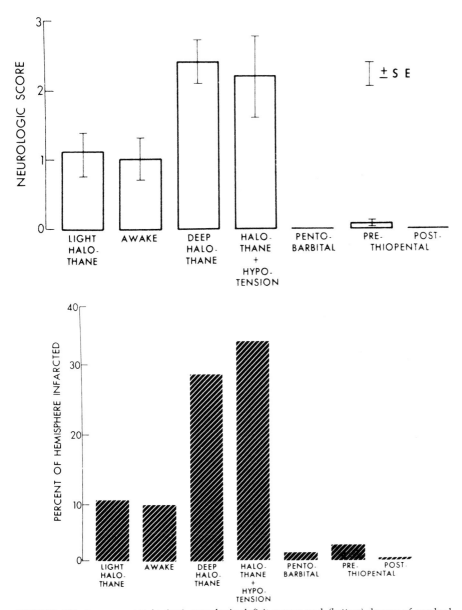

FIGURE 122. Improvement in *(top)* neurologic deficit scores and *(bottom)* degree of cerebral infarction after experimental internal carotid occlusion in dogs with barbiturate anesthesia compared to other forms of anesthesia. (From Smith, et al,[37] with permission.)

emia.[37,38] Barbiturate anesthesia reduced neurologic disability and the severity of cerebral infarction following occlusion of the internal carotid arteries in dogs[37] (Fig. 122). The protection afforded was specific to barbiturates and not shared by other anesthetics.

Uncontrolled trials of patients with differing cerebral pathologies are inconclusive,[39,40] and no properly conducted double-blind study has been undertaken. Serious obstacles deter effective barbiturate therapy.[41] Only special intensive care centers can care for patients with this degree of deep prolonged anesthesia and, since neurologic contact with the

MANAGEMENT

233

patient is lost, no satisfactory method for monitoring the effective dose of the drug is available. Blood and CSF levels of the drug are unreliable, and specialized EEG monitoring is of controversial value. The question must remain unanswered until a properly conducted study is performed.

Naloxone

Rapid but transient reversal of neurologic deficits in two patients with cerebral ischemia given 0.4 mg naloxone intravenously was reported by Baskin and Hosabuchi,[42] an effect that did not occur with placebo. The same authors[43] later reported reversal of neurologic deficits in gerbils with ischemic stroke given intraperitoneal naloxone. Intraperitoneal morphine in these animals induced hemiparesis lasting 4 to 24 hours, reversed within 5 minutes of naloxone administration. The higher concentration of "beta-endorphin–like material" in the ischemic hemisphere was proposed as the cause of the hemiparesis. Opiate antagonists might hypothetically reverse this effect in the absence of actual cellular necrosis.

Prostacyclin Therapy

Prostacyclin (PGI_2) is a prostaglandin metabolite of arachidonic acid synthesized by vascular endothelial cells, causing vasodilation and platelet antiaggregation.[44,45] These actions are the opposite of another arachidonic acid metabolite, thromboxane A_2, and a prostacyclin-thromboxane balance has been suggested (see Fig. 25). When this mechanism becomes disrupted, an excess of vasoactive prostaglandins are produced. Prostacyclin may also be "cytoprotective," since it reduces the size of myocardial infarction, decreasing oxygen demand of the tissue and the effect of endotoxic shock.[45]

Therapeutic experimental prostacyclin infusions are so far disappointing, affecting neither infarct size nor regional CBF, though there was diminished blood-brain barrier leakage.[46] The beneficial results of prostacyclin infusion in an uncontrolled study of stroke patients[47] have not yet been confirmed by a controlled randomized trial.

Fluorocarbons

Fluorocarbons, through their increased oxygen-carrying and viscosity-decreasing capacity, reduce the size of experimental cerebral infarction, producing encouraging clinical responses.[48–50]

Therapy of Unproven Value

Routine Oxygen Therapy

Administration of oxygen under normal circumstances will not increase the oxygen-carrying power of the blood, which is already maximal. Supersaturating the blood with oxygen (hyperbaric oxygen therapy) to reverse ischemic cell damage produces partial resolution of the neurologic deficit while the patient is in the hyperbaric chamber, but this effect lasts only hours.[51] Toxic effects occur after prolonged use of high concentrations of oxygen,[52] making it unjustifiable unless evidence of therapeutic value is forthcoming.

Thrombolytic Therapy

Systemic and intracerebral hemorrhage occurring during streptokinase and urokinase therapy in "thrombotic" stroke soon prohibited their use. These drugs are more dangerous than heparin[53] and are without demonstrated benefit in ischemic stroke.[54]

Dextran 40

Low molecular weight dextran decreases blood viscosity and platelet aggregation and improves the cerebral microcirculation and cerebral blood flow.[55] In a randomized, controlled but unblinded study of this drug in patients with ischemic stroke, morbidity and mortality apparently decreased,[56] but the improvements noted were often in insubstantive variables such as "mentation" and "reflexes." In a double-blind study there was improved mortality after severe stroke but no benefit in less severe stroke, and survivors in the drug and placebo groups were equally disabled at 6 months.[57] The authors concluded that dextran 40 affected cerebral swelling in the acute stage. The small numbers of patients used in these studies makes them liable to erroneously positive results.

Cerebral Vasodilators

Since ischemic stroke is due to deficient regional cerebral perfusion, cerebral vasodilators have obvious therapeutic potential. Carbon dioxide is the most potent vasodilator, though papaverine and other drugs are also effective.[4,54,58-60] "Intracerebral steal" may accompany this increased perfusion since normal cerebral vessels vasodilate, stealing blood from ischemic areas that are unresponsive because they are already maximally dilated[61] (Fig. 123). Cerebral perfusion did not change in regional ischemia following CO_2 inhalation, so that vasodilator therapy is not only

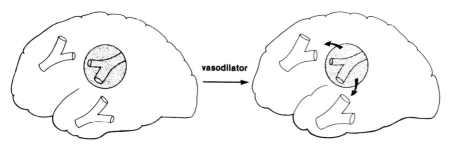

vasodilator

normal vessels dilate

FIGURE 123. Diagrammatic illustration of intracerebral steal when vasodilator drugs are used in patients with regional cerebral ischemia.

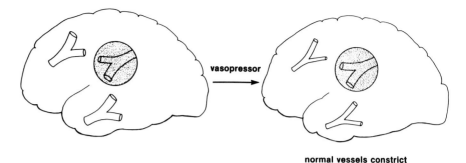

FIGURE 124. Principle of hyperventilation therapy.

useless but may *increase* ischemic damage.[62] In an open controlled trial of papaverine, there was no difference in mortality but improved status of survivors.[63]

Vasoconstrictor Therapy

Vasoconstrictors should shunt blood into areas of regional ischemia, since only normal cerebral vessels will vasoconstrict. Attempts to treat stroke with prolonged hyperventilation failed to change mortality or morbidity and were accompanied by serious pulmonary complications[64] (Fig. 124). Drug-induced metabolic alkalosis using tris (hydroxymethal) aminomethane produced no beneficial effect.[65] Theophylline trials in ischemic stroke have also proven negative.[66]

Steroid Therapy

In spite of largely negative experimental and clinical results,[67–70] steroid therapy is still widely prescribed for "stroke." There are errors in study design in all published series,[71–73] all were without CT scanning, and few used double-blind randomized techniques (Table 43). A subgroup of stroke patients might derive benefit from steroid therapy, but these would still represent a tiny minority. A multicenter trial large enough to identify such a potential benefit would also produce serious complica-

TABLE 43. Summary of Double-Blind Randomized Trials of Steroid Therapy in Stroke

Author	Number	"Stroke"	Dexamethasone		Outcome
			Dose	Time	
Dyken et al, 1956[68]	36	Infarction	? (cortisone)	21 days	Worse
Rubinstein, 1965[84]	19	Infarction & hemorrhage	52 mg	3 days	Better
Patton et al, 1972[85]	31	Infarction & hemorrhage	200 mg	17 days	Better
Bauer and Tellez, 1973[69]	54	Infarction	120 mg	10 days	Unchanged
Norris, 1976[70]	53	Infarction	140 mg	12 days	Worse
Mulley et al, 1978[86]	118	?	192 mg	14 days	Unchanged
Norris and Hachinski, 1985[87]	113	Infarction	480 mg	12 days	Unchanged

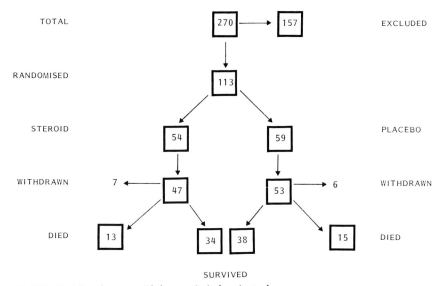

FIGURE 125. Megadose steroid therapy in ischemic stroke.

tions in sufficient patients to question its justification. The hyperglycemia that occurs so frequently with this drug might be the cause of the adverse effect in treated patients.

Steroid therapy may be dangerous as well as ineffective. Dyken and White[68] terminated their study prematurely, since more patients died in the drug group; and Norris[70] found no effect on mortality, although survivors of the steroid group fared worse because of infections and uncontrollable diabetes. In a later study in the Toronto Unit of high-dose steroids in cerebral infarction with autopsy and CT confirmation, there was no significant effect on mortality or morbidity (Fig. 125).[74]

TREATMENT OF INTRACEREBRAL HEMORRHAGE

Supratentorial Hemorrhage

Cerebral hemorrhage usually occurs over the course of a few minutes and does not generally progress,[75,76] but serial CT studies indicate that sometimes slow but disastrous leakage of blood occurs over several hours[77] (Fig. 126). Death from acute cerebral hemorrhage is secondary to transtentorial herniation, so surgery must be performed during this acute stage if the patient has recovery potential (Table 44).

The guide to surgical management suggested by Hier and associates,[75] although well reasoned, is not supported by controlled data. Hemorrhages within the vascular centrencephalon destroy compact structure and tend to cause major damage. Their central location makes them inaccessible without inflicting further injury. No series has yet shown improved morbidity in operated patients. The potential advantages of decreased mortality compare uneasily with the crippling disability of most survivors. By contrast, lobar hematomas tend to occur in less crucial locations, are more accessible, and have a better prognosis. However, surgery is justified only when hemorrhage causes increased intracranial

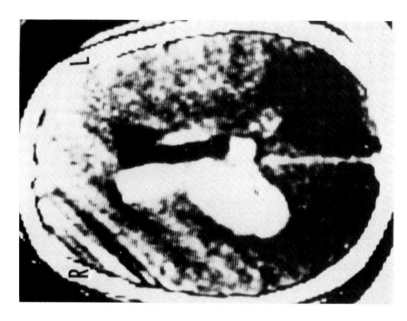

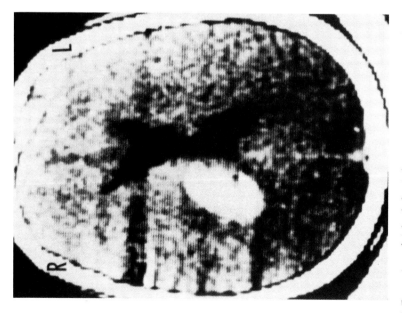

FIGURE 126. Expansion of right thalamic hematoma over the course of 15 minutes during which time the patient lapsed into stupor and became densely hemiparetic. (From Kelley, et al.[79] with permission.)

TABLE 44. Comparison Between Mechanisms of Death During the First Week and Second to Fourth Weeks in 180 Patients with Supratentorial Lesions

Cause of death	Infarction		Hemorrhage	
	1st wk	2nd–4th wk	1st wk	2nd–4th wk
Transtentorial herniation	36	6	42	2
Pneumonia	0	28	1	2
Cardiac	7	17	0	2
Pulmonary embolism	0	4	0	0
Sudden death	2	8	0	0
Septicemia	1	4	0	0
Unknown	0	12	1	3
Brainstem extension of hematoma	—	—	1	1
Total	46	79	45	10

pressure or poses a danger of herniation, since all hematomas tend to be reabsorbed eventually.

CT scanning alone can differentiate hypertensive intracerebral hemorrhages from those resulting from underlying vascular lesions such as saccular aneurysms in 90 percent of cases, lessening the need for arteriography.[78]

Infratentorial Hemorrhage

Reports of successful evacuation of pontine hemorrhage are anecdotal,[79,80] and it is difficult to determine how such therapy changes the natural history of the disease (Fig. 127).

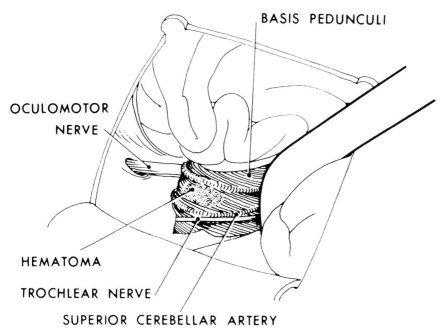

BASIS PEDUNCULI

OCULOMOTOR NERVE

HEMATOMA

TROCHLEAR NERVE

SUPERIOR CEREBELLAR ARTERY

FIGURE 127. Subtemporal approach to removal of midbrain hematoma. (From Humphreys, RP: *Computerized tomographic definition of mesencephalic hematoma with evacuation through pedunculotomy—Case report.* J Neurosurg 49:749, 1978, with permission.)

Cerebellar Hemorrhage

The case for urgent surgical evacuation of cerebellar hemorrhage is less controversial. In the pre-CT era, evacuation after diagnosis was often recommended[81,82] but CT facilitates detection, serial examination, and a more conservative policy. Fatal acute hydrocephalus may occur as late as 1 month after a cerebellar hemorrhage,[83] making this lesion the most unpredictable and yet the most remediable of intracerebral hematomas.

CONCLUSION

Numerous treatment regimens are advocated for stroke, yet even the few effective methods are of limited value. An attitude of therapeutic nihilism has been generated by ignorance of underlying pathophysiology and uncritical evaluation of therapy.

Re-evaluation of established but unproven treatments by critical application of methodologic strategies justifies their rejection, and revelation of the basic mechanisms of acute cerebrovascular damage by new technology is leading to a more selective approach in finding new therapies.

The role of surgery in acute stroke is limited to decompression of lobar hemorrhage and cerebellar infarcts and hematomas that raise intracranial pressure and threaten herniation.

REFERENCES

1. FISHER, CM, KARP, H, AND ADAMS, RD: *Cerebrovascular diseases.* In HARRISON, TR, ET AL: *Principles of Internal Medicine,* ed 3. McGraw-Hill, New York, 1958.

2. CAPLAN, LR, AND SERGAY, S: *Positional cerebral ischemia.* J Neurol Neurosurg Psychiatry 39:385, 1976.

3. NORRIS, JW, AND HACHINSKI, VC: *Intensive care management of stroke patients.* Stroke 7:573, 1976.

4. OLESEN, J: *Cerebral blood flow methods for measurement, regulation, effects of drugs and changes in disease.* Acta Neurol Scand 50(Suppl 57):1, 1974.

5. PLUM, F: *What causes infarction in ischemic brain? The Robert Wartenberg Lecture.* Neurology 33:222, 1983.

6. BLACK, SE, HACHINSKI, VC, AND NORRIS, JW: *Seizures after stroke* (abstr). Can J Neurol Sci 9:291, 1982.

7. MAZUREK, MF, ET AL: *Vasopressin and inappropriate antidiuresis in acute neurovascular illness* (abstr). Can J Neurol Sci 8:297, 1981.

8. THOMAS, DJ, ET AL: *Cerebral blood-flow in polycythemia.* Lancet 2:161, 1977.

9. DENHAM, MJ, FARRAN, H, AND JAMES, G: *The value of 125-I fibrinogen in the diagnosis of deep vein thrombosis in hemiplegia.* Age Ageing 2:207, 1973.

10. WARLOW, CP, OGSTON, D, AND DOUGLAS, AS: *Deep vein thrombosis of the legs after strokes, part 1: Incidence and predisposing factors.* Br Med J 1:1178, 1976.

11. McCARTHY, ST, ET AL: *Low-dose heparin as a prophylaxis against deep-vein thrombosis after acute stroke.* Lancet 2:800, 1977.

12. MEYER, JS: *Medical and surgical treatment of cerebrovascular disease.* In MEYER, JS (ED): *Modern Concepts of Cerebrovascular Disease.* Spectrum Publications, New York, 1975, p 159.

13. BRUCE, DA, ET AL: *Regional cerebral blood flow, intracranial pressure, and brain metabolism in comatose patients.* J Neurosurg 38:131, 1973.

14. MEYER, JS, ET AL: *Treatment with glycerol of cerebral edema due to acute cerebral infarction.* Lancet 2:993, 1971.

15. MATHEW, NT, ET AL: *Double-blind evaluation of glycerol therapy in acute cerebral infarction.* Lancet 2:1327, 1972.

16. CLASEN, RA, PANDOLFI, S, AND CASEY, D, JR: *Furosemide and pentobarbital in cryogenic cerebral injury and edema.* Neurology 24:642, 1974.

17. EASTON, JD, AND SHERMAN, DG: *Management of cerebral embolism of cardiac origin.* Stroke 11:433, 1980.

18. CARTER, AB: *Prognosis of cerebral embolism.* Lancet 2:514, 1965.

19. WELLS, CE: *Cerebral embolism—the natural history, prognostic signs and effects of anticoagulation.* Arch Neurol Psychiatry 81:667, 1959.

20. FURLAN, AJ, ET AL: *Hemorrhage and anticoagulation after nonseptic embolic brain infarction.* Neurology 32:280, 1982.

21. DALEY, R, ET AL: *Systemic arterial embolism in rheumatic heart disease.* Am Heart J 42:566, 1951.

22. SZEKELY, P: *Systemic embolism and anticoagulant prophylaxis in rheumatic heart disease.* Br Med J 1:1209, 1964.

23. BEAN, WB: *Infarction of the heart. 3. A clinical course and morphological findings.* Ann Intern Med 12:71, 1938.

24. EBERT, RV: *Anticoagulants in acute myocardial infarction: Results of a cooperative clinical trial.* JAMA 225:724, 1973.

25. MILLIKAN, CH, AND MCDOWELL, FH: *Treatment of progressing stroke.* Stroke 12:397, 1981.

26. CARTER, AB: Ingravescent cerebral infarction. Q J Med 29:611, 1960.

27. MARSHALL, J: *The Management of Cerebrovascular Disease.* J & A Churchill, London, 1968.

28. CAPLAN, LR: *Are terms such as completed stroke or RIND of continued usefulness?* Stroke 14:431, 1983.

29. MILLIKAN, CH: *Anticoagulant therapy of cerebrovascular disease.* In MILLIKAN, CH, SIEKERT, RG, AND WHISNANT, JP (EDS): *Cerebral Vascular Diseases.* Grune & Stratton, New York, 1965, p 181.

30. DE BOER, AC, ET AL: *Plasma betathromboglobulin and serum fragment E in acute partial stroke.* Br J Haematol 50:327, 1982.

31. SIBLEY, WA, MORLEDGE, JH, AND LAPHAN, LW: *Experimental cerebral infarction: Effect of dicumarol.* Am J Med Sci 234:663, 1957.

32. WOOD, NW, ET AL: *Relationship between anticoagulants and hemorrhage and cerebral infarction in experimental animals.* Arch Neurol Psychiatry 79:390, 1958.

33. WHISNANT, JP, ET AL: *Effect of anticoagulants on experimental cerebral infarction.* Circulation 20:56, 1959.

34. KOLLER, RL: *Recurrent embolic cerebral infarction and anticoagulation.* Neurology 32:283, 1982.

35. SHAPIRO, HM, ET AL: *Rapid intraoperative reduction of intracranial pressure with thiopentone.* Br J Anaesth 45:1057, 1973.

36. WILHJELM, BJ, AND ARNRED, I: *Protective action of some anesthetics against anoxia.* Acta Pharmacol Toxicol 22:93, 1965.

37. SMITH, AL, ET AL: *Barbiturate protection in acute focal cerebral ischemia.* Stroke 5:1, 1974.

38. BLEYAERT, AL, ET AL: *Thiopental amelioration of brain damage after global ischemia in monkeys.* Anesthesiology 49:390, 1978.

39. ROCKOFF, MA, MARSHALL, LF, AND SHAPIRO, HM: *High-dose barbiturate therapy in humans: A clinical review of 60 patients.* Ann Neurol 6:194, 1979.

40. WOODCOCK, J, ROPPER, AH, AND KENNEDY, SK: *High dose barbiturates in non-traumatic brain swelling: ICP reduction and effect on outcome.* Stroke 13:785, 1982.

41. MILLER, JD: *Barbiturates and raised intracranial pressure.* Ann Neurol 3:189, 1979.

42. BASKIN, DS, AND HOSOBUCHI, Y: *Naloxone reversal of ischemic neurological deficits in man.* Lancet 2:272, 1981.

43. HOSOBUCHI, Y, BASKIN, DS, AND WOO, SK: *Reversal of induced ischemic neurologic deficit in gerbils by the opiate antagonist naloxone.* Science 215:69–71, 1982.

44. MOSKOWITZ, MA, AND COUGHLIN, SR: *Basic properties of the prostaglandins.* Stroke 12:696, 1981.

45. MONCADA, S: *Biology and therapeutic potential of prostacyclin.* Stroke 14:157, 1983.

46. AWAD, I, ET AL: *Treatment of acute focal cerebral ischemia with prostacyclin.* Stroke 14:203, 1983.

47. GRYGLEWSKI, RJ, ET AL: *Treatment of ischaemic stroke with prostacyclin.* Stroke 14:197, 1983.

48. PEERLESS, SJ, ET AL: *Protective effect of Fluosol-DA in acute cerebral ischemia.* Stroke 12:558, 1981.

49. Peerless, SJ: *The use of perfluorochemicals in the treatment of acute cerebral ischemia.* Prog Clin Biol Res 122:353, 1983.

50. Biro, GP: *Current status of erythrocyte substitutes.* Can Med Assoc J 129:237, 1983.

51. Meyer, JS, and Mathew, NT: *Medical management in cerebral ischemia.* In Ingelfinger, FJ, et al (eds): *Controversy in Internal Medicine 2.* WB Saunders, Philadelphia, 1974, p 771.

52. Mertin, J, and McDonald, WI: *Hyperbaric oxygen for patients with multiple sclerosis.* Br Med J 288:957, 1984.

53. Meyer, JS, et al: *Therapeutic thrombolysis in cerebral thrombus-embolism. Randomized evaluation of intravenous streptokinase.* In Millikan, CH, Siekert, RG, and Whisnant, J (eds): *Cerebral Vascular Diseases.* Grune & Stratton, New York, 1965, p 200.

54. Meyer, JS: *Medical and surgical treatment of cerebrovascular diseases.* In Meyer, JS (ed): *Modern Concepts of Cerebrovascular Disease.* Spectrum Publications, New York, 1975, p 159.

55. Hass, WK: *Drug effects in regional cerebral blood flow in focal cerebrovascular disease.* J Neurol Sci 19:461, 1979.

56. Gilroy, J, Barnhart, MI, and Meyer, JS: *Treatment of acute stroke with Dextran 40.* JAMA 210:293, 1969.

57. Matthews, WB, et al: *A blind controlled trial of Dextran 40 in the treatment of ischemic stroke.* Brain 99:193, 1976.

58. Kety, SS, and Schmidt, CF: *The effects of active and passive hyperventilation in cerebral blood flow, cerebral oxygen consumption, cardiac output and blood pressure of normal young men.* J Clin Invest 25:107, 1946.

59. McHenry, LC, et al: *Effect of papaverine on regional blood flow in focal vascular disease of the brain.* N Engl J Med 282:1167, 1970.

60. Gottstein, U, and Paulson, OB: *Effect of intracarotid aminophylline infusion on the cerebral circulation.* Stroke 3:560, 1972.

61. Lassen, NA, and Palvolgyi, R: *Cerebral steal during hypercapnia and the inverse reaction during hypocapnia observed by the 133-Xenon technique in man.* Scand J Clin Lab Invest 22 (Suppl 102):13D, 1968.

62. Høedt-Rasmussen, K, et al: *Regional cerebral blood flow in acute apoplexy: The 'luxury perfusion syndrome' of brain tissue.* Arch Neurol 17:271, 1967.

63. Meyer, JS, et al: *Improvement in brain oxygenation and clinical improvement in patients with strokes treated with papaverine hydrochloride.* JAMA 194:957, 1965.

64. Christensen, MS, et al: *Cerebral apoplexy (stroke) treated with or without prolonged artificial hyperventilation. 1. Cerebral circulation, clinical course, and cause of death.* Stroke 4:568, 1973.

65. Meyer, JS, et al: *Abnormal hemispheric blood flow and metabolism in cerebrovascular disease. ii. Therapeutic trials with 5% CO_2 inhalation, hyperventilation and intravenous infusion of THAM and mannitol.* Stroke 3:157, 1972.

66. Britton, M: *Lack of effect of theophylline on the outcome of acute cerebral infarction.* Acta Neurol Scand 62:116, 1980.

67. Joint Committee for Stroke Resources: *iv. Brain edema in stroke.* Stroke 8:512, 1977.

68. Dyken, M, and White, PT: *Evaluation of cortisone in the treatment of cerebral infarction.* JAMA 132:1531, 1956.

69. Bauer, RB, and Tellez, H: *Dexamethasone as a treatment in cerebrovascular disease. 2. A controlled study in acute cerebral infarction.* Stroke 4:547, 1973.

70. Norris, JW: *Steroid therapy in acute cerebral infarction.* Arch Neurol 33:69, 1976.

71. Norris, JW, and Hachinski, VC: *Steroid therapy of stroke: Designing the ideal study.* In Meyer, JS, Lechner, H, and Reivich, M (eds): *Cerebral Vascular Disease 3.* Excerpta Medica, Amsterdam, 1980, p 27.

72. Spence, JD, and Donner, A: *Problems in design of stroke treatment trials.* Stroke 13:94, 1982.

73. Capildeo, R, Haberman, S, and Rose, FC: *Stroke trials: The facts.* In Rose, FC (ed): *Advances in Stroke Therapy.* Raven Press, New York, 1982, p 53.

74. Norris, JW, and Hachinski, VC: *Megadose steroid therapy in ischemic stroke.* Stroke 16:18, 1985.

75. Hier, DB, et al: *Hypertensive putaminal hemorrhage.* Ann Neurol 1:152, 1977.

76. Fisher, CM: *Clinical syndromes in cerebral hemorrhage.* In Fields, WS (ed): *Pathogenesis and Treatment of Cerebrovascular Disease.* Charles C Thomas, Springfield, IL, 1961, p 218.

77. KELLEY, RE, ET AL: *Active bleeding in hypertensive intracerebral hemorrhage: Computed tomography.* Neurology 32:852, 1982.

78. HEYWARD, RD, AND O'REILLY, GVA: *Intracerebral hemorrhage. Accuracy of computerised transverse axial scanning in predicting the underlying aetiology.* Lancet 1:1, 1976.

79. DURWARD, QJ, BARNETT, HJM, AND BARR, HWK: *Presentation and management of mesencephalic hematoma.* J Neurosurg 56:123, 1982.

80. MCKISSOCK, W, RICHARDSON, A, AND WALSH, L: *Spontaneous cerebellar hemorrhage: A study of 34 consecutive cases treated surgically.* Brain 83:1, 1960.

81. NORRIS, JW, EISEN, AA, AND BRANCH, CL: *Problems in cerebellar hemorrhage and infarction.* Neurology 19:1043, 1969.

82. HEIMAN, TD, AND SATYA-NURTI, S: *Benign cerebellar hemorrhages.* Ann Neurol 3:366, 1978.

83. BRILLMAN, J: *Acute hydrocephalus and death one month after non-surgical treatment for acute cerebellar hemorrhage.* J Neurosurg 50:374, 1979.

84. RUBINSTEIN, MK: *The influence of adrenocortical steroids on severe cerebrovascular accidents.* J Nerv Ment Dis 141:291, 1965.

85. PATTON, BM, ET AL: *Double-blind study of the effects of dexamethasone on acute stroke.* Neurology 22:377, 1972.

86. MULLEY, G, WILCOX, RG, AND MITCHELL, JRA: *Dexamethasone in acute stroke.* Br Med J 2:994, 1978.

87. NORRIS, JW, AND HACHINSKI, VC: *High-dose steroid therapy in cerebral infarction.* (In press.)

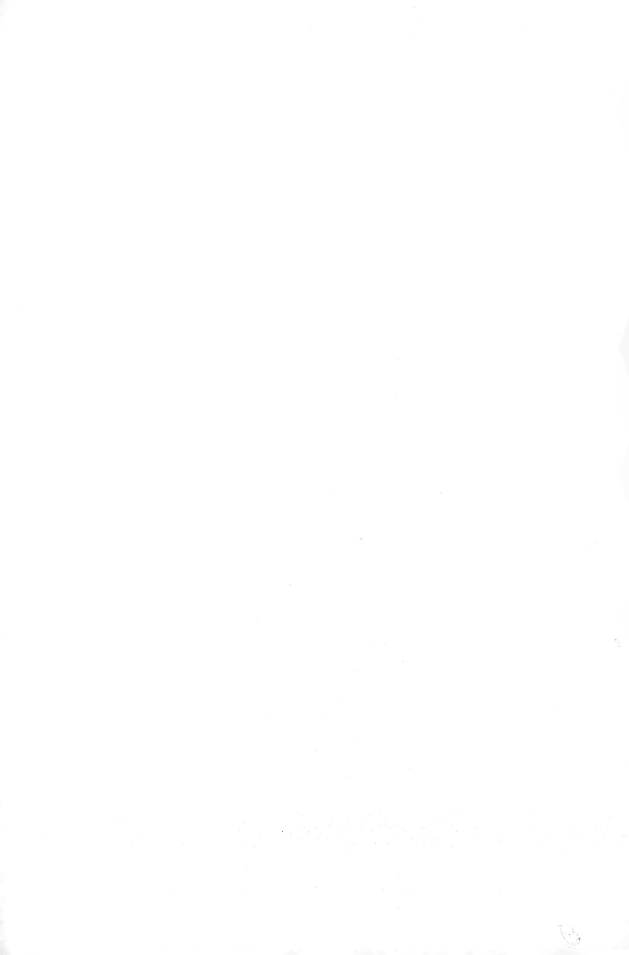

Chapter 13

PROGNOSIS

The duration of palsy is very different in different cases.
John Cooke, 1823

The brain functions with infinite complexity but fails in a few predictable ways, making prognosis possible. Prognosis relies on accurate diagnosis, and yet, the classification, diagnostic fashions, treatment, and nature of stroke have all been changing.[1] The International Classification of Disease lacks precision for stroke, and its periodic changes have consisted of juggling a mixture of anatomy, etiology, and obsolete terms.[2]

The incidence of intracranial hemorrhage has been overestimated because of changing diagnostic conventions, because cerebral infarction and hemorrhage were often confused prior to CT scanning, and because of a true decline in stroke incidence.[1] Lacunar infarction is estimated at 19 percent of strokes in some series[3] but is not even mentioned in others.[4] Further ambiguity is generated by the decline of stroke with the improved treatment of hypertension,[5] while the decline of rheumatic heart disease is highlighting other causes of cerebral embolism such as mitral valve prolapse.[6]

Changes in the nature and treatment of stroke complicate analysis of the natural history of cerebrovascular disease and oblige us to rely more on recent series of well-studied cases than on previous studies that were classics in their time but no longer provide contemporary, accurate data.

MORTALITY FOLLOWING STROKE

Early mortality has a bimodal distribution. A peak in the first week is largely due to cerebral causes (transtentorial herniation) and a second peak during the second and third weeks results from systemic complications. Cardiac complications remain a deadly threat throughout the first month (see Table 44; see Fig. 7). The overall mortality is 20 percent and is greater for cerebral hemorrhage than cerebral infarction.[7]

Death in the *chronic* phase most commonly results from myocardial infarction and is more frequent than in the general population. In the Framingham Study, the 5-year survival rate for brain infarction was reduced from 85 percent to 35 percent in men and from 70 percent to 50 percent in women if the patient had pulmonary disease, congestive failure, or hypertension. Hypertension alone reduced the survival rate from 85 percent to 51 percent in men but not in women.[8] Myocardial infarction is the commonest cause of death in stroke patients.[1]

NEUROLOGIC FACTORS

Site of the Lesion

Within the Brain

In an outcome study of 1013 stroke patients admitted to the Toronto Unit, survival curves showed higher mortality for hemispheric hemorrhage than for brainstem hemorrhage, and showed a poorer prognosis for patients with hemispheric infarction than for those with brainstem infarction (Table 45; Fig. 128).[9]

The prognosis also differs, depending on which hemisphere is damaged. In right-hemisphere stroke, recovery from left-sided neglect and anosognosia is usually more rapid than recovery from hemianopia and hemiparesis.[10] Improvement of aphasia, a prominent feature of most left-hemisphere strokes, is greatest for Broca's aphasia and good in conduction aphasia, but poor in Wernicke's aphasia and dismal in most cases of global aphasia.[11] Patients with left hemiplegia tend to do less well than do those with right hemiplegia,[12] although individual variability is great.

Vascular Location

The prognosis of individual lesions in arteries has to be interpreted along with other prognostic factors such as the patient's age, and the presence

TABLE 45. Mortality at 30 Days by Stroke Type in 1073 Consecutive Patients Admitted with Completed Stroke

Stroke Type	Died	Total	Mortality
Infarction			
Supratentorial	125	814	15%
Infratentorial	28	153	18%
Hemorrhage			
Supratentorial	55	93	58%
Infratentorial	4	13	31%
Total	212	1073	20%

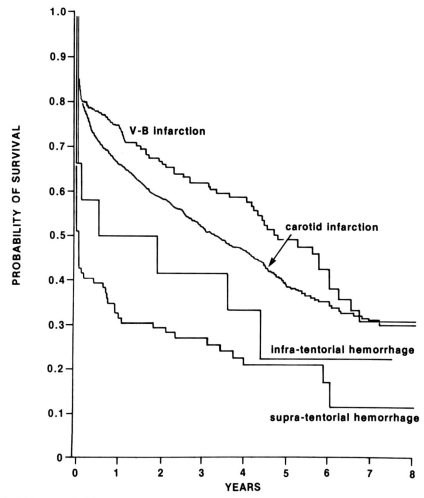

FIGURE 128. Probability of survival according to location and type of stroke. (From Chambers et al,[9] with permission.)

of other lesions, cardiac disease, and vascular risk factors (e.g., hypertension and diabetes).

Patients with *internal carotid artery* occlusion have a relatively benign prognosis, the subsequent stroke rate being 3 percent per year, two-thirds in the territory of the occluded carotid artery.[13] Côté and colleagues[14] found a 5 percent incidence of stroke distal to the occluded artery and half their patients continued to have TIAs in the territory of the occluded artery. Patients with intracranial internal carotid disease have a poorer prognosis, the ipsilateral stroke rate being 7.6 percent per year and mortality 8 to 17 percent per year.[15,16]

Middle cerebral artery occlusion usually results from cerebral embolism[17,18] and only about one quarter of patients recover significantly.[19,20] Middle cerebral artery stenosis most often results from local atherosclerotic disease. About 80 percent of patients make a good recovery, and estimates of recurrence vary from 0 to 24 percent and mortality from 0 to 29 percent in 6 years.[21,22]

The only report of long-term outcome of *vertebral artery* stenosis is unrepresentative since 52 of 96 patients were also selected for carotid endarterectomy.[23] Of 23 patients having stroke, only two had brainstem infarcts and these had concomitant basilar artery stenosis. Occlusion of the vertebral artery at its origin usually leads to minimal or no symptoms, whereas distal occlusion more frequently results in brainstem infarction.[24] Patients with *basilar artery* stenosis and occlusion have a poor prognosis, many dying.[25]

Nature of the Lesion

Patients with cerebral hemorrhage have worse survival than do those with infarction (Fig. 128), and patients with lacunar infarcts have a better prognosis than do those with thromboembolic infarcts.[26,27] Intracerebral hemorrhage often devastates the brain, but at times it compresses rather than destroys cerebral tissue. Central (deeply placed) hemorrhages have a poorer prognosis than lobar hemorrhages.[28]

The quality of life 1 year after stroke also depends on etiology. When patients admitted to the Toronto Unit were classified according to their degree of disability, those with vertebrobasilar infarcts fared best, followed by those with carotid territory infarction, infratentorial hemorrhage, and supratentorial hemorrhage (Fig. 129). Seven years after cerebral infarction, 31 percent of patients needed assistance with activities of daily living, 20 percent needed assistance with ambulation, and 71 percent had decreased vocational capacity.[9]

Severity of the Lesion

The larger the lesion and the greater the neurologic impairment, the worse the prognosis (Table 46). Gowers observed in 1888 that, the

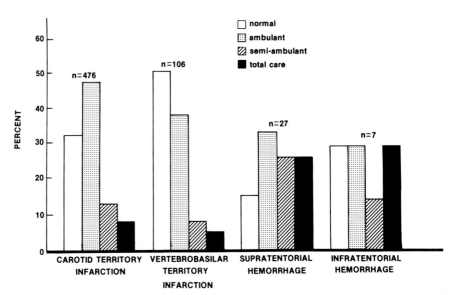

ACUTE STROKE

FIGURE 129. Functional state at 1 year of patients in the Toronto series. (From Chambers et al,[9] with permission.)

TABLE 46. Factors that Negatively Influence the Prognosis of Stroke

NEUROLOGIC FACTORS
Site of lesion
  Within the brain
    Hemisphere vs. brainstem
    Right hemisphere vs. left hemisphere
  Vascular location
    Intracranial carotid
      vs. middle cerebral artery stenoses and occlusions
      vs. cervical carotid occlusion
    Basilar vs. vertebral artery lesions
Nature of lesion
  Hemorrhage vs. infarct
  Hemispheric vs. centrencephalic infarct
  Centrencephalic vs. hemispheric hemorrhage
Severity of lesion
  Decreased level of consciousness
  Forced gaze deviation
  Dense hemiplegia
  Loss of movement in distal limbs
  Dense hemisensory impairment
  Slow recovery rate
  CT—Hypodense lesion
  Isotope brain scan—Increased uptake
Number of lesions
  Recurrent stroke

GENERAL FACTORS
Age
Cardiac disease
Polycythemia
Hyperglycemia
Hyperthermia
Hypertension?

COMPLICATING FACTORS
Cardiac complications
Infections
  Pneumonia
  Urinary tract infection
  Septicemia
Deep venous thrombosis and pulmonary embolism
Depression
Seizures
Recurrent stroke
Multi-infarct dementia

sooner the patient begins to show signs of recovery, the greater the eventual recovery.[30] The preservation or early appearance of distal movement in a limb usually implies that useful function will return, presumably through some maintenance of corticospinal pathways.

Impaired consciousness, forced gaze deviation, and dense hemiplegia indicate a poor prognosis.[31] Abnormal uptake on radioisotope brain scan is also said to indicate a poor prognosis[32] and correlates well with other signs of a poor prognosis, such as forced gaze, dense hemiplegia, and severe aphasia.[33]

Number of Lesions

The effect of a second cerebral lesion often exceeds the deficit expected from each lesion alone, illustrating a multiplicative effect of cumulative

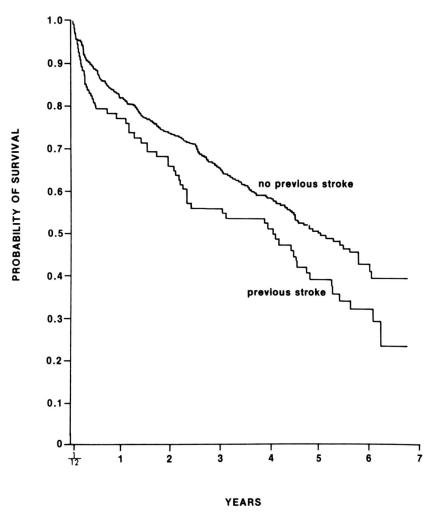

FIGURE 130. Probability of survival after first or subsequent stroke. (From Chambers et al,[9] with permission.)

brain damage. Patients with recurrent stroke also have a lowered life expectancy, compared with patients with a first cerebral infarct (Fig. 130).[9]

Other neurologic factors such as handedness may play a role in prognosis. Aphasia and apraxia were less severe in left-handed than in right-handed patients with unilateral brain damage.[34] Brain asymmetries may also prove important in prognosis. Patients with global aphasia and atypical cerebral hemispheric asymmetries recovered better than patients with typical or no asymmetries.[35]

Mechanisms of Recovery

Stroke surprises not for the damage it inflicts, but for the recovery it allows, perhaps a reflection of the *reversibility of ischemia*. Brain damage in cerebral infarction is uneven and an injured area may have perfusion low enough to lose cellular function but not life in an ischemic "penumbra."[36] As regional blood flow returns to normal, through the dissolution of an embolus or from increased collateral blood flow, the affected tissue regains function. Positron emission tomography data suggest that, in the initial 48 hours of cerebral infarction, blood flow is below the tissue's metabolic requirements, "misery perfusion."[37] After 72 hours, cerebral blood flow is often in excess of metabolic requirements, termed "luxury perfusion."[38] In embolic stroke, the embolus may disintegrate or lyse, so the ultimate deficit is less than the initial assessment would indicate.

It is uncertain whether *cerebral edema* is itself harmful or whether it merely reflects the degree of cerebral injury. Clinically and experimentally, cerebral edema is maximal by the third day after cerebral infarction and disappears by the third week.[39] Even if cerebral edema is intrinsically harmless, compression of adjacent unimpaired tissue may cause functional loss, which reverses once the edema resolves.

Diaschisis describes depressed blood flow and metabolism contralateral to an infarcted hemisphere.[40-42] It is diffuse but maximal in the area mirroring the infarct.[43] Positron emission tomography shows decreased oxygen and glucose metabolism in the contralateral cerebellar hemisphere,[37,43] although the clinical effect is uncertain. Diaschisis may result from sudden disconnection of functional pathways, impairing function and secondarily decreasing metabolism and cerebral blood flow.

Profound *abnormalities in neurotransmitters* such as alterations in the noradrenergic systems may follow cerebral infarction.[44] The cholinergic system resists ischemia, but all systems are probably affected in varying degrees.[45] Leakage of neurotransmitters from nerve endings may block receptor sites and interfere with neuronal signals and function. Some substances, especially catecholamines, are vasoactive, leading to further ischemia and dysfunction.[46] Neuropharmacologic agents may improve neurotransmitter function.[47]

Redundancy and *reorganization* in the central nervous system may also play a role in recovery. Although the exquisite organization and microspecialization unraveled in the visual cortex[48] does not suggest redundancy, a hierarchy of function has been demonstrated in the motor system.[49] The cerebellum can readjust motor programs very quickly following injury.[50] When one system is damaged, another may compensate but never entirely substitute for the original function.

GENERAL FACTORS

Only a fraction of the functional capacity of the brain is used daily and, as the organism ages, its reserve diminishes and the ability to compensate for injury decreases.[51] Mortality increases with *age* and in the presence of ischemic or hypertensive *cardiac disease* for all types of stroke (Figs. 131,132). *Hypertension* prior to stroke increases mortality.[52,53] In the Toronto Unit raised blood pressure exerted only a minor effect on survival, perhaps because of better treatment of hypertension after stroke.[9]

Polycythemia is a risk factor for stroke[54] and, when stroke occurs, causes it to be more severe.[55] Evidence for an adverse effect of *hyperglycemia* on stroke is persuasive[33,56,57] but inconclusive. Diabetes did not affect survival of patients in the Toronto Unit.[9] Brain metabolism

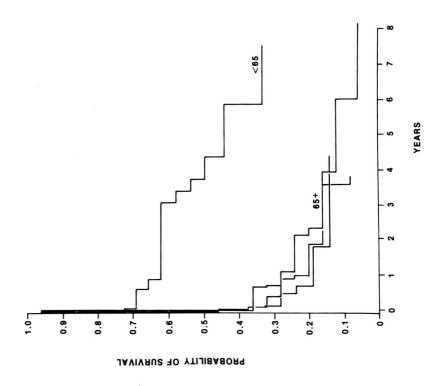

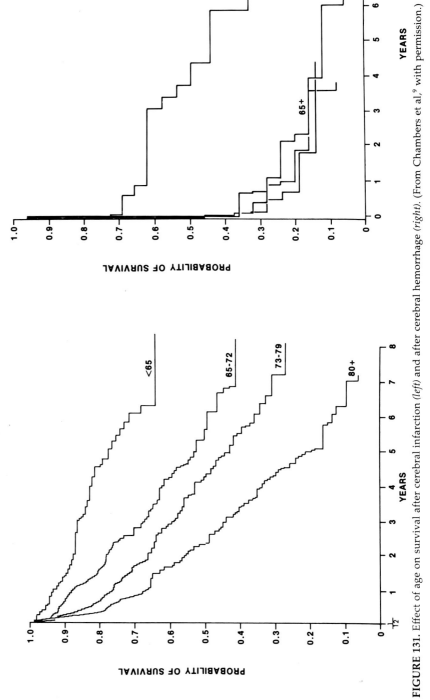

FIGURE 131. Effect of age on survival after cerebral infarction *(left)* and after cerebral hemorrhage *(right)*. (From Chambers et al,[9] with permission.)

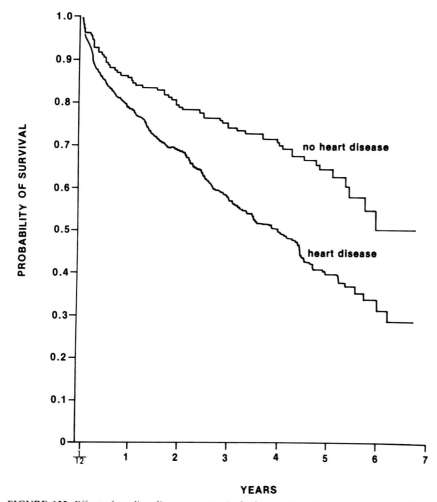

FIGURE 132. Effect of cardiac disease on survival after stroke. (From Chambers et al,[9] with permission.)

increases by 5 to 7 percent for each 1°C of *temperature*.[58] When raised metabolism cannot be matched by increased blood flow because of arterial occlusion, further brain damage probably occurs. Temperature increases as small as 0.5°C during the first week following cerebral infarction may carry a bad prognosis.[59]

COMPLICATING FACTORS

Cardiac complications often accompany stroke. In the Toronto Unit, half of patients with minor stroke dying from noncerebral causes in the first 30 days succumbed to a cardiac cause.[7] The risk of cardiac complications remained constant throughout this time (see Fig. 7).

Unlike fatal cardiac complications, *pneumonia* and *sepsis* occurred in relatively immobile patients with little hope of useful recovery. *Thrombophlebitis* and *pulmonary embolism* occurred in relatively immobile patients and also in the functionally independent (see Table 43).

Stroke may cause not only physical disability but also intellectual, emotional, and personality changes. *Depression* burdens about half of stroke patients and lasts at least 6 months, with major depressive symptoms increasing during this time.[60,61] Stroke may disrupt a person's self-image, decrease learning capacity, and cause dependence and social embarrassment, leading to a reactive depression. Post-stroke depression may also have an organic basis. Patients with left-hemispheric lesions are most prone to depression, its incidence and severity being directly related to the proximity of the lesion to the left frontal pole. Patients with right-hemispheric lesions showed the opposite trend—patients with right posterior damage were more depressed than were those with right anterior lesions, who were unduly cheerful or apathetic.[61]

Seizures developed in 9 percent of 827 patients admitted to the Toronto Unit during their first admission or during 2 to 5 years' followup. Only patients with hemispheric lesions developed seizures. The likelihood of seizures in acute stroke increases with a potential source of cardiac emboli and with involvement of the sensorimotor cortex. Seizures were initially focal in 7 percent, remained focal in 41 percent of these, but became generalized in the remainder. Seizures are a feature of acute stroke: 42 percent of seizures occurred in the first day, 62 percent in the first week, and 87 percent during the first year. Only 18 percent of patients had recurrent seizures. Early mortality was not associated with seizures.[62]

Recurrent Stroke

Stroke is the greatest risk factor for stroke. The recurrence rate in cerebral infarction approaches 10 percent per year,[63,64] compared with 5 percent per year following TIA.[6] The prevalence of cerebral infarction is greater than that of TIA,[65] making stroke patients the largest group at risk and most in need of secondary prevention. Preliminary evidence suggests

TABLE 47. An Ischemic Score*

Feature	Score
Abrupt onset	2
Stepwise deterioration	1
Fluctuating course	1
Nocturnal confusion	1
Relative preservation of personality	1
Depression	1
Somatic complaints	1
Emotional incontinence	1
History of hypertension	1
History of strokes	2
Evidence of associated atherosclerosis	1
Focal neurologic symptoms	2
Focal neurologic signs	2

(From Hachinski, VC, et al: *Cerebral blood flow in dementia.* Arch Neurol 32:634, 1975, with permission.)
*Patients attaining 7 points or more are likely to have either multi-infarct dementia or a vascular component to their mental impairment.

that control of hypertension[66] and the use of antiplatelet agents[67,68] can decrease recurrent stroke. Stroke patients remain at high risk of myocardial infarction and are more likely to die from heart disease than from subsequent stroke.[1]

Multiple strokes may cause progressive intellectual impairment but *multi-infarct dementia* is rarely responsible when a patient presents with mental impairment alone.[69,70] Vascular disease may contribute in up to one third of dementia patients.[71,72] Patients with multi-infarct dementia can be identified using an ischemic score (Table 47). Prognosis in multi-infarct dementia varies, largely depending on the severity and underlying cause of the illness.[73]

REHABILITATION

No evidence supports the view that treatment affects the outcome of the brain lesion although specialized treatment reduces complications and favors recovery.[74] The concept of stroke rehabilitation remains appealing,[75,76] but most studies are marred by selection bias and lack of controls. Unfortunately, "experts in stroke rehabilitation abound, but none of them has ever proven anything about rehabilitation to the satisfaction of anybody else."[77]

While the objective value of specific rehabilitative measures is the subject of study and debate, the need and value of the physician's support to the patient and family are obvious. Our own experience is that early rehabilitation decreases the number of complications and has psychologic and social benefits, although biologic effects and cost benefits remain to be demonstrated. The outcome in any individual is subject to measureless combinations of biologic individuality, motivation, and personality. Agnes de Mille, in her book *Reprieve*, illustrates how someone who suffered repeated strokes and medical complications recovered to return to a stage career, an outcome unforeseen medically.[78] In predicting outcome after stroke, there is safety in numbers but hazard in forecasting for individuals.

CONCLUSION

Accurate diagnosis must precede prognosis. A reasonably confident prognosis can be made within the first few days by assessing neurologic, general, and complicating factors. The severity of the stroke is the single most important factor and is usually reflected in impaired consciousness.Coma portends a poor prognosis in stroke regardless of etiology. Forced gaze deviation, major motor and sensory deficits, hypodense lesions on CT scan, or abnormal uptake on radioisotope scan are poor prognostic signs. Increasing age and associated heart disease, polycythemia, hyperglycemia, hyperthermia, and perhaps hypertension contribute to a poor outcome.

Mortality in stroke is about 20 percent in the first month and is higher for cerebral hemorrhage than for infarction. Most deaths in the first week result from transtentorial herniation, while sepsis and pulmonary embolism predominate in the second and third weeks. Cardiac death remains a menace throughout, striking the mildly and severely impaired alike.

Recovery varies with the severity and etiology of the stroke and is best for brainstem infarction, intermediate for cerebral infarction, and poorest for hemorrhage, but all stroke patients remain at risk of recurrent stroke and myocardial infarction.

REFERENCES

1. WHISNANT, JP: *The role of the neurologist in the decline of stroke*. Ann Neurol 14:1, 1983.
2. KURTZKE, JF: *ICD 9: A regression*. Am J Epidemiol 109:383, 1979.
3. MOHR, JP, ET AL: *The Harvard Cooperative Stroke Registry: A prospective study*. Neurology 28:754, 1978.
4. WOLF, PA, KANNEL, WB, AND VERTER, J: *Current status of risk factors for stroke*. Neurol Clin 1:317, 1983.
5. FISHER, CM: *Lacunar strokes and infarcts: A review*. Neurology 32:871, 1982.
6. BARNETT, HJM: *Further evidence relating mitral-valve prolapse to cerebral ischemic events*. N Engl J Med 302:139, 1980.
7. SILVER, FL, ET AL: *Early mortality following stroke: A prospective view*. Stroke 15:492, 1984.
8. SACCO, RL, ET AL: *Survival and recurrence following stroke, the Framingham Study*. Stroke 13:290, 1982.
9. CHAMBERS, BR, ET AL: *Prognostic profiles in acute stroke*. (In press).
10. HIER, DB, MONDLOCK, J, AND CAPLAN, LR: *Recovery of behavioral abnormalities after right hemisphere stroke*. Neurology 33:345, 1983.
11. KERTESZ, A, AND MCCABE, P: *Recovery patterns and prognosis in aphasia*. Brain 100:1, 1977.
12. ADAMS, GF, AND HURWITZ, LJ (EDS):*Cerebrovascular Disability and the Ageing Brain*. Churchill-Livingstone, Edinburgh, 1974.
13. FURLAN, A, ET AL: *Long-term prognosis after carotid artery occlusion*. Neurology 30:986, 1980.
14. CÔTÉ, R, ET AL: *Internal carotid occlusion: A prospective study*. Stroke 14:898, 1983.
15. MARZEWSKI, DJ, ET AL: *Intracranial internal carotid artery stenosis: Longterm prognosis*. Stroke 13:821, 1982.
16. CRAIG, DR, ET AL: *Intracranial internal carotid artery stenosis*. Stroke 13:825, 1982.
17. LHERMITTE, F, ET AL: *Ischemic accidents in the middle cerebral artery territory*. Arch Neurol 19:248, 1968.
18. LHERMITTE, F, ET AL: *Nature of occlusions of the middle cerebral artery*. Neurology 20:82, 1970.
19. LASCELLES, RG, AND BURROWS, EH: *Occlusion of the middle cerebral artery*. Brain 88:85, 1965.
20. ALLCOCK, JM: *Occlusion of the middle cerebral artery: Serial angiography as a guide to conservative therapy*. J Neurosurg 27: 353, 1967.
21. CORSTON, RN, KENDALL, BE, AND MARSHALL, J: *Prognosis in middle cerebral artery stenosis*. Stroke 15:237, 1984.
22. HINTON, RC, ET AL: *Symptomatic middle cerebral artery stenosis*. Ann Neurol 5:152, 1979.
23. MOUFARRIJ, NA, ET AL: *Vertebral artery stenosis: Long-term follow-up*. Stroke 15:260, 1984.
24. FISHER, CM, ET AL: *Atherosclerosis of the carotid and vertebral arteries—extracranial and intracranial*. J Neuropathol Exper Neurol 24:455, 1965.
25. CAPLAN, LR: *Vertebrobasilar disease—time for a new strategy*. Stroke 12:111, 1981.
26. FISHER, CM, ET AL: *Acute hypertensive cerebellar hemorrhage: Diagnosis and surgical treatment*. J Nerv Ment Dis 140:38, 1965.
27. FISHER, CM: *Lacunes: Small, deep cerebral infarcts*. Neurology 15:774, 1965.
28. ROPPER, AH, WECHSLER, LR, AND WILSON, LS: *Carotid bruit and the risk of stroke in elective surgery*. N Engl J Med 307:1388, 1982.
29. GRESHAM, GE, ET AL: *Residual disability in survivors of stroke. Framingham Study*. N Engl J Med 293:954, 1975.

30. GOWERS, WR: *A Manual of Diseases of the Nervous System (1888).* Classics of Medicine Library, Birmingham, AL, 1981.

31. OXBURY, JM, GREENHALL, RCD, AND GRAINGER, KMR: *Predicting the outcome of stroke: Acute stage after cerebral infarction.* Br Med J 3:125, 1975.

32. NARVA, EV: *Radionuclide brain scanning and rapid sequential scintiphotography in patients with cerebral infarction.* Dissertation. University of Turku, Finland, 1980.

33. CARONNA, JJ, AND LEVY, DE: *Clinical predictors of outcome in ischemic stroke.* Neurol Clin North Am 1:103, 1983.

34. KIMURA, D, AND HARSHMAN, RA: *Sex differences in brain organization for verbal and non-verbal functions.* In DEVRIES, GJ, ET AL (EDS): *Progress in Brain Research,* Vol 61. Elsevier, Amsterdam, 1984.

35. SCHENKMAN ET AL: *Cerebral hemisphere asymmetry in CT and functional recovery from hemiplegia.* Neurology 33:473, 1983.

36. ASTRUP, J, SIESJÖ, BK, AND SYMON, L: *Thresholds in cerebral ischemia—the ischemic penumbra.* Stroke 12:723, 1981.

37. BARON, JC, ET AL: *Noninvasive tomographic study of cerebral blood flow and oxygen metabolism in vivo.* Eur Neurol 20:273, 1981.

38. LASSEN, NA, ET AL: *The luxury-perfusion syndrome and its possible relation to acute metabolic acidosis localised within the brain.* Lancet 2:1113, 1966.

39. KATZMAN, R, ET AL: *iv. Brain edema in stroke.* Stroke 8:512, 1977.

40. SKINHØJ, E, ET AL: *Bilateral depression of CBF in unilateral cerebral diseases.* Acta Neurol Scand 41:161, 1965.

41. MEYER, JS, ET AL: *Diaschisis resulting from acute unilateral cerebral infarction: Quantitative evidence for man.* Arch Neurol 23:241, 1970.

42. SLATER, R, ET AL: *Diaschisis with cerebral infarction.* Stroke 8:684, 1977.

43. HEISS, WD, ET AL: *Decreased glucose metabolism in functionally inactivated brain regions in ischemic stroke and its alteration by activating drugs.* In MEYER, JS, ET AL (EDS): *Cerebral Vascular Disease.* Raven Press, New York, 1983, p 162.

44. MOSKOWITZ, MA, AND WURTMAN, RJ: *Acute stroke and brain monoamines.* In SCHEINBERG, P: *Cerebrovascular Diseases.* Raven Press, New York, 1976, p 153.

45. SIESJÖ, BK: *Brain energy metabolism.* John Wiley & Sons, Chichester, 1978.

46. WURTMAN, RJ, AND ZERVAS, NT: *Monoamine neurotransmitters and the pathophysiology of stroke and central nervous system trauma.* J Neurosurg 40:34, 1974.

47. FEENEY, DM, GONZALEZ, A, AND LAW, WA: *Amphetamine, haloperidol and experience interact to affect rate of recovery after motor cortex injury.* Science 217:855, 1982.

48. HUBEL, DH: *Exploration of the primary visual cortex, 1955–78.* Nature 299:515, 1982.

49. GOLDBERGER, ME, AND MURRAY, M: *Locomotor recovery after deafferentation of one side of the cat's trunk.* Exp Neurol 67:103, 1980.

50. GOLDBERGER, ME, AND GROWDEN, JH: *Pattern of recovery following cerebellar deep nuclear lesions in monkeys.* Exp Neurol 39:307, 1974.

51. SCHEFF, SW (ED): *Aging and Recovery of Functions in the Central Nervous System.* Plenum Press, New York, 1984.

52. KANNEL, WB, ET AL: *Vascular disease of the brain: Epidemiological aspects, the Framingham study.* Am J Publ Health 55:1355, 1965.

53. RABKIN, SW, MATHEWSON, FAL, AND TATE, RB: *The relation of blood pressure to stroke prognosis.* Ann Intern Med 89:15, 1978.

54. WOLF, PA, KANNEL, WB, AND VERTER, J: *Current status of risk factors for stroke.* Neurol Clin 1:317, 1983.

55. HARRISON, MJG: *Hematocrit et accident vasculair cerebral.* Presse Med 12:3095, 1983.

56. PULSINELLI, WA, ET AL: *Hyperglycemia augments ischemic brain damage: A neuropathologic study in the rat.* Neurology 32:1239, 1982.

57. LONGSTRETH, WT, DIEHR, P, AND INUI, TS: *Prediction of awakening after out-of-hospital cardiac arrest.* N Engl J Med 308:1378, 1983.

58. NEMOTO, EM, AND FRANKEL, HM: *Cerebraloxygenation and metabolism during progressive hyperthermia.* Am J Physiol 219:1784, 1970.

59. HINDFELT, B: *The prognostic significance of subfebrility and fever in ischemic cerebral infarction.* Acta Neurol Scand 53:72, 1976.

60. ROBINSON, RG, ET AL: *A 2-year long study of post-stroke mood disorders: Findings during the initial evaluation.* Stroke 14:736, 1983.

61. ROBINSON, RG, ET AL: *Mood disorders in stroke patients: Importance of location of the lesion.* Brain 107:81, 1984.

62. BLACK, SE, HACHINSKI, VC, AND NORRIS, JW: *Seizures after stroke* (abstr). Can J Neurol Sci 9:291, 1982.

63. BAKER, RN: *Prognosis among survivors of ischemic stroke.* Neurology 18:933, 1968.

64. FREEDMAN, M, NORRIS, JW, AND HACHINSKI, VC: *Outcome of cerebral infarction.* Can J Neurol Sci 5:339, 1978.

65. WIEBERS, DO, AND WHISNANT, JP: *Epidemiology.* In WARLOW, C, AND MORRIS, PJ (EDS): *Transient Ischemic Attacks.* Marcel Dekker, New York and Basel, 1982, p 1.

66. BEEVERS, DG, ET AL: *Antihypertensive treatment and the course of established cerebrovascular disease.* Lancet 2:1409, 1973.

67. CANADIAN COOPERATIVE STUDY GROUP: *A randomized trial of aspirin and sulfinpyrazone in threatened stroke.* N Engl J Med 299:53, 1978.

68. BOUSSER, MG, ET AL: *"AICLA" controlled trial of aspirin and dipyridamole in the secondary prevention of atherothrombotic cerebral ischemia.* Stroke 14:5, 1983.

69. HACHINSKI, VC, LASSEN, NA, AND MARSHALL, J: *Multi-infarct dementia. A cause of mental deterioration in the elderly.* Lancet 2:207, 1974.

70. BRUST, JCM: *Vascular dementia—still overdiagnosed.* Stroke 14:298, 1983.

71. TOMLINSON, BE, BLESSED, G, AND ROTH, M: *Observations on the brains of demented old people.* J Neurol Sci 11:205, 1970.

72. WELLS, CE: *Role of stroke in dementia.* Stroke 9:1, 1978.

73. HACHINSKI, VC, ET AL: *Cerebral blood flow in dementia.* Arch Neurol 32:632, 1975.

74. KENNEDY, FB, ET AL: *Stroke intensive care—an appraisal.* Am Heart J 80:188, 1977.

75. TRUSCOTT, BL, ET AL: *Early rehabilitative care in community hospitals: Effect on quality of survivorship following a stroke.* Stroke 5:623, 1974.

76. FEIGENSON, JS, ET AL: *Stroke rehabilitation: Effectiveness, benefits and cost—Some practical considerations.* Stroke 10:1, 1979.

77. ISAACS, B: *Problems and solutions in rehabilitation of stroke patients.* Geriatrics 33(7):87, 1978.

78. DE MILLE, A: *Reprieve.* Doubleday, New York, 1981.

Chapter 14

PREVENTION

*Resist beginnings; too late is the medicine prepared
when the disease has gained strength by long delays.*

Ovid

Prevention is incomparably more effective than the treatment of stroke, and the decline of stroke documented in recent years reflects prophylaxis, not cure. Opportunities for prevention exist in the asymptomatic phase, in the "warning" phase of stroke, and even after the patient has suffered a stroke (Table 48).[1] Those 10 percent of people who will suffer half of all strokes can be identified by assessing risk factors[2] (Tables 49, 50).

PREVENTION IN THE ASYMPTOMATIC PHASE

Treatment of Risk Factors

Hypertension

No risk factor is more powerful or more prevalent than hypertension; it applies to systolic and diastolic blood pressure, to ischemic and hemorrhagic stroke, to males and females, and at all ages.[2] Risk of stroke has a direct relationship with blood pressure, even within the normal range (Fig. 133). In persons 40 years or older, the prevalence of hypertension is about 30 percent[3] but decreasing, the decline coinciding with the effective, widespread use of antihypertensive medication. The proportion of patients using antihypertensive drugs rose markedly from 1956 to 1968, especially among women[3] which may explain the earlier decline in stroke incidence in this group (Fig. 134). Also, patients treated systematically in a hypertension detection and followup program had fewer strokes than

TABLE 48. Therapeutic Opportunities in the Prevention of Stroke

1. Asymptomatic phase
     Treatment of risk factors
     Management of asymptomatic bruits and stenoses

2. Warning phase
     Diagnosis and management of TIAs and minor strokes

3. Recurrence phase
     Management to prevent further strokes

TABLE 49. Risk Factors for Stroke

1. Hypertension (diastolic and systolic)
2. Cardiac disease
     Ischemic/hypertensive
       Coronary heart disease
       Myocardial infarction
         Acute—Endocardial damage → thrombi
         Chronic—Akinetic segments → thrombi
       Congestive heart failure
       Left ventricular hypertrophy
         On ECG
         On chest x-ray
     Valvular
       Rheumatic heart disease
       Prolapsing mitral valve
       Endocarditis
         Infectious
         Marantic
       Aortic stenosis
       Prosthetic heart valves
       ? Calcified mitral annulus
     Arrhythmias such as
       Atrial fibrillation
       Sick sinus syndrome
3. Diabetes
4. Erythrocytosis
5. Cigarette smoking
6. Other
     Physical inactivity
     Hyperlipidemia
     Heredity
     Environmental factors

TABLE 50. Incidence of Risk Factors in 820 Patients with Completed Stroke Admitted to the Toronto Unit

Risk Factor	Cerebral Infarction (742)	Cerebral Hemorrhage (78)	Matched Controls (98)
Cardiac disease	75%	63%	12%
Hypertension	50%	48%	22%
Diabetes	18%	11%	0%
Peripheral vascular disease	20%	13%	12%
Cervical bruit	22%	9%	2%
TIAs	33%	18%	0%

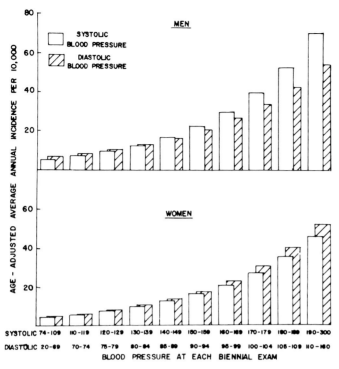

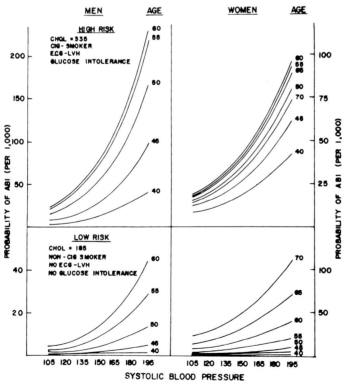

FIGURE 133. *Top,* Incidence of atherothrombotic brain infarction according to systolic versus diastolic blood pressure at biennial exam; men and women, aged 45 to 74 years.

Bottom, Risk of atherothrombotic brain infarction in 8 years according to systolic blood pressure in each sex. (Framingham Study: 18-year followup.) (From Kannel, WB,[2] with permission.)

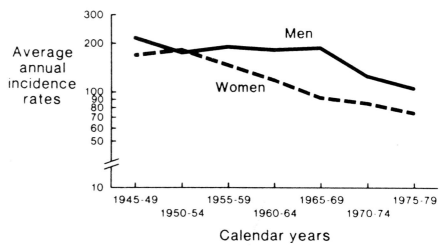

FIGURE 134. Differential decline of stroke incidence in women. (From Whisnant, JP,[3] with permission.)

did those patients who were referred to their physicians (35 percent and 45 percent, respectively, in the group aged 60 to 69 years).[3]

Cardiac Disease

Many patients with cerebrovascular disease have cardiac abnormalities, and myocardial infarction is the commonest cause of death in patients with stroke, TIA, and asymptomatic bruits.[4,5]

Patients with *ischemic and hypertensive heart disease* have a fivefold increase in stroke. Congestive heart failure carries a ninefold increased risk of stroke, particularly in the presence of left ventricular hypertrophy and coronary heart disease. Left ventricular hypertrophy is also an index of stroke risk.[6] Patients with *valvular heart disease,* including rheumatic heart disease, infectious or marantic endocarditis, prolapsing mitral valve, calcified mitral annulus, calcified aortic stenosis, and prosthetic heart valves are at increased risk of stroke.[7]

Cardiac arrhythmias also are associated with the risk of stroke. Half the patients monitored with bedside ECG or Holter (long-term) ECG monitoring had cardiac arrhythmias, and the incidence was equal in hemorrhagic and ischemic stroke patients[8,9] (Table 51). Most arrhythmias were harmless ectopics, but serious treatable arrhythmias such as atrial fibrillation or sick sinus syndrome occurred in 17 percent of patients.[10] Chronic atrial fibrillation alone carries more than a fivefold increased risk for stroke and a 17-fold risk when associated with rheumatic heart disease.[11] Over one third of patients with atrial fibrillation have systemic emboli at autopsy.[12] In 150 patients with atrial fibrillation, 31 percent had a stroke or peripheral embolism,[13] and only 20 percent had cardiac valvular disease, the commonest associated condition being hypertension. Most of the cerebral infarcts were large, disabling, and unheralded by TIAs. Although the treatment of atrial fibrillation with anticoagulants remains controversial,[14,15] safer, lower-dose anticoagulation[16] demands new studies in symptomatic and asymptomatic atrial fibrillation and serious consideration in individual cases.

Even mild *diabetes mellitus* predisposes to vascular disease.[17] Diabetes increased stroke risk 2.6 times in men and 3.1 times in women in the Framingham Study.[6] Eighteen percent of patients with cerebral infarction in the Toronto Unit were diabetic (see Table 50). Cerebral infarcts tend to be larger in the presence of hyperglycemia,[18] but the effect of controlling diabetes and acute hyperglycemia remains uncertain.

Polycythemia predisposes to stroke. Hematocrit relates to stroke risk, beginning within the normal range,[19] partly from associated hypertension[20] but mainly due to increased viscosity. Thomas and associates[21] showed an inverse relationship between viscosity and cerebral blood flow. Whether the increased cerebral blood flow resulting from venesection compensates for the decreased oxygen-carrying capacity of the blood is debatable.[22,23]

Smoking represents a small risk for stroke. In the Framingham Study, the association was only for men younger than 65.[6] Cessation of smoking remains worthwhile, as smoking is a significant risk factor for coronary heart disease, a common companion of and risk factor for cerebrovascular disease.

Physical inactivity may increase risk of stroke,[24] but current evidence only justifies exercise as a general health measure with a possible effect on preventing myocardial infarction.

Hyperlipidemia bears little risk for stroke and only a weak relationship among increased cholesterol, cholesterol-rich betalipoproteins, and triglyceride pre-betalipoproteins, and stroke under the age of 55 years has been observed.[2]

Strokes cluster in families. Studies of *heredity* showed a higher frequency of stroke among siblings of stroke patients than among the siblings of their spouses.[25] The familial incidence of hypertension, diabetes, and heart disease may account for this,[6] but genetic or unrecognized factors may explain the remaining risk.

Environmental factors such as diet may promote or protect against stroke; for instance, Eskimos consuming fish that contains unsaturated long-chain fatty acids, a prostacyclin-promoting factor, may acquire protection against vascular disease.[26]

Stroke Risk Factors in the Young

Although similar risk factors apply at all ages, some predominate in the young (Table 51).

Multiple Risk Factors

A combination of risk factors may represent a worse threat for stroke than the sum of the individual hazards.[6,27] For example, the likelihood of stroke in the presence of hypertension rises steeply in the presence of other risk factors (Fig. 135). Risk factors may interact, be independent, or be mutually dependent on common factors.

TABLE 51. Risk Factors for Stroke in the Young (as Discussed in Chapter 9)

1. Cardiac disease
    Valvular heart disease, especially
       mitral valve prolapse
    Cardiomyopathies
    Atrial myxoma
2. Hypertension
3. Migraine
4. Hyperlipidemia
5. Oral contraceptives
6. Cigarette smoking
7. Trauma
8. Drug abuse
9. Alcohol
10. Neurosyphilis

Management of Risk Factors

All risk factors are not equal. Hypertension is most powerful and demands early, consistent, and vigorous treatment. Cigarette smoking, while not a strong determinant of stroke, compounds the risk in young women and carries a strong risk for coronary artery disease. Treating hypertension and stopping smoking offer good opportunities for prevention in both the patient and the family, since family members are seldom as motivated about their own risk as when someone close has a stroke. While managing other risk factors is desirable, compliance in one or two high-yield areas is more beneficial than attempting a comprehensive but difficult regimen.

Asymptomatic Bruits and Stenoses

Cervical bruits are associated with an increased risk of stroke and heart disease.[28,29] Women have a higher incidence of asymptomatic bruits but are at lesser risk of developing stroke.[29] The risk of stroke is not confined to the side of the bruit, and the stroke may be hemorrhagic rather than ischemic.[28] Only half of patients with a neck bruit have underlying stenosis,[30] and two thirds of carotid stenoses occur without bruits.[31] Also, patients with cervical bruits are two to three times as likely to suffer myocardial infarction as stroke.[28,29] Cervical bruits may be markers rather than risk factors for stroke. Although reports on asymptomatic bruits are many, the epidemiologically sound ones are few. Natural history studies of asymptomatic bruits suggest that the risk for stroke is between 0.7 percent[28] and 2.3 percent per year.[29] Preliminary results from a prospective study of asymptomatic carotid bruits at the Mayo Clinic suggest an annual stroke rate of about 2.5 percent per year.[3] Studies reporting a higher incidence have not made adjustments for associated but unreported hypertension, cardiac disease, and other risk factors. While a high-pitched systolic and diastolic midcervical bruit usually signals carotid stenosis, the causes of neck noises are many; they include hyperkinetic states, referred bruits from thyroid, thorax, and other adjacent structures, and innocent venous hums, particularly in the young. Non-

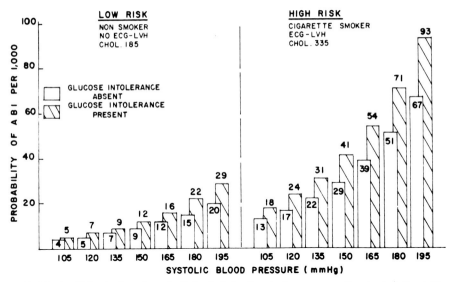

FIGURE 135. Risk of atherothrombotic brain infarction in 8 years according to diabetic status and level of other risk factors; 55-year-old women. (Framingham Study: 18-year followup.) (From Kannel, WB,[2] with permission.)

invasive methods of diagnosing carotid stenosis and other lesions are now available, facilitating much-needed prospective, randomized natural history studies of different cervical bruits and lesions.[30,31] Meanwhile, only vigorous treatment of associated risk factors can be justified in the vast majority of patients.[32,33]

Anesthesia and surgery do not pose additional risks of stroke for patients with carotid bruits. Ropper and associates[34] studied 753 patients over the age of 55 years who underwent elective nonneurologic surgery. Fourteen percent of patients had carotid bruits, and 0.7 percent developed stroke with no difference in stroke incidence in patients with or without bruits.

Asymptomatic carotid stenoses also have a relatively benign prognosis. Of 73 patients undergoing endarterectomy for a symptomatic carotid lesion, 3 percent had a stroke over an average of 4 years in the contralateral asymptomatic but stenosed carotid artery.[35] This incidence is similar to that of stroke in the territory of the operated carotid artery (5 percent) and of vertebrobasilar stroke (4 percent).

Carotid endarterectomy increased alarmingly, from 7.4 per 100,000 to 24 per 100,000, in the last decade in the United States.[36] With more widespread availability of digital subtraction angiography and better carotid Doppler imaging, this is likely to increase further. In 1982, 85,000 carotid endarterectomies were performed in the United States, with a reported mortality of 2.8 percent—stroke usually occurring two to five times as frequently as death.[37] This outcome is worse than with medical management and worse than the natural history.

Risk factors for stroke and ischemic heart disease should be treated, since patients with asymptomatic cervical bruits and stenoses are at greater risk of suffering a myocardial infarction than a cerebral infarct.[29] Close followup is necessary to detect transient ischemic attacks. Evaluation of carotid bruits by noninvasive methods or digital intravenous angiography may be helpful to rule out a vascular cause but may complicate decision-making if it shows stenosis. The annual incidence of stroke in patients with asymptomatic bruits ranges from 0.7[28] to 2.5 percent,[3] which is below the combined morbidity of angiography and endarterectomy (3 percent) in the best hands.[38]

PREVENTION OF STROKE IN THE WARNING PHASE

Transient Ischemic Attacks (TIAs)

In community surveys, fewer than 10 percent of patients report TIAs prior to cerebral infarction,[38] whereas about 35 percent of patients with stroke will have a prior history of TIA[3] (see Table 49).

In community surveys, the risk of developing stroke after TIAs is about six times that of the normal population.[39] Most information about the natural history of TIA in clinical series derives from control groups of anticoagulant or antiplatelet trials. In the Canadian Cooperative Study of Antiplatelet Agents, the cumulative risk for stroke and death was 13 percent in the first year and 22 percent and 30 percent in the second and third years, respectively, with higher risks for men.[40] The stroke risk of 5 percent annually following TIA can materialize at any time, continuing indefinitely.[41]

The frequency of TIAs bears no predictable relationship to the likelihood of stroke.[42,43] Patients with vertebrobasilar symptoms have TIAs more frequently than do those with carotid TIAs but their prognosis is better. Fields [44] found a higher mortality rate among patients with carotid TIA than among those with vertebrobasilar TIAs. Gender does not help predict risk for stroke in individual cases, but women generally have a more benign prognosis after TIAs than men have.[45]

The incidence of TIAs depends on increasing age and the assiduity with which the symptom is sought. Whisnant and coworkers[39] found an age-specific incidence of 2 per 100,000 in a largely Caucasian midwestern population. Blacks may have fewer TIAs prior to stroke, even when underreporting in this racial group is considered.[46] In hospital populations, the ratio of men to women is usually 2 to 1, whereas in general population studies the rate is somewhat lower.

Treat Risk Factors

Scrupulous management of risk factors (Table 52), particularly hypertension, probably has greater impact on the prognosis of TIA patients than all surgical procedures combined. Consequently, every patient deserves the closest attention to any risk factors that may be present, no matter what further surgical or medical therapy is considered.

Carotid Endarterectomy

Patients with a hemodynamically significant carotid stenosis (more than 80 percent stenosed) but without good collateral circulation may risk stroke. Carotid endarterectomy is performed in patients with an ulcer-

TABLE 52. Management of TIAs

1. Treat risk factors
2. Consider surgery
   - Carotid endarterectomy
   - (Unproven, good rationale)
     - Factors favoring consideration
       - Appropriate carotid stenosis that on angiography is
         - Hemodynamically significant
         - Ulcerated
         - Shows intraluminal thrombus
       - Experienced surgeon with a known record
       - Experienced angiographer with a known record
     - Factors militating against consideration
       - Age >70 years
       - Serious associated disease
       - Widespread cervicocerebral vascular disease
   - Vertebrobasilar system surgery
   - (Unproven, poor rationale, experimental)
   - Extra-/intracranial arterial bypass
   - (Unproven, reasonable rationale for selected cases, being evaluated)
3. Consider antiplatelet agents and anticoagulation
   - Antiplatelet agents
     - Aspirin 325 mg 4 times daily
       - (only antiplatelet agent of proven value in TIA/minor stroke)
     - Dipyridamole (being evaluated)
     - Ticlopidine hydrochloride (being evaluated)
   - Anticoagulants
     - Heparin ⎤
     - Coumadin ⎦ for cardiac emboli

ated carotid stenosis to prevent platelets, thrombi, and debris from embolizing to the brain.

Clinical symptoms and angiographic appearances correlate poorly in patients with TIA.[42,43] Asymptomatic individuals may have carotid stenoses and occlusions,[47] and TIAs may be caused by cardiac and other etiologies, making it difficult to decide whether a stenosed carotid artery is responsible for the patient's symptoms.

Carotid endarterectomy reduced the later incidence of stroke in a controlled study of patients with unilateral carotid lesions,[48] but, if the results are calculated from the time of randomization rather than from discharge, surgically treated patients fared no better than the medically treated group. Surgical mortality and morbidity bias the results against surgery acutely, and followup was too short to show a definite long-term benefit for surgery.[14]

Series reporting procedure rather than patient complication rates underreport the risks of the procedure. Younger healthier patients predominate in most surgical series, favoring better outcomes, yet the results of many surgical series are worse than the natural history.[14]

Carotid endarterectomy should only be considered if the combined morbidity and mortality from arteriography and surgery procedure is below 3 percent.[38] Patients with an ulcerated lesion may have a worse prognosis than those with stenosis alone, justifying higher morbidity and mortality from arteriography and surgery, if this evidence is confirmed.[49,50] Surgical decisions should always relate to the angiographic and surgical complication rates of *the particular center.*

The results of *surgery on the vertebrobasilar system* are even more difficult to evaluate. Diagnosis of vertebrobasilar TIAs remains the most difficult, since the attacks mimic nonspecific dizziness, syncope, and even forgetfulness, disorientation, and other symptoms more suggestive of Alzheimer's dementia than of cerebrovascular disease. Patients with vertebrobasilar TIAs probably have a more benign prognosis than do those with carotid TIAs,[44,51] and surgery on the vertebrobasilar system carries greater technical risks. Surgical procedures on the vertebrobasilar system remain unproven. Even the subclavian steal syndrome remains largely a radiologic phenomenon that seldom manifests clinically or is severe enough to justify the major surgery involved. The diagnosis of vertebrobasilar ischemia is so uncertain, the natural history so benign, and the surgery so risky that medical management remains the treatment of choice.

Extracranial-Intracranial Arterial Anastomosis

Patients with TIA or minor stroke and those with internal carotid occlusions, inaccessible cervical lesions, intracranial internal carotid lesions, or middle cerebral lesions are involved in a trial of this procedure in North America, Europe, Japan, and Taiwan.[52] All patients are treated with aspirin and the best available medical care. The usual surgical procedure involves anastomosis of the temporal artery with a branch of the middle cerebral artery. The results of this study are not yet available.

Antiplatelet Agents

The Canadian Cooperative Trial showed that aspirin, 1300 mg per day, decreases the risk of stroke and death in men with "threatened stroke" by 49 percent but was ineffective in women. Sulfinpyrazone was ineffective in preventing stroke. Subsequent prospective studies have confirmed the usefulness of aspirin[53,54] and the ineffectiveness of dipyridamole in preventing stroke. A large trial of aspirin-dipyridamole combined versus aspirin alone failed to show any benefit from dipyridamole.[55]

Aspirin inhibits the enzyme cyclo-oxygenase; this interferes with the metabolism of arachidonic acid, the precursor of both thromboxane-A_2, which promotes platelet aggregation and vasoconstriction, and prostacyclin PGI_2, which disaggregates platelets and inhibits release of vasoconstrictors such as serotonin. The dose of aspirin that achieves maximum inhibition of thromboxane-A_2 with minimal inhibition of prostacyclin in PGI_2 remains undetermined. For example, bleeding time in men and women is prolonged by 300 mg but not by 3.9 g aspirin per day.[56] Other hematologic variables are also altered by use of one aspirin per day,[57] but the only clinically proven dose for preventing stroke is four plain aspirin (1300 mg) per day, and this should be the dose used until more information from clinical trials emerges. A current British study[58] comparing two dosages of aspirin may provide much-needed data on dosage and on whether aspirin helps to prevent stroke in women.

Of available antiplatelet agents, only aspirin has been shown to reduce the risk of stroke and death in patients with TIAs and minor strokes. Two issues remain outstanding, gender and dosage. The apparent ineffectiveness of aspirin in women with TIA may be artifactual,[59] or it may be a reflection of a lower stroke incidence in women with TIA.[60]

However, the results of experimental studies[61,62] and clinical trials indicate a male but not female response to antiplatelet agents in hip replacement,[63] and in arteriovenous shunts used in dialysis. Men with rheumatoid arthritis treated with aspirin for 15 years have a decreased incidence of myocardial infarction and stroke, but this effect was absent in women.[64] Bousser and colleagues[54] found that aspirin did benefit women; however, there were few women in this trial. At present, the possible benefits of aspirin outweigh the actual risks and, since the effects remain controversial, its use in women may be justified.

Ticlopidine is another powerful antiplatelet agent that is at present undergoing an extensive trial in North America.

Anticoagulants

No controlled study of anticoagulants has been performed since the 1960s. Only four trials were randomized, and all were negative.[65] The methodology of clinical trials was not well developed at that time, and common shortcomings included insufficient numbers, heterogeneity of the patients studied, and lack of awareness or control of associated risk factors.[65]

In the Cooperative Study of TIAs,[46] physicians treated the patients according to their best judgment and found no difference in outcome between the patients treated with anticoagulants and those treated with other therapy. Anticoagulants are often used for TIAs of cardiac origin, but antiplatelet agents may be more appropriate to specific entities such as symptomatic mitral valve prolapse.[7]

PREVENTION IN THE RECURRENCE PHASE

Stroke as a Risk for Stroke

There is increased risk of stroke in patients who have already had a stroke. About 10 percent of patients have a recurrent stroke within a year.[66] In Marquardsen's series,[67] the recurrence rate was 8.9 percent in men and 10.6 percent annually in women during 10 years' followup. Patients with a history of heart failure or ECG abnormalities at the time of the first stroke had an annual recurrence rate of 15 percent. If the patient's diastolic blood pressure exceeded 120 mm Hg, the recurrence rate reached 20 percent annually.

The benefits of treating risk factors such as ischemic heart disease, diabetes, and polycythemia after first stroke are unproven. Control of hypertension decreased mortality and stroke recurrence in a randomized study of 99 patients.[68] The recurrence rate of stroke in patients with uncontrolled hypertension was 55 percent compared with 6 percent in patients whose blood pressure was well controlled.[69]

In considering carotid surgery for patients recovered from partial stroke, the severity of the stroke and the uncertain results of preventive cerebrovascular surgery should be taken into account.[14]

Antiplatelet agents are unproven in preventing recurrent stroke. Although Bousser and colleagues[54] included patients with completed stroke, the great majority of patients had TIA and minor stroke. Ticlopidine hydrochloride is currently undergoing a trial in the prevention of recurrent cerebral and myocardial infarction.

Trials of *anticoagulants* in stroke carried out in the 1960s are suboptimal in design,[65] but results suggest that anticoagulant therapy is ineffective after stroke and is associated with higher mortality and morbidity from bleeding. The evidence is persuasive that patients with stroke from cardiac embolism benefit from anticoagulation,[37] but the timing remains a subject of debate.[70-79]

CONCLUSION

No treatment of acute stroke can compete with its prevention in effect and economy. The most powerful stroke risk factor is hypertension, both systolic and diastolic. This applies to both sexes, to all types of stroke, and to all ages. More benefit has accrued from the recognition and treatment of hypertension as a risk factor for stroke than all other therapeutic efforts combined. TIA, heart disease, diabetes, polycythemia, and cigarette smoking are also treatable risk factors. Prevention does not deny the importance of acute care (since stroke will never be wholly avoidable) but emphasizes the need to disclose and delineate further risk factors for stroke.

The value of preventive surgery for cerebrovascular disease remains unproven. The decision to operate depends on the evaluation of potential benefits weighed against actual risks demonstrated at a particular center. Among antiplatelet agents, only aspirin has proven value in preventing stroke and death, while anticoagulants are only justified in preventing cardiac emboli.

Prevention should be considered not only for patients but also for their families, who are at increased hazard of stroke. Prevention consists of treating risk factors in the asymptomatic phase, in responding to the warning of TIA or minor stroke, and in recognizing stroke as the greatest risk for recurrent stroke.

REFERENCES

1. HACHINSKI, VC: *Prognostic indicants in cerebrovascular disease.* In REIVICH, M, AND HURTIG, HI (EDS): *Cerebrovascular Diseases.* Raven Press, New York, 1983, p 41.
2. KANNEL, WB: *Epidemiology of cerebrovascular disease.* In ROSS RUSSELL, RW (ED): *Cerebral Arterial Disease.* Churchill-Livingstone, Edinburgh, 1976, p 1.
3. WHISNANT, JP: *The decline of stroke.* Stroke 15:160, 1984.
4. HEYMAN, A, ET AL: *Risk of ischemic heart disease in patients with transient ischemic attacks.* Neurology 34:626, 1984.
5. ADAMS, HP, KASSELL, NF, AND MAZUZ, H: *The patient with transient ischemic attacks—Is this the time for a new therapeutic approach?* Stroke 15:371, 1984.
6. WOLF, PA, KANNEL, WB, AND VERTER, J: *Current status of risk factors for stroke.* Neurol Clin 1:317, 1983.
7. BARNETT, HJM: *Heart in ischemic stroke—A changing emphasis.* Neurol Clin 1:291, 1983.
8. NORRIS, JW, FROGGATT, GM, AND HACHINSKI, VC: *Cardiac arrhythmias in acute stroke.* Stroke 9:392, 1978.
9. MYERS, MG, ET AL: *Cardiac sequelae of acute stroke.* Stroke 13:838, 1982.
10. NORRIS, JW: *Effects of cerebrovascular lesions on the heart.* Neurol Clin 1:87, 1983.

11. WOLF, PA, ET AL: *Epidemiologic assessment of chronic atrial fibrillation and risk of stroke: The Framingham study.* Neurology 28:973, 1978.

12. HINTON, RC, ET AL: *Influence of etiology of atrial fibrillation on incidence of systemic embolism.* Am J Cardiol 40:509, 1977.

13. SHERMAN, DG, ET AL: *Thromboembolism in patients with atrial fibrillation.* Arch Neurol 41:708, 1984.

14. STARKEY, I, AND WARLOW, CP: *The secondary prevention of stroke in patients with atrial fibrillation.* Arch Neurol (in press).

15. SHERMAN, DG, HART, RG, AND EASTON, JD: *The secondary prevention of stroke in patients with atrial fibrillation.* Arch Neurol (in press).

16. HULL, R, ET AL: *Different intensities of oral anticoagulant therapy in the treatment of proximal-vein thrombosis.* N Engl J Med 307:1676, 1982.

17. FULLER, JH, ET AL: *Coronary heart-disease risk and impaired glucose tolerance.* Lancet 1:1373, 1980.

18. PLUM, F: *What causes infarction in ischemic brain? The Robert Wartenberg lecture.* Neurology 33:222, 1983.

19. KANNEL, WB, ET AL: *Hemoglobin and the risk of cerebral infarction: The Framingham study.* Stroke 3:409, 1972.

20. TOGHI, H, ET AL: *Importance of the haematocrit as a risk factor in cerebral infarction.* Stroke 9:369, 1978.

21. THOMAS, DJ, ET AL: *Effect of hematocrit on cerebral blood-flow in man.* Lancet 2:941, 1977.

22. PAULSON, OB, ET AL: *Influence of carbon monoxide and of hemodilution on cerebral blood flow and blood gases in man.* J Appl Physiol 35:111, 1973.

23. WADE, JPH: *Transport of oxygen to the brain in patients with elevated hematocrit values before and after venesection.* Brain 106:513,1983.

24. HERMAN, B, ET AL: *An evaluation of risk factors for stroke in a Dutch community.* Stroke 13:334, 1982.

25. ALTER, M, ET AL: *Cerebral infarction, clinical and angiographic correlations.* Neurology 22:590, 1972.

26. EDITORIAL: *Eskimo diets and diseases.* Lancet 1:1139, May 1983.

27. PAFFENBERGER RS, JR, AND WILLIAMS, JL: *Chronic disease in former college students. v. Early precursors of fatal stroke.* Am J Publ Health 57:1290, 1967.

28. WOLF, PA, ET AL: *Asymptomatic carotid bruit and risk of stroke: The Framingham Study.* JAMA 245:1442, 1981.

29. HEYMAN, A, ET AL: *Risk of stroke in asymptomatic persons with cervical arterial bruits: A population study in Evans County, Georgia.* N Engl J Med 302:838, 1980.

30. MOORE, WS, ET AL: *The use of ophthalmosonometryin the diagnosis of carotid artery stenosis.* Surgery 82:107, 1977.

31. CHAMBERS, BR, AND NORRIS, JW: *The case against surgery for asymptomatic carotid stenosis.* Stroke 15:964, 1984.

32. CHAMBERS, BR, AND NORRIS, JW: *Outcome of patients with asymptomatic neck bruits.* (In press.)

33. HACHINSKI, VC: *Asymptomatic carotid stenosis: Rationale for management.* Arch Neurol (in press.)

34. ROPPER, AH, WECHSLER, LR, AND WILSON, LS: *Carotid bruit and the risk of stroke in elective surgery.* N Engl J Med 307:1388, 1982.

35. DURWARD, QJ, FERGUSON, GG, AND BARR, HWK: *The natural history of asymptomatic carotid bifurcation plaques.* Stroke 13:459, 1982.

36. MOHR, JP: *Asymptomatic carotid artery disease.* Stroke 13:431, 1982.

37. DYKEN, ML, AND POKRAS, R: *The performance of endarterectomy for disease of the extracranial arteries of the head.* Stroke 15:948, 1984.

38. HASS, WK, AND JONAS, S: *Caution: falling rock zone. Analysis of the medical and surgical management of threatened stroke.* Proc Inst Med Chic 33:80, 1980.

39. WHISNANT, JP, MATSUMOTO, N, AND ELVEBACK, LR: *Transient cerebral ischemic attacks in a community. Rochester, Minnesota—1955 through 1969.* Mayo Clin Proc 48:194, 1973.

40. CANADIAN COOPERATIVE STUDY GROUP: *A randomized trial of aspirin and sulphinpyrazone in threatened stroke.* N Engl J Med 299:53, 1978.

41. BARNETT, HJM: *Progress towards stroke prevention: The Robert Wartenberg lecture.* Neurology 30:1212, 1980.

42. CONNEALLY, PM, ET AL: *Cooperative study of hospital frequency and character of transient ischemic attacks. viii. Risk factors.* JAMA 240:742, 1978.

43. PESSIN, MS, ET AL: *Clinical and angiographic features of carotid transient ischemic attacks.* N Engl J Med 296:358, 1977.

44. FIELDS, WK: *Discussion.* In REIVICH, M, AND HURTIG, HI (EDS): *Cerebrovascular Diseases.* Raven Press, New York, 1983, p 86.

45. DYKEN, ML: *Transient ischemic attacks and stroke: Aspirin trials.* In BANG, NU, ET AL (EDS): *Thrombosis and Atherosclerosis.* Year Book Medical Publishers, Chicago, 1982, p 393.

46. DYKEN, ML, ET AL: *Cooperative study of hospital frequency and character of transient ischemic attacks. i. Background, organization and clinical survey.* JAMA 237:882, 1977.

47. FARIS, AA, ET AL: *Radiologic visualization of neck vessels in healthy men.* Neurology 13:386, 1963.

48. FIELDS, WS, ET AL: *Joint study of extracranial arterial occlusion. v. Progress report of prognosis following surgery or non-surgical treatment for transient cerebral ischemic attacks and cervical carotid artery lesions.* JAMA 211:1993, 1970.

49. MOORE, WS, ET AL: *Natural history of nonstenotic, asymptomatic ulcerative lesions of the carotid artery.* Arch Surg 113:1352, 1978.

50. DIXON, S, ET AL: *Natural history of nonstenotic, asymptomatic ulcerative lesions of the carotid artery, a further analysis.* Arch Surg 117:1493, 1982.

51. MARSHALL, J: *Management of Cerebrovascular Disease,* ed 3. Blackwell Scientific, Oxford, 1976.

52. BARNETT, HJM: *The collaborative EC/IC bypass study.* In ITO, Z, KUTSUZAWA, T, AND YASUI, N (EDS): *Cerebral Ischemia.* Excerpta Medica, Amsterdam, 1982, p 7.

53. GUIRAUD-CHAUMEIL, B, ET AL: *Prévention des récidives des accidents vasculaires cérébraux ischemiques par les anti-agrégants plaquettaires. Résultats d'un essai thérapeutique contrôlé de 3 ans.* Rev Neurol 138:367, 1982.

54. BOUSSER, MG, ET AL: *"AICLA" controlled trial of aspirin and dipyridamole in the secondary prevention of atherothrombotic cerebral ischemia.* Stroke 14:5, 1983.

55. AMERICAN-CANADIAN CO-OPERATIVE STUDY GROUP: *Persantine aspirin trial in cerebral ischemia.* Stroke (in press.)

56. O'GRADY, J, AND MONCADA, S: *Aspirin: A paradoxical effect on bleeding time.* Lancet 2:780, 1978.

57. JAFFE, EA, AND WEKSLER, BB: *Recovery of endothelial cell prostacyclin production after inhibition by low doses of aspirin.* J Clin Invest 63:532, 1979.

58. TOGNONI, G, AND GARATTINI, S (EDS): *Drug Treatment and Prevention in Cerebrovascular Disorders.* Elsevier-North Holland, Amsterdam, 1979.

59. KURTZKE, JF: *Controversy in neurology: The Canadian Study on TIA and aspirin. A critique of the Canadian TIA Study.* Ann Neurol 5:597, 1979.

60. DYKEN, ML: *Transient ischemic attacks and aspirin, stroke and death: Negative studies and type II error.* Stroke 14:2, 1983.

61. KELTON, JG, ET AL: *Sex differences in the antithrombotic effects of aspirin.* Blood 52:1073, 1978.

62. PRESTON, FE, ET AL: *Inhibition of prostacyclin and platelet thromboxane A_2 after low-dose aspirin.* N Engl J Med 304:76, 1981.

63. HARRIS, WH, ET AL: *Aspirin prophylaxis of venous thromboembolism after total hip replacement.* N Engl J Med 297:1246, 1977.

64. LINOS, A, ET AL: *Effect of aspirin on prevention of coronary and cerebrovascular disease in patients with rheumatoid arthritis, a long-term follow-up study.* Mayo Clin Proc 53:581, 1978.

65. JOINT COMMITTEE FOR STROKE RESOURCES (GENTON, E, ET AL): *xiv. Cerebral ischemia: The role of thrombosis and of antithrombotic therapy.* Stroke 8:150, 1977.

66. FREEDMAN, M, NORRIS, JW, AND HACHINSKI, VC: *Outcome of cerebral infarction—A Canadian experience.* Can J Neurol Sci 5:339, 1978.

67. MARQUARDSEN, J: *Natural history and prognosis of cerebrovascular disease.* In ROSS RUSSELL, RW (ED): *Vascular Disease of the Central Nervous System,* ed 2. Churchill-Livingstone, Edinburgh, 1983.

68. CARTER, AB: *Hypotensive therapy in stroke survivors.* Lancet 1:485, 1970.

69. BEEVERS, DG, ET AL: *Antihypertensive treatment and the course of established cerebral vascular disease.* Lancet 2:407, 1973.

70. KOLLER, RL: *Recurrent embolic cerebral infarction and anticoagulation.* Neurology 32:283, 1982.

71. FURLAN, AJ: *Hemorrhage and anticoagulation after nonseptic embolic brain infarction.* Neurology 32:280, 1982.

72. SHIELDS, RW, JR, ET AL: *Anticoagulant-induced hemorrhage in acute cerebral embolism* (abstr). Ann Neurol 12:75, 1982.

73. SHERMAN, DG, ET AL: *Thromboembolism in patients with atrial fibrillation.* Arch Neurol 41:708, 1984.

74. CEREBRAL EMBOLISM STUDY GROUP: *Immediate anticoagulation of embolic stroke: A randomized trial.* Stroke 14:668, 1983.

AN EPILOGUE

Traveller, there are no paths.
Paths are made by walking.
Juan de Mairena

Faced with a patient with established stroke, the physician today remains as helpless as ever. The use of potentially injurious and unproven drugs marks scant progress over the application of leeches and the liberation of evil spirits by craniotomy. Current optimism in stroke management stems from the increasing realization that stroke is not one entity but many, that cerebral ischemia is a continuum, and that the opportunities for stroke prevention are improving.

The power of CT scanning was so dramatic in delineating brain lesions that studies done without it need validation. Even as CT techniques were refined, magnetic resonance imaging appeared, offering even more versatility and accurate definition of previously invisible or obscure lesions. Imaging techniques have radically changed the classification of stroke, forcing a new look at old dogmas. Lacunar strokes may account for many clinical syndromes previously attributed to sizable cerebral lesions,[1] "TIAs" are not uncommonly caused by small infarcts,[2] and cerebral hemorrhage commonly masquerades as ischemic stroke.[3] The present terminology of stroke needs revision. A more pragmatic classification is preferable, including information about the location, nature, and cause of the lesion.

Noninvasive cardiac imaging has also affected cerebrovascular diagnosis. The cardiac chambers were seldom visualized when dangerous angiography, inaccurate isotope scanning, and M-mode echocardiography were the only alternatives. Two-dimensional echocardiography has identified the heart as a common source of emboli,[4-6] and mitral valve prolapse has displaced rheumatic heart disease as a common cause of ischemic stroke, especially in young adults.[7]

The concept of ischemic stroke as a continuum has emerged from determinations of biochemical, structural, and perfusion thresholds of ischemia. The neurologic deficit reflects maximal dysfunction, but not necessarily maximal damage, since some tissue will lose function but not life. The viability of this "penumbra" surrounding a cerebral infarct depends on the final balance of adverse and beneficial factors.[8]

The reversible role of calcium in ischemic cellular damage[9] and the inconstant but dramatic reversal of neurologic deficits following the administration of certain drugs offers hope.[10] The use of fluorocarbons provides evidence that decreasing viscosity while increasing oxygen-carrying capacity to the brain may be beneficial.[11-13]

Physicians should be skeptical of the many unproven treatments, but always be willing to evaluate them, since so little effective therapy is available. Anyone is entitled to an opinion about therapy, but no one has the right to impose it on patients without some rational balance of favorable and adverse probabilities. While the development of effective treatment begins with a single laboratory or clinical observation, demonstration of its effectiveness is a costly, laborious, systematic effort by many people. The use of computers has multiplied with profligate ease, simplifying individual steps while complicating the process. More and more of what is quantifiable, repeatable, or recordable will become available on computers, leaving the intangibles to the physician. The challenge will not be information, but its use. Although randomized, double-blind, controlled studies remain the standard, their expense and effectiveness are being questioned,[12] and other approaches are being explored.[13] It is nevertheless clear that we cannot revert to clinical impressions or uncontrolled observations because of the heterogeneity of stroke, the inherent bias in clinical experience and the changing epidemiology of cerebrovascular disease.[14]

How people live influences how they die.[15] Healthier lifestyles can be coaxed by government policy[16] and financial advantage.[17] Studies aimed at prevention promise most in future therapy. Until the etiology of atherosclerosis is better understood, therapeutic strategies are limited to the treatment of known risk factors, the search for new ones, and the evaluation of drugs that may reverse plaque progression.[18] Increased diagnosis of asymptomatic extracranial vascular disease by noninvasive techniques is a mixed blessing,[1] as the risk of stroke in these patients is less than the current surgical risk.[19-21] Carotid endarterectomy rates are rising disturbingly in the United States,[1,22] encouraged by the increasing availability of DSA and improved carotid Doppler imaging. An operation may bestow benefit, but can become an unintended distraction. Patients and doctors may focus on the dramatic moment of surgery, neglecting the more pedestrian and prolonged tasks of controlling risk factors, which ultimately may be more important.

Many patients with ischemic stroke first have TIAs,[1,23] but, sadly, both patients and physicians commonly disregard these valuable warnings. Identification of these potential stroke victims could be increased by further public and professional education and TIA clinics or questionnaires.[24]

Both stroke and our perspective of it are changing.[25] The dynamic nature of stroke dictates that our assumptions about it be re-evaluated constantly. As one challenge is met, another arises. Physicians caring for stroke are engaged not only in learning how best to treat their patients, but in learning about the brain. Theirs is an unending but rewarding quest.

REFERENCES

1. MOHR, JP: *Lacunes*. Stroke 13:3, 1982.

2. LADURNER, G, ET AL: *A correlation of clinical findings and CT in ischaemic cerebrovascular disease*. Eur Neurol 18:281, 1979.

3. KINKEL, W: *Computerized tomography in clinical neurology*. In BAKER, AB, AND BAKER, LH (EDS): *Clinical Neurology*, Vol 1. Harper & Row, Philadelphia, 1983, p 1.

4. ASINGER, RW, ET AL: *Incidence of left-ventricular thrombosis after acute transmural myocardial infarction*. N Engl J Med 305:297, 1981.

5. MELTZER, R, AND ROELANDT, J: *Letter to the Editor: 2-D echo for left ventricular thrombi*. Chest 80:118, 1981.

6. EZEKOWITZ, MD, ET AL: *Comparison of Indium-111 platelet scintigraphy and two-dimensional echocardiography in the diagnosis of left ventricular thrombi*. N Engl J Med 306:1509, 1982.

7. HART, RG, AND EASTON, JD: *Mitral valve prolapse and cerebral infarction*. Stroke 13:429, 1982.

8. ASTRUP, J, SIESJÖ, BK, AND SYMON,L: *Thresholds in cerebral ischemia—The ischemic penumbra*. Stroke 12:723, 1981.

9. HASS, WK: *The cerebral ischemic cascade*. Neurol Clin 1:345, 1983.

10. FADEN, AI: *Opiate antagonists in the treatment of stroke*. Stroke 15:575, 1984.

11. PEERLESS, SJ, ET AL: *Protective effect of Fluosol-DA in acute cerebral ischemia*. Stroke 12:558, 1981.

12. FEINSTEIN, AR: *An additional basic science for clinical medicine. II. The limitations of randomized trials*. Ann Intern Med 99:544, 1983.

13. KOLATA, G: *A new kind of epidemiology*. Science 224:481, 1984.

14. DYKEN, ML, AND CALHOUN, RA: *Changes in stroke mortality: Effects on evaluating and predicting outcome for therapeutic studies*. In REIVICH, M, AND HURTIG, HI (EDS): *Cerebrovascular Diseases*. Raven Press, New York, 1983, p 51.

15. BERKMAN, LF, AND BRESLOW, L: *Health and ways of living: The Alameda County study*. Oxford University Press, 1983.

16. DOLL, R: *Prospects for prevention*. Br Med J 286:445, 1983.

17. MOSER, M, RAFTER, J, AND GAJEWSKI, J: *Premium reductions. A motivating factor in long-term hypertensive treatment*. JAMA 251:756, 1984.

18. SPENCE, JD: *Effects of hydralazine vs propranolol on blood velocity patterns in patients with carotid stenosis*. Clin Sci 65:91, 1983.

19. NORRIS, JW, AND D'ALTON, JG: *Outcome of patients with asymptomatic carotid bruits*. In REIVICH, M, AND HURTIG, HI (EDS):*Cerebrovascular Diseases*. Raven Press, New York, 1983, p 63.

20. DURWARD, QJ, FERGUSON, GG, AND BARR, HWK: *The natural history of asymptomatic carotid bifurcation plaques*. Stroke 13:459, 1982.

21. CHAMBERS, BR, AND NORRIS, JW: *The case against surgery for asymptomatic carotid stenosis*. Stroke 15:964, 1984.

22. DYKEN ML, AND POKRAS, R: *The performance of endarterectomy for disease of the extracranial arteries for the head*. Stroke 15:948, 1984.

23. PESSINS, MS, ET AL: *Mechanisms of acute carotid stroke*. Ann Neurol 6:245, 1979.

24. WILKINSON, WE, ET AL: *Use of a self-administered questionnaire for detection of transient cerebral ischemic attacks. 1. Survey of elderly persons living in a retirement facility*. Ann Neurol 6:40, 1979.

25. WHISNANT, JP: *The role of the neurologist in the decline of stroke*. Ann Neurol 14:1, 1983.

AN EPILOGUE

INDEX

An *italic* number indicates a figure.
A "t" indicates a table.

279

Cerebral venous infarction, 157–158
Cerebrovascular accident (CVA), 3
Cervical bruits. *See* Bruits
Chagas' disease, 146, *148*, 167
Chest x-ray, 192
Chiropractic manipulation, 151
Clinical manifestations of stroke
  differential diagnosis of, 97–99
  history, 79–81
  interpretation of, 97
  neurologic, 85–97
  neurovascular, 82–85
  physical, 81–82
Clinical manifestations of transient ischemic
    attack, 67–70
  differential diagnosis of, 70–76
CO_2. *See* Carbon dioxide
Collagen vascular diseases, 151–152
Collateral blood flow, 27, 31, *32*, 85
Coma
  stroke and, 95–97, 120
  subarachnoid hemorrhage and, 159
Computerized tomography. *See* CT scan-
    ning
Conduction aphasia, 93
Confusion, 98
Conscious patient, approaches to
  cortical dysfunction, 91–94
  cranial nerve impairment, 91
  dysarthria and dysphagia, 91
  gaze deviation, 89–91
  hemiparesis, 85–87
  hemisensory involvement, 88–89
  incoordination, 87
  memory impairment, 95, 98
  right-hemisphere syndromes, 94–95
Consciousness, 98, 249
Contraceptive pill, 156, 158
Cortical dysfunction, 91–94
Cranial bruits, 83
Cranial nerve impairment, 91
Creatine kinase, 191
Critical gray matter flow, 54, 57
CT scanning
  complications and limitations of, 197–198
  diagnosis of stroke and, 3, 4, 79, 99, 193–
      197, 275
  dynamic, 220
CVA. *See* Cerebrovascular accident
Cytoplasmic vacuolation, 54
Cytotoxic edema, 53, 126

Deep venous thrombosis (DVT), 23–24. *See
    also* Pulmonary embolism
Dementia, 4, 8
Deteriorating stroke
  brainstem hemorrhage and, 133–134
  cardiac causes of, 134
  cerebellar hemorrhage and, 129, 132–133
  cerebral edema in, 126
  definition of, 4, 5, 123–125
  drugs and, 137
  hemispheric hemorrhage and, 129
  hemorrhagic infarction and, 124–129
  post-stroke depression and, 134–135
  progressive thrombosis in, 125–126

rebleeding in, 129
  syndrome of inappropriate antidiuretic
      hormone, 135–136
Deterioration, 97
  from drugs, 137
Dextran 40, 235
Diabetes mellitus, 2, 81, 82, 263
Diagnosis of stroke
  accuracy, 18–20
  differential, 97–99
  history, 79–81
  interpretation and, 97
  laboratory evidence and, 6
  physical examination, 79, 81–97
Diagnosis of transient ischemic attack
  differential, 70–76
  physical examination and, 70
  symptoms and, 67–68
  unusual presentations of, 68–70
Diagnostic tests. *See* Laboratory inves-
    tigation
Diaschisis, 251
Diastolic blood pressure, 259
Diet, 2, 8
Differential diagnosis of stroke, 97–99
Differential diagnosis of transient ischemic
    attack, 70–76
Digital subtraction arteriography
  IA-DSA, 214
  IV-DSA, 209–214
Dipyridamole, 268
Disseminated intravascular coagulopathy,
    157
Doppler ultrasonography, 215–218
Drop attacks, 69
Drug(s), 137, 152
Duplex scanning, 218
DVT. *See* Venous thrombosis
Dysarthria, 91
Dysphagia, 91

ECG. *See* Electrocardiography
Echocardiography, 218–219
Eclampsia, 156
Edema. *See* Cerebral edema; Ischemic
    edema
Electrocardiography
  changes in stroke, 180–183, 191
  long-term, 192, 262
Electroencephalography, 192–193
Electrolytes, 191
Embolism. *See also* Cerebral embolism
  cardiac, 142
  paradoxical, 146, 179–180
  pulmonary, 23–24, 230, 253
Endocarditis
  infective, 176–178
  nonbacterial thrombotic, 178–179
Endoperoxides, 50–51
Enhancement, 193–194
Environmental factors, 263
Epidemiology
  age and sex, 7
  geography, 6–7
  long-term trends, 8–10
  social factors, 7–8

Erythrocyte sedimentation rate, 189, 190
Etiology
    of deteriorating stroke, 125–129
    of young stroke, 142–159
    quality of life and, 248
Evoked responses, 219–220
Examination
    appearance of patient, 81–82
    deteriorating stroke and, 137–139
    interpretation of, 97
    neurologic, 85–97
    neurovascular, 82–85
Extracranial/intracranial bypass surgery, 8, 268

FACIAL weakness, 91
Falciparum malaria, 151, 190
Fibrinogen, 57
Fibrinoid degeneration, 29
Fibromuscular dysplasia, 152, 154
Fibrous dysplasia, 151
Fluent aphasia, 93, 120
Fluorocarbons, 234
Fortification spectra, 70
Free fatty acids, 51
Free radicals, 50–51

GAZE, wrong-way, 91
Gaze deviation, 89–91, 249
Geographic location, incidence and, 1, 6–7
Gerstmann's syndrome, 94
Glucose metabolism, 34–35

HANDEDNESS, 82, 85, 92, 250
Headache(s)
    stroke and, 81, 97
    transient ischemic attack and, 68
Hematocrit, 57, 190
Hematologic disorders, 156
Hematologic factors in cerebral ischemia
    blood viscosity, 57–58
    platelet abnormalities, 58
Hematology investigation, 190
Hemianopia, 80, 91
Hemiparesis, 6, 85–87, 249
Hemiplegic gait, 106
Hemisensory involvement, 88–89
Hemispheric hemorrhage, 129
Hemispheric lesions, 96, 246
Hemodynamic infarction, 97
Hemodynamic stroke, 180
Hemodynamic transient ischemic attack, 69, 180
Hemoglobin electrophoresis, 219
Hemoglobinopathy, 156
Hemorrhage
    cerebral, 81, 91, 118, 120
    hemispheric, 129
    intracranial, 195
    prognosis of patient with, 248
Hemorrhagic infarction, 127–129
Hemorrhagic stroke. See also Cerebral hemorrhage
    deterioration of patient with, 129–134
    infratentorial, 120
    supratentorial, 118–120

Heredity, 81, 263
Herniation, 97
Heroin, 152
History of patient with stroke, 79–81, 97
Hot stroke, 215
Hyaline degeneration, 29
Hydrocephalus, 129, 132, 133
Hyperglycemia, 191, 251. See also Diabetes mellitus
Hyperlipidemia, 263
Hypertension
    centrencephalic microaneurysm and, 29
    diet and, 8
    family history and, 81
    prognosis of stroke and, 251
    risk factor for stroke, 1, 2, 3, 82, 259–262
Hypertensive encephalopathy
    cerebral ischemia and, 34
    transient ischemic attack and, 73–74
    young stroke and, 159
Hypertensive heart disease, 262
Hypertensive hemorrhage, 29
Hypoglycemia, 74, 99, 191, 229
Hypotension, 31, 97, 180
Hysterical hemiparesis, 74
Hysterical monoparesis, 74

IA-DSA, 214
ICD. See International Classification of Disease
Idiopathic hypertrophic subaortic stenosis, 146
^{125}I-fibrinogen scanning, 23–24. See also Phlebography
Immunoglobulins, 57
Impedance plethysmography (IPG), 24
Inattention, 106
Inappropriate ADH syndrome, 191
Incidence
    age and sex affecting, 7
    geographic location and, 1, 6–7
    mortality and, 8–9
    social factors affecting, 7–8
    stroke in young and, 141–146, 156
Incomplete ischemia, 58, 60
Incoordination, 87
Infarction(s). See also Cerebral infarction
    hemodynamic, 97
    lacunar, 29, 225
    lateral pontine, 108
    myocardial, 81, 146, 246
    venous, 157–158
Infection, 146, 151, 229
Infective endocarditis, 176–178, 190
Infratentorial hemorrhage, 120, 239
Intensive care for stroke, 14. See also Acute stroke unit
Internal carotid artery(ies), 29
    occlusion of, 104–105, 247
International Classification of Disease (ICD), 4, 10, 225
Intracerebral hemorrhage, 159
Intracerebral steal, 46
Intracranial hemorrhage, 195
IPG. See Impedance plethysmography
Ischemia. See Cerebral ischemia
Ischemic edema, 95–97

RC
388.5
·H33
1985

47.50